How Everyday Products Make People Sick

How Everyday Products Make People Sick

TOXINS AT HOME AND IN THE WORKPLACE

Paul D. Blanc, M.D.

UNIVERSITY OF CALIFORNIA PRESS

BERKELEY   LOS ANGELES   LONDON

University of California Press, one of the most distinguished university presses in the United States, enriches lives around the world by advancing scholarship in the humanities, social sciences, and natural sciences. Its activities are supported by the UC Press Foundation and by philanthropic contributions from individuals and institutions. For more information, visit www.ucpress.edu.

University of California Press
Berkeley and Los Angeles, California

University of California Press, Ltd.
London, England

Library of Congress Cataloging-in-Publication Data

Blanc, Paul David, 1951–.
    How everyday products make people sick : toxins at home and in the work-place / Paul David Blanc.
        p.   cm.
    Includes bibliographical references and index.
    ISBN-13: 978–0-520–24881–6 (cloth : alk. paper).
    ISBN-10: 0-520–24881–3 (cloth : alk. paper).
    ISBN-13: 978–0-520–24882–3 (pbk. : alk. paper).
    ISBN-10: 0-520–24882–1 (pbk. : alk. paper).
    1. Toxicology—Popular works.   2. Environmental health—History.   3. Occupational diseases—History.   4. Health risk assessment.   5. Product safety.   I. Title.
RA1213.B53   2007
615.9—dc22   2006011268

Manufactured in the United States of America

15   14   13   12   11   10   09   08   07
10   9   8   7   6   5   4   3   2

This book is printed on New Leaf EcoBook 50, a 100% recycled fiber of which 50% is de-inked postconsumer waste, processed chlorine free. EcoBook 50 is acid free and meets the minimum requirements of ANSI/ASTM D5634–01 (*Permanence of Paper*).

CONTENTS

Illustrations follow page 44

ACKNOWLEDGMENTS

A NUMBER OF INSTITUTIONS and individuals have provided assistance in the research and writing of this book. Institutional support has come from the Burroughs Wellcome Fund through a travel award for research at the Wellcome Institute for the History of Medicine; the Rockefeller Foundation through a Bellagio Program Residence; and the American Academy in Rome through a visiting fellowship. I also want to personally thank Arlene Shaner for assistance at the historical collections of the New York Academy of Medicine; Heidi Heilmann for assistance at the Lane Medical Library, Stanford University; Valerie Wheat for her assistance at the University of California San Francisco special collections; Dr. Gina Solomon of the Natural Resources Defense Council, particularly for background material on manganese; Dr. Bruce Bernard of the National Institute for Occupational Safety and Health, especially for additional background on ergonomic issues; and Dr. Brian Dolan, Dr. Kjell Torén, Dr. Rick Stryker, Yudie Fishman, Louise Swig, W. Thomas Davey III, and Gary B. Sokol for critical reviews of the manuscript, and Robin Whitaker for her diligent editing.

ALS   amyotrophic lateral sclerosis (Lou Gehrig's disease)

BASF   Badische Anilin-und-Soda Fabrik

BMAA   β-n-methylamino-L-alanine (a cycad toxin)

Buna-S   *bu*tadiene *na*trium [sodium]–*S*tyrene copolymer (an artificial rubber)

CA   copper azole

CBA   copper boron azole

CCA   chromated copper arsenate

CDC   Centers for Disease Control and Prevention

CPSC   Consumer Product Safety Commission

DMF   dimethylformamide

DNP   dinitrophenol

EDF   Environmental Defense Fund

EPA   Environmental Protection Agency

FDA   Food and Drug Administration

GHB   gamma hydroxybutyrate

GR-S   government rubber-styrene

IARC   International Agency for Research on Cancer

JAMA   *Journal of the American Medical Association*

MCA   Manufacturing Chemists' Association

MDI   methylene diphenyl diisocyanate

MMT   methylcyclopentadienyl manganese tricarbonyl (aka HiTec 3000)

MMWR   *Morbidity and Mortality Weekly Report*

MPTP   1-methyl-4-phenyl-1,2,3,6-tetrahydropyridine (a heroin substitute)

MRI   magnetic resonance imaging

MTBE   methyl tertiary butyl ether

NIH   National Institutes of Health

NIOSH   National Institute for Occupational Safety and Health

OSHA   Occupational Safety and Health Administration

Perna   *Per*chlor*na*phthalin

PVC   polyvinyl chloride

RADS   reactive airway dysfunction syndrome

SARS   severe adult respiratory syndrome

TNT   trinitrotoluene

2,4,5-T 2,4,5-tricholorophenoxyacetic acid

UNITE   Union of Needletrades, Industrial, and Textile Employees

INTRODUCTION

WHEN SOMEONE INQUIRES ABOUT my professional work and I reply, "Occupational and environmental medicine," an awkward pause usually follows. To fill in the gap, I'll elaborate, "That's the treatment of diseases that people get from their work or as a result of pollution." Sometimes bringing up a specific problem clarifies matters. Officers of the Immigration and Naturalization Service (since March 1, 2003, the Bureau of Citizenship and Immigration Services), for example, seem to relate easily to carpal tunnel syndrome, likely because of their own experience with keying in data and hand stamping documents for hours at a stretch.

People often ask whether my field is a new branch of health care, along the lines of modern subspecialties such as sports medicine, genetic counseling, and bariatrics (the treatment of obesity). That such issues could even become the stuff of popular song only serves to further reinforce the impression that occupational medicine, so topical, must also be novel, too. Dire Straits' 1982 ironic rock-n-roll ballad "Industrial Disease" was nothing if not a processional anthem meant to be played at the arrival of yet one more late twentieth-century health obsession:

Doctor Parkinson declared "I'm not surprised to see you here
you've got smoker's cough from smoking, brewer's droop from
    drinking beer
I don't know how you came to get the Bette Davis knees
but worst of all young man you've got Industrial Disease."

he wrote me a prescription he said "you are depressed
but I'm glad you came in to see me to get this off your chest
come in and see me later—next patient please
send in another victim of Industrial Disease."[1]

In fact, occupational and environmental disease is not new at all. In my work as a poison control physician, I have been called on to consult on cases arising from toxic chemical exposures. In my medical research, I carry out investigations of current-day health problems, such as illness among welders from metal fumes and asthma among workers in professions exposed to allergy-producing dusts. In both settings, I always encounter the same recurring phenomenon. Time and time again, I am astonished to learn that what I first believed was a novel finding in fact had already been reported by others often ten, twenty, or thirty years earlier, sometimes as long as a century or more ago.

I have learned through trial and error that this distant history may be documented somewhere but is all too often exceedingly hard to find. Such information is frequently omitted from textbooks. Even specialized review articles in scientific journals rarely follow the past trails of evidence in order to track down how, when, and why a specific man-made illness may have first occurred and what attempts, if any, were made to control the disease at its initial outbreak. Coming on the same story told and retold again and again, albeit with a different cast of characters, I had to ask myself, *Why is this the case?*

Over time, I have come to understand that the pivotal difference between industrial injuries or illnesses and environmental contamination episodes on the one hand and most other medical problems on the other hand is that a human perpetrator usually is not involved in the latter. It is one thing to isolate a deadly microbe but quite another to identify, by name, a life-threatening place of employment or clearly pinpoint a hazardous environmental epicenter. Ibsen understood this contradiction in *An Enemy of the People,* his play describing the ostracism of a medical doctor after he threatens the local tourist-based economy by revealing pollution of the town's bathing spring and seashore by industrial tannery waste.[2] Arguably, similar forces also were at play, acting in a way that we ended up with an illness named Legionnaire's disease rather than Bellevue-Stratford Hotel pneumonia.[3]

As I began to explore further the backgrounds of different and seemingly unrelated occupational and environmental case studies, another common thread began to emerge. First, the story of each newly introduced hazard and the disease outbreak that resulted from it was mirrored in a parallel process of medical discovery, as intriguing as the tale of any microbe hunter tracking infectious disease. Second and more surprising still, I was also finding a remarkably similar pattern of delay, deferral, and outright defeat when it came to prevention. Not only did the perpetrators go unnamed; they usually went on with business unrestrained.

Following out the various ramifications of each of these episodes, I could well appreciate the old adage "Everything is connected to everything." In its way, this is the absolute inverse of the bromide "The solution to pollution is dilution," a favorite utterance of a rather reactionary public health professor I once had. By this he meant that a smokestack, if tall enough, could solve any problem. Acid rain falling in New England but originating from midwestern power plants is a potent refutation of this proposition. Acid rain also underscores the truism that risks do not evaporate outside the factory door. There is no absolute boundary point between "occupational" and "environmental" risks. Hazardous materials certainly do not recognize a separation between the workplace and the wider environment. Each such product passes though its own life cycle, from invention through technological refinement, then on to mass production, until it reaches obsolescence. Along the way, to paraphrase the advertising slogan of the chemical industry, *something it makes will touch your life.*

My impetus in writing this book is to tell a story that has not yet been told but needs to be heard. This is not the saga of one exceptional manufacturer, notorious for the particularly brazen manner in which it flouts occupational and environmental protections. Such industries do exist and are instructive in their way, but they are not central to this tale. Rather, this is the story of the run-of-the-mill, the unexceptional—no more or less damaging than a scofflaw manufacturer. It is the narrative accompanying many of the everyday objects that surround us: a tube of glue in a kitchen drawer, a bottle of bleach on the laundry room counter, a rayon scarf on a closet shelf, a brass knob on a door, or the wooden plank in an outside deck.

This is also a story that does not transpire in a simple linear sequence of events. It focuses on disparate problems that do not dovetail neatly in place and time but are nonetheless intertwined over time. Seemingly disconnected matters, on closer inspection, turn out to be linked by a common thread of related technological developments or through the shared experience of common historical figures. These problems, despite their wide separation in time and location, emerge and reemerge as similar issues.

In taking away a central lesson from these case histories, I find their most telling point is the repeated way in which new hazards are recognized, yet the effective prevention of further illness and injury is so often thwarted. Recognizing this basic pattern should be a prerequisite for those who intend to protect the public through legislative policy meant to reduce risks, whether encountered on the job, at home, or in the wider environment. Without our taking this recurring history into account, no isolated remediation or narrowly prescriptive regulatory reform is likely to be effective in any truly sustained way.

Above all else, in telling a story that transpires over differing time periods in many places and is related to a wide mix of technologies and toxins, I found it paramount not to lose sight of the key unifying connection that links each and every episode that I recount. That connection is the bond among the women and men of every age who, going about their lives as best they could, have fallen victim to hazards that need not have been placed in their paths.

Almost fifty years before Dire Straits' "Industrial Disease" hit the airways, the folk musician Josh White released a song inspired by one of the largest single outbreaks of occupational illness ever to occur in the United States. This episode took place in West Virginia in the 1930s, when a Union Carbide subcontractor hired migrant laborers to carve out a water-diversion tunnel in rock containing a high grade of silica.[4] Within months, hundreds succumbed to the fatal lung disease silicosis. Josh White's song "Silicosis Blues" goes in part:

> Now silicosis, you're a dirty robber and a thief,
> Yes, silicosis, you're a dirty robber and a thief
> Robbed me of my right to live and all you brought poor me was grief.
> I was there diggin' that tunnel for just six bits a day
> I was diggin' that tunnel for just six bits a day
> Didn't know I was diggin' my grave—silicosis was eatin' my lungs
>   away.[5]

These problems, still with us today, stretch back in time long before 50 years ago, when Josh White composed "Silicosis Blues," or even before 150 years ago. A medieval Jewish prayer, still recited annually on the Day of Atonement, includes the admonition, "Man earns his bread at the peril of his own life."[6]

May it not always be so.

ONE

The Forgotten Histories of "Modern" Hazards

MERCURY POISONING

A few years ago, I was asked to provide a medical consultation for a four-month-old boy who was admitted to the hospital because of possible appendicitis. He was of an unusually young age for such a problem, but the precipitant of the problem was more unusual still. A few weeks before, the parents of the boy had noticed symptoms of colic in the infant and treated him with the remedy that had been used in their home village in rural Mexico for generations: they gave him some quicksilver to drink.

One might wonder how this village had gone on for very many generations with this kind of folk wisdom, but, in fact, quicksilver (another name for pure elemental mercury) isn't taken up through the stomach or intestines very quickly. By other routes mercury is indeed quite hazardous; for example, if inhaled, it rapidly enters the body through the lungs, and in forms such as salts and their by-products it is well absorbed through the gut. But in most cases, when quicksilver is taken by mouth it passes right through the system. It may not cure colic, but it doesn't do too much harm, either.

Mercury, however, is a curious substance. Because of its properties, it may not pass. It is a fluid, but it is also very heavy, much more so than water. For this reason, liquid mercury tends to settle to the lowest spot it can. The appendix, hanging as a little tail off the intestines, is just such a low spot. In the case of this child, the appendix filled up like a thermometer. By X-ray, the dense mercury in his abdomen lit up like a metallic worm. He was suffering from a mercury-impacted appendix that, in the end, required surgical removal.[1]

Toxic substances have become so much an everyday fact of modern life as to verge on being perceived as a cliché of risk rather than as a true and substantive threat. We may find it incredible that anyone could use quicksilver as a folk remedy. Then again, many of my peers, members of a generation who were children or adolescents in the 1950s and 1960s, can report at least one experience of playing with mercury in the schoolyard or, better yet, mixing up tiny puddles of it in their own basements.

Times do change. To an important extent, so too do the toxins to which we are exposed. These changes involve more than simply evolving perceptions of what constitutes an unacceptable risk. To keep up with an expanding inventory of hazards requires tracking unusual if not arcane information sources. On my preferred reading list is a twelve-page newsletter published every week by the federal Centers for Disease Control in Atlanta. Its upbeat name is the *Morbidity and Mortality Weekly Report*. The cognoscenti refer to it simply as the *MMWR*.

In the pages of the *MMWR*, for example, one can learn of such cases as that of a child in a Michigan suburb who was struck with a bizarre illness. His hands turned pink and began to scale, he began to drool, and his mood became irascible and difficult to manage. An unusual infection was considered as one possible explanation, but this was excluded by laboratory testing. No hereditary condition fit his bizarre constellation of abnormalities. But the child's syndrome does have a name. The illness is called pink's disease. It was, at one time, a well-known entity.

This syndrome, including both the odd skin changes and ominous nervous system findings, is exactly how mercury poisoning is manifest in a child afflicted with chronic poisoning. This child's parents had not given him mercury to drink as a home remedy, nor had he been experimenting with quicksilver in the family room. An exhaustive battery of questions revealed little. When asked of any recent changes at home, the parents could report only that the interior of the house had recently been repainted. There was nothing extraordinary in that: a standard commercial indoor latex paint had been applied. Yet when the child was tested, he had extremely high mercury levels. The rest of the family was tested as well. They, too, were poisoned, albeit less severely.

What, then, was the source of their toxic exposure? The answer lay in the seemingly innocuous house paint. As it turns out, it contained excessive amounts of an approved chemical additive intended to prevent mildew. That additive is called phenyl mercuric acetate, a form of mercury not previously associated with human illness. Nonetheless, enough mercury had vaporized from the paint to cause harm. Trapped within the indoor environment, it turned the suburban house into an ideal exposure chamber, leading to mercury poisoning in the entire family.[2]

The links between the first child, with mercury in his appendix, and the second, suffering the effects of mercury inhalation, are stronger than they might appear at first. The link is not simply that the same toxin was involved in each case. The more important tie is that a single, ancient hazard is still present in our everyday environment, not only in an old and traditional form but also in an entirely new combination. This is a scenario repeated all too often in the last decade, the last fifty years, and stretching back over a span of centuries.[3]

REVISIONIST ENVIRONMENTAL HISTORY

The pages that follow will detail the stories of many of these recycled and reinvented hazards. These stories call into question what we may take as a given: that because our modern ecological concept of the "environment" is relatively new, the toxic threats that drive our understanding of this construct are also of recent origin. The superficial timeline of environmental history, it is true, supports this mistaken view. When I first began my training in public health, focusing on occupational safety and health, the United States was preparing for its bicentennial. The Occupational Safety and Health Administration and the Environmental Protection Agency were both less than ten years old. Earth Day was an idea in its infancy. The pockmarked geography of our poisonous landscape had not yet erected the familiar signposts of Love Canal or Chernobyl, catastrophes that were to follow in the later 1970s and 1980s. The environmental map, as we know it today, was then largely terra incognita.

We've come a long way since then. Ironically it's just far enough to see the emergence of what can best be labeled a *revisionist* history of both the movement for environmental protection and even the environment itself.[4] Central to this revisionism is an inclination to debunk and discard almost any concern that may be raised over the risks of toxic substances. Whether a hazard is identified on the basis of laboratory studies, is linked to an outbreak of human illness, or is detected as a more subtle ecological threat on a global scale, the revisionist response invariably minimizes the risk.

Revisionist environmental theory justifies attacks on key pieces of environmental legislation. For example, in 2000 the American Enterprise Institute–Brookings Joint Center on Regulatory Studies revisited the question of lead's adverse effects on childhood intelligence. The report issued did not dispute that the metal was toxic but found that the economic benefit to parents was only eleven hundred to nineteen hundred dollars per IQ point gained through lead abatement. The spare-the-lead-and-spoil-the-child conclusion the report reached reads, "This analysis suggests lead standards will redistribute resources from parents to their children, because the benefits to parents are less than the costs of the standards. The Environmental Protection Agency and the Department of Housing and Urban Development should reconsider their lead standards."[5]

New versions of environmental history instruct us that our fetish over toxins is likely to be seen by future generations for the absurdity that it surely must be. The environment can take care of itself, we are falsely reassured, just as it has always done. Woody Allen humorously mined this vein in his film *Sleeper* a number of years ago, portraying a character waking up in the not-too-distant future only to discover a world in which cigarettes and high cholesterol diets have been found to be health promoting. Allen's film was healthy satire, but the revisionists would have us take it as a documentary. They promote as established fact the dangerous misconception that environmental concerns are purely modern creatures born of our narcissistic age.

Perhaps this distorted view merely reflects a general shortsightedness we all share to one extent or another. William Faulkner observed that the old do not perceive the past to stretch back linearly. Rather, they look back through a very narrow corridor of sequentially ordered recent history, which then opens out onto a wider expanse of time, as if a large meadow where more distant and less distant events, like cattle, graze comfortably together. The timeline of environmentalism can be similarly perceived, even by those closest to the movement itself. About as far away as anyone can make out in this landscape stands the distant figure of Rachel Carson, heroically holding aloft a copy of *Silent Spring*. In the cosmology of environmentalism, one cannot even extrapolate beyond this point: we arbitrarily fix the date of the ecological big bang as the year 1962.[6]

Thus, for all intents and purposes, *Silent Spring* becomes a holy text, a Veda of the environmental movement's own creation myth. DDT serves as totemic a role in this mythology as Jackie's pillbox hat serves for the myth of a Kennedy Camelot (from precisely the same time period). Back beyond 1960, in environmental time, there is only an expanse of apocryphal prehistory in which vague rumor or impressionistic allusion links scattered images or anecdotes of contamination with possible real historical events. A connection is sometimes made between the expression "mad as a hatter" and mercury poisoning, which occurs in the hat trade from use of the toxin to make felt from rabbit fur and can result in mental derangement. The theory that widespread lead poisoning may have contributed to the decline of the Roman Empire is recycled with a certain frequency. Otherwise, all seems unformed and void, even to most environmentalists themselves.[7]

In fact, the true environmental record is far from a blank slate. There is a rich and well-documented history of injury and illness, much of it concentrated in the workplace or in neighborhoods contaminated from spillage just beyond the factory door. This history has a clear and important message to transmit. It shows us how time and again innovative processes have been introduced into large factories or small workshops, novel products have entered the marketplace, and new contaminants have been released into the environment. Each time these have occurred, episodes of disease, disability, and death have ensued. This is not a new story beginning in 1960 or even in 1690. It is an old, sad tale that gets told over and over but seems somehow to be forgotten after each new recitation. The revisionist recounting of the anti-environmental time line intentionally undermines it, characterizing the issues involved as little more than a modern fad that will soon pass and be forgotten. The environmentalist sense of the movement's history, cut off from much of its own past, often has the same net effect.

We must reclaim our lost history so that, going forward, we can accurately judge the steps we must take to address the public health and safety threats before us today. These threats predictably arise as the unintended by-products of the ways in which we make and use consumer goods and produce and transport basic commodities and industrial materials alike. This does not mean that health and safety risks are unavoidable. Rather, past experience teaches that the amelioration of these problems will require strategies geared to their complex social, economic, and technological interrelationships.

This chapter reexamines some of the deceptively simple but incorrect assumptions that we have about what is, in fact, "new" in our environment, whether at work, at home, or in the wider ecosystem. We can easily start with a list of our hypermodern concerns that seem to be of recent origin: pollution in the water and air; asbestos fibers in our workplaces and schools; carpal tunnel syndrome from our keyboards; sick building syndrome from our sealed-in International Style offices; and the vague toxicity of "burnout" from the day-to-day stress of modern life.

WATER POLLUTION

Nothing is more prototypically modern than the specter of massive water pollution from an oil tanker spill. Thus the *Exxon Valdez* sails on in the public mind as a kind of latter-day, environmental *Flying Dutchman*. This symbolism was epitomized by the tanker's Hollywood reappearance as a postapocalyptic, floating palace of evil in the 1995 film *Waterworld*.

I had always assumed that much before 1970, and certainly before 1960, people had little or no awareness of the possibility of significant ocean pollution from any man-made source, particularly from petroleum transport. Completely by accident, I came across a small pamphlet in a secondhand bookstall that forced me to rethink this chronology. It was a copy of a groundbreaking report submitted to the Council of the Royal Society in Great Britain, one of the world's leading scientific institutions. Entitled *The Pollution of the Sea and Shore by Oil,* its twenty-two pages lay out with great foresight this emerging environmental threat. The report is dated October 1936.[8]

The author of the pamphlet, a university chemist named Neil K. Adam, gathered his information from a wide variety of sources, including ninety-three beaches in England, personally inspected over a single summer. Of these beaches, he found that eleven were heavily polluted and twenty-one were moderately so. Adam identified "wrecks of oil burning ships or oil tankers . . . holed so as to allow the oil to escape" as a major source of pollution. He also described in great detail the effects of oil spills on bird life:

> Birds are washed, or in some cases swim, ashore, with their feathers more or less covered with the tarry residues from fuel oil; they are often alive when they come ashore, but it is usually hopeless to try to save them. If there is any quantity of oil on them, they cannot fly, and it is stated that they cannot swim or dive either; they must die of starvation. . . . Cleaning oil off birds is extremely difficult; solvents such as petrol remove the natural grease so that water penetrates the feathers and the bird dies of cold.

To further document these effects, Adam reviewed the files of the Royal Society for the Prevention of Cruelty to Animals in Britain. One inspector of the society regularly sent reports for the same thirteen-mile stretch of beach. In the twelve months ending 31 August 1936, the inspector had counted over fourteen hundred oiled birds.

Despite its far-sighted environmental message, *The Pollution of the Sea and Shore by Oil* remains an obscure document. I have never seen it cited, and other than my own copy, I have been able to identify only two copies held in major libraries. This should not be all that surprising. The report's cover is clearly marked in a printed, underlined subtitle, *For Private Circulation Only.*

Recognition of the environmental threat resulting from the chemical contamination of freshwater rivers goes back considerably further than awareness of the threat of ocean discharges. Indeed, freshwater pollution was a stimulus for the formation of some of the earliest public action forerunners of modern environmental groups. One of these was Britain's Fisheries Preservation Association, whose 1868 pamphlet *On the Pollution of the Rivers of the Kingdom* reads as if it could have been drafted by the Sierra Club.[9]

If our modern concerns over water pollution are not so very new after all, then what about air pollution? Consider the following scenario: A toxic cloud menacingly overshadows an entire community, even though scientists have previously assured the public that such an event is highly unlikely if not impossible. The federal government rapidly dispatches a public health team to the site in Pennsylvania. The team of scientists try to come to grips with the new mix of hazards they encounter but conclude that, without long-term research, the effects of such exposures cannot be adequately understood. This is not a description of Three Mile Island circa 1980. It involves a small factory town called Donora, near Pittsburgh. The date is 1948. For four days in October of that year, a meteorological inversion trapped deadly air pollutants over the town, making hundreds ill and killing a score of the town's inhabitants.[10]

Donora put the United States on the international air pollution map, but this episode was far less dramatic than the large-scale catastrophe that had already taken place in December 1930 in Belgium's industrial Meuse Valley.[11] Scientists from around the world studied and commented on that event, too. It became clear that the Meuse factory smokestacks had released a combination of materials that had settled in over the valley, directly leading to the fatalities observed among its inhabitants. One of the few U.S. scientists who studied the Belgian disaster was a Harvard researcher named Philip Drinker, a major public hygiene expert of the time. In 1939, less than ten years before the Donora episode, Drinker wrote in a scientific journal article entitled "Atmospheric Pollution," "Naturally, we want to know whether such an accident could occur in industrial America. Our stacks emit the same gases as did the Belgian, but fortunately, so meteorologists tell us, we have no districts in which there is even a reasonable chance of such a catastrophe taking place."[12]

The United States was not the only country lulled into complacency by a false sense of safety. In the winter of 1952 the "Killer Fog of London," as it came to be known, proved to be a far larger air pollution disaster.[13] The exact number of persons who succumbed as a result of this smog episode has not been determined, but even conservative estimates set the lower limit at thirty-five hundred to four thousand deaths. The crisis took governmental leaders by surprise. Harold Macmillan, minister of housing at the time but later to become prime minister, at first even tried to block any official inquiry, professing that acts of nature can be neither predicted nor prevented.

Yet the 1952 event did not occur without a prelude. In 1948, a similar winter fog fell over London, albeit not as densely, leaving only three hundred dead.[14] In the four-year interval, the British government embarked on a campaign to encourage the consumption of low-grade, pollutant-containing (high-sulfur) domestic coal, so that better quality fuel stuffs could be exported, as a strategy to ease the post–World War II national debt. Simultaneously, London was phasing out its fleet of electric omnibuses, replacing them with diesel-driven vehicles. Were this not enough, large coal-burning power plants along the River Thames within the heart of London were also just coming on line.

In December 2002, the London School of Hygiene and Tropical Medicine hosted a scientific conference to mark the fiftieth anniversary of the Killer Fog. During a question and answer period, a young researcher recounted a story that his father had told him only a few days before, on learning of the meeting and his son's participation in it.[15] The father, then a young man just out of school, was working at the time as an assistant in a funeral parlor in the East End of London. As soon as the 1952 Killer Fog began, his bosses prepared for extra business, predicting that the lad would soon have extra pocket money for the girl he was dating. Another, more "scientific" prediction of catastrophe is equally relevant to the story. Following the earlier Belgian smog disaster but before the London fogs occurred, one of the leading scientific investigators of the Belgian episode warned in 1936, "Wherever fogs of several days are frequent, public authorities are anxious to know the causes of this catastrophe. . . . This apprehension was quite justified when we think that, proportionally, the public services of London, e.g., might be faced with the responsibility of 3200 sudden deaths if such a phenomenon occurred there."[16]

Nor did the Belgian crisis of 1936 provide Britain with its earliest inkling of the smog episodes to come. On several occasions, large increases in the death rate in London were noted to be tightly linked to the dense fogs of the nineteenth century, the most lethal of which occurred in London in January and February of 1880.[17] These episodes became a fact of everyday life. The deadly pall of London smoke even came to be transfigured into a recurring backdrop to the urban impressionist painting of that era. Indeed, some have argued that such pollution is a central thematic link, if not an aesthetic underpinning, for much of that work.[18]

A number of Victorian hygienists, recognizing the seriousness of the problem of air pollution nearly a century before the 1952 Killer Fog, began to tally its environmental and health impacts and to analyze systematically the chemical constituents of air pollution, including the role of sulfur dioxide in what we now call acid rain.[19]

The following is taken from the notes of a Dr. Thomas Scattergood, who, in 1886, delivered a lecture titled "The Air We Breathe in Large Towns" to the Working Man's Institute. Referring to sulfur dioxide, Scattergood tells his audience, "This gas (from sulfur coal) diffused in the air is rapidly changed into the acid oil of vitriol [sulfuric acid], making the atmosphere almost always acid. . . . This is washed out of the air by rain, which is thereby made generally acid."[20]

In addition to identifying acid rain as a major aftereffect of burning sulfur-containing fossil fuel, Scattergood included the following among the "evils arising from smoke": decreased sunlight causing loss of warmth, increased expense cleaning the dirt left by pollution, and the destruction of plant life. He was all for prevention at the individual level, specifically advising his listeners, "In securing the complete burning of fuel with as little smoke as possible, the stoker or fireman, not only economizes his employer's expenses, but does far more than this as benefits his fellow workmen and himself."

Although scientific methods were first applied to the issue of London's air pollution in the nineteenth century, it was recognized as a public health problem long before Victorian times.[21] In the year 1316, during the period when coal was first brought into London in quantity, Parliament petitioned King Edward II to ban its use because it was seen as a public nuisance. Edward decreed that those who burned coal should be fined, and, on second offense, the burner of coal was to have his furnace demolished, a fairly definitive abatement strategy.

Coal use declined for a time but slowly picked up again because the decree was eventually ignored and then forgotten. By the seventeenth century, the coal smoke problem in London had become severe. In fact, the first book ever devoted solely to the subject of air pollution was published in 1661. It was written about coal smoke and titled *Fumifugium: or, the Inconvenience of the Aer, and Smoake of London Dissipated.*[22] The author of *Fumifugium,* John Evelyn, was also a major diarist of his age (he was a friend as well as a contemporary of Pepys). He kept his diary from 1620 to 1706. Evelyn's diary entry for 25 November 1699 includes the following passage (in Evelyn's idiosyncratic spelling): "There happen'd this weeke so thick a mist and fog that people lost their way in the streetes, it being so intense that no light of candles or torches yielded any (or but very little) direction. I was in it and in danger. . . . It began about 4 in the afternoone, and was quite gon by 8, without any wind to disperse it. At the Thames they beat drums to direct the watermen to make to the shore."[23]

Evelyn zeroed in on the source of London's air contamination being coal-smoke generated by the key industrial polluters of his day, especially lime burners in the cement trade. Evelyn was more a country gentleman and gardener than a scientist. *Fumifugium* was a polemical tract, not a treatise. Yet if his language lacked scientific precision, he made up for it in dramatic phrasing. Referring to the furnaces of the polluters, Evelyn wrote in *Fumifugium,* "Whilst these are belching it forth their sooty jaws, the City of London resembles the face rather of *Mount Aetna,* the *Court of Vulcan, Stromboli,* or the Suburbs of *Hell,* than an Assembly of Rationale Creatures."[24]

ASBESTOS

Evelyn recognized the problem of ambient pollution, even in the seventeenth century, because it was so obvious. It was as plain as a smoke-darkened day. By the same token, water pollution may also have been self-evident to our forebears. Thus, one could argue that these examples are not relevant to subtler threats, such as those that arise in the work or home environment today. Would not our modern litany of high-tech occupational and environmental illnesses be as unfathomable to previous generations as retroviral infection or mad cow disease?

If novel agents and modern conditions only recently began to exert their adverse effects and if, furthermore, these effects are so subtle that only current medical science is sufficiently sophisticated to allow their diagnosis, then an even more explicit question needs to be asked: *Doesn't the very recognition that such problems exist at all demand prerequisites that could not have been met in early times?* Simply put, the answer is no.

Asbestos is a case in point. Asbestos is a natural, not an artificial, material. In fact, its heat-resistant properties have been known since antiquity. Asbestos use on a commercial scale, both in Europe and North America, dates back more than a hundred years.[25] For example, late nineteenth-century advertisements by H. W. Johns (later Johns-Manville) extolled the benefits of this company's asbestos roofing and made even bigger claims for its new line of asbestos-containing paint:

> This article is now well known in all parts of the country as the only reliable standard low-priced Roofing. . . . Do not be deceived by worthless materials, which are represented by unscrupulous parties as genuine ASBESTOS ROOFING. . . .
>
> ASBESTOS FIRE-PROOF PAINT; 75 cents per Gallon, white or light tints; for the protection of Factories, Bridges, Boiler Rooms, and other wooden structures in danger of ignition from sparks, cinders, or flames. It is also an economical and desirable substitute for white lead, for preserving the class of Outbuildings, Fences, etc., which are usually left unpainted.[26]

If asbestos has been around for such a long time, its history should have been sufficient for linking several generations of disease victims to this toxic agent. Why does it seem, then, that the risks of asbestos went unnoticed until the 1970s? The actual history of asbestos disease tells a different story. Asbestos-related lung disease has been well described in medical reports for more than seventy-five years. In areas of heavy manufacture and use, asbestosis, progressive lung scarring from asbestos, was endemic and recognized as such. The first known death from asbestos-caused lung scarring occurred in 1900, although the details were preserved only in evidence given to a governmental compensation committee.[27] Over the next two decades, asbestos-related lung disease was regularly documented in reports of the British chief inspector of factories and workshops, yet it was not until 1924 that the next fatal case was published.[28] By August 1927, the term *asbestosis* entered the English medical lexicon via a short announcement, carried by the *British Medical Journal,* of presentations made at the annual meeting of the Section of Preventive Medicine of the British Medical Association.[29] The journal later ran as a prominent series the three papers based on those presentations.[30]

Soon knowledge of asbestosis was not isolated to the medical arena. In *Tragic America,* his 1931 commentary on the social and economic status of the American working class, Theodore Dreiser specifically cites asbestosis as an example of a worker's health risk to which factory owners in New Jersey were completely indifferent.[31] New Jersey was a center of asbestos processing ever since H. W. Johns had first opened shop in the nineteenth century.

Although the link between asbestos exposure and cancer (as opposed to lung scarring) was first reported somewhat later, this notice still dates back to 1935, fifty years before any substantive controls were introduced. By 1960 the *Index Medicus* had a separate subject heading for asbestosis with fifteen scientific citations under eight separate subheadings.[32] Paul Brodeur's 1974 landmark work *Expendable Americans* fully documents the extent to which the health risks of asbestos were pinpointed early on, even though protective action was successfully derailed by the asbestos industry.[33] Brodeur makes clear that the machinations of Johns-Manville make those of Philip Morris seem naive and ineffectual by comparison.

Today, despite a century of well-documented deadly experience, worldwide production of asbestos products is as great as ever. Although the use of asbestos in many applications in the United States and European countries has been strictly curtailed or banned altogether, much of the rest of the world lags far behind in protective regulation for asbestos.[34]

CARPAL TUNNEL SYNDROME

Carpal tunnel syndrome may be even better than asbestos as an example of "what's old is new again." Many have had some connection with asbestos, often because of old insulation materials at home, work, or school, but few are likely to be personally acquainted with someone with actual asbestos-related lung disease. In contrast, most people directly know someone who has had carpal tunnel syndrome or may even have been diagnosed themselves with this condition. Given its current frequency, why is it that until ten or fifteen years ago hardly anyone had ever heard of carpal tunnel syndrome? Surely this is a prime example of a truly modern or even a post-modern industrial illness.

Carpal tunnel syndrome refers to a painful condition of the hands that often begins with a sensation of "pins and needles." In its most severe manifestation, it can progress to profound loss of sensation and muscle atrophy of the hand. The symptoms of carpal tunnel syndrome reflect damage to a major nerve in the hand as it enters through a narrow anatomic passageway in the wrist, the "carpal tunnel." Although carpal tunnel syndrome can have a variety of causes, in working persons the main factor leading to this condition is physical insult on the job. Carpal tunnel syndrome is caused by repetitive motion of the hands, particularly with the wrists extended (rather than flexed) or with their repeated application of a torquelike twisting force.

As it turns out, the computer keyboard provides a highly effective means for sustaining the kind of repetitive strain that induces carpal tunnel syndrome. Certain other kinds of keyboard equipment induce even more injuries. One of the most notorious is the electronic letter-sorting machinery currently used by U.S. Postal Service workers to key in zip codes and thereby direct streams of envelopes. Because the machine keyboard used in letter-sorting technology is engineered to require much force and is poorly positioned for the hands, my colleagues and I have treated a large cohort of postal workers beleaguered with carpal tunnel syndrome related to mail sorting. Carpal tunnel syndrome, however, is not exclusively the result of the ergonomic design limitations of keypunching and other keyboard devices. The grocery store price-scanning apparatus that requires repeated wrist torque (grasping cans and jars in particular) is also an effective agent of carpal tunnel syndrome.

Given the changing characteristics of the workplace involving these equipment-oriented tasks, we should not be surprised that carpal tunnel syndrome has exploded on the scene, spreading like a computer virus. But this disease too, just like asbestosis, is not new. Carpal tunnel syndrome is one of a family of conditions known collectively as either *cumulative trauma disorders* or *repetitive strain injuries*.[35] These conditions share a common and critical aspect: they are caused by the repeated use of certain parts of the body, be it the arms, feet, legs, or, in the case of carpal tunnel syndrome, the hands. In each case, overuse damages key nerves or tendons. Overuse may be promoted by a piece of mechanical equipment, but any job-related physical activity performed over and over again is capable of causing similar problems.

Carpal tunnel syndrome is presumed to be a modern disease, in part, because the name is new. In truth, the same syndrome has been around for a long while but has simply gone by many different names over time. A prime example of carpal tunnel syndrome by another name is *seamstress's cramp*. Seamstress's cramp was first described in the nineteenth century. Then, as now, this huge class of workers was predominantly female. In Victorian times, the plight of the needle trades was prominent enough to be a matter of both public concern and parliamentary investigation and was much written about.

An 1845 three-pence pamphlet by Ralph Barnes Grindrod is illustrative of the genre. Its title is *Slaves of the Needle; an Exposure of the Distressed Condition, Moral and Physical, of Dress-Makers, Milliners, Embroiderers, Slop Workers &c.*[36] This pamphlet details a number of cumulative trauma syndromes among the workers named, describing injury to the hands and feet and to the back and other muscles, as well as emphasizing severe eyestrain. Grindrod also quotes in full Thomas Hood's "Song of the Shirt," which had been published anonymously in *Punch* two years before. It is worth noting the poem's opening lines:

With fingers weary and worn,
With eyelids heavy and red

Seamstress's cramp, along with all of the other cumulative trauma disorders of the needle trade, was not a condition that first originated in nineteenth-century Britain, any more than carpal tunnel syndrome originated in the office towers of twentieth-century America. The following is from a centuries-old traditional weaver's song from Tajikistan describing a form of repetitive strain injury to the ankle:

My eyes are full of tears from broken threads:
From dawn till dusk I push my foot into the hole on which the loom
    stands.
I live as if walking on thistles and needles.[37]

Carpal tunnel syndrome may be our cumulative trauma disorder du jour, but one can choose particular injuries linked to specific vocations from a much longer à la carte menu of diseases. The major medical journals regularly publish letters from practitioners that semihumorously document disabilities such as *espresso machine operator's arm* or *video game player's finger.*

In fact, applying catchy syndrome names to cumulative trauma disorders represents a long-standing medical tradition. In much of this sport of disease naming, an underlying theme of social role and class distinction is far from subtle.[38]

New vocations linked to changing technologies have always provided the most popular monikers. *Telegrapher's cramp* is a name created by an earlier generation of practitioners, as is *scrivener's palsy* (writer's cramp), which pertains to a condition that suddenly became epidemic among nineteenth-century copy clerks using metal-tipped pens newly introduced in place of softer quills. *Carpet-layer's knee* is a modern term that is in current orthopedic use, whereas *chauffeur's knee,* which at one time referred to the partial destruction of the right knee from repetitive forcing of the crank, has become understandably archaic. The early medical umbrella categorization of these colorful syndromes was either "trade palsies" or "occupational neuroses." One of the first medical descriptions of such a condition was published in England in 1806.[39]

Clinicians may find a subtle pleasure in naming these disorders, but those afflicted take little comfort. For the very reason that these syndromes often arise as a result of core job activities, the injuries worsen with continued employment and its related trauma. Whether the condition is called carpal tunnel syndrome or zip code hand, the typical U.S. Postal Service mail sorter contracting it has few options. Typically, the employee is temporarily assigned to "casing," a tedious task of hand filing oversized items or other letters that fail electronic reading. When the injured worker returns to his or her previous task of machine-driven mail sorting, symptoms flare again. If no suitable alternative duties can be found and the worker continues sorting, the condition progresses unchecked, leading to long-term disability. If the worker cannot sort and has no other work, the only alternative is also disability.

In all likelihood, cumulative trauma injuries have troubled humankind ever since we first differentiated ourselves by making and using tools. Skeletal findings from Neolithic remains suggest cumulative trauma from stonework.[40] The documentary evidence of repetitive strain injury spans written human history. The ancient Egyptian Papyrus Sallier II mentions the mason whose "arms are worn out with work" and the weaver who is so "doubled up with his knees to his stomach, he cannot breathe."[41] Workplace injuries are not an inevitable part of modern work life or the unavoidable cost of doing business; the view that they are implies that any ergonomic critique (for example, of computer design) is tantamount to back-to-the-cave agitation by latter-day Neanderthals preferring the risks of stonework. Mechanization, when designed and used appropriately, however, can ameliorate the onset of these problems and, when wrongly applied, can facilitate them. Machine operation has never been the sine qua non for cumulative trauma.

The salient risk factor for repetitive strain injury is not high-tech, nor is it low-tech; it is simply overuse. Loss of control over the pace of work is a harbinger of cumulative trauma; piecework, its greatest sponsor. Thus, it can be associated with the sewing treadle and cutting table, the nineteenth-century paradigm, or the modern computer keyboard. The office worker, especially the employee whose efficiency is graded on the number of key-strokes made per minute, may have a set of symptoms that have been given a new name, but the essentials are unchanged. It is still the "Song of the Shirt." The lyrics may be different, but the tune is the same.

Despite this long history, it was not until 1998 that the U.S. National Institute for Occupational Safety and Health (NIOSH) published its first "white paper," full-length report on cumulative trauma disorders. The review was intended to set the stage for the promulgation of new OSHA standards but was immediately attacked by industry and trade associations. The prestigious National Academy of Sciences was called upon to re-review the entire matter, including, one by one, the more than one thousand studies cited in the original NIOSH document.[42] Despite unprecedented outside pressure that attempted to forestall its re-review, the academy found no fault with any of the previous major conclusions of NIOSH.[43]

A week before Thanksgiving 2000, to vociferous congressional and business criticism, the outgoing Clinton administration finally proposed workplace rules intended to prevent carpal tunnel syndrome and other repetitive strain injuries. By then, the government estimated that 1.8 million U.S. workers suffered from the effects of such damage. Promising to actively fight the standard, the U.S. Chamber of Commerce spokesperson responded, "We don't think there is any scientific basis to say how many repetitions are too many, how much weight is too much."[44]

A few months later, after just one day of consideration, the incoming U.S. Congress in 2001 negated the new rules.[45] In their place, the secretary of labor under the new Bush administration promulgated a set of rules for industry's self-monitoring of cumulative trauma. The principal guidelines were entirely voluntary.

Sick building syndrome serves as another ideal illustration for the presumed recent history of environmental illness, perhaps even better than carpal tunnel syndrome. After all, our modern office buildings, with their sealed windows and environmentally controlled atmospheres, are entirely a phenomenon of the last thirty to forty years. The very term *HVAC,* engineering patois for "heating, ventilation, and air-conditioning," resonates as some kind of high-tech offspring spawned by the post–World War II military-industrial complex. Sick building syndrome refers to a constellation of non-specific physical complaints, including headache, stomach upset, and malaise (medical jargon for just not feeling very good). Sick building syndrome is typically associated with large building complexes, particularly newly constructed or recently renovated ones.

No one has identified a universal, quantifiable cause of sick building syndrome. In some sick buildings, trace air contaminants given off by a variety of different materials, such as wall-to-wall carpeting, laminated furniture, and architectural detailing, have been the suspected contributors to an outbreak of symptoms. The most common factor in sick building syndrome, however, appears to be insufficient ventilation. Ventilation can be quantified in a fairly straightforward way in terms of *air exchanges.* A well-ventilated room (no less than an entire floor of a building or the entire building itself) should have enough new air brought into it and standing air discharged from it to constitute an entire exchange of its air volume many times each day.

Prior to 1980, the phrase "sick building syndrome" had not appeared in a single medical-scientific journal article title. Between 1980 and 1985, it appeared twice; between 1985 and 1990, twelve times. In the ensuing decade through 2000, at least 121 different research articles included this syndrome name in their titles.[46] Nonetheless the apparent fixation on sick buildings is not a modern preoccupation at all. Just as with carpal tunnel syndrome, it's simply the name that is new.

The importance of good air for good health has a very long medical tradition. By and large in most early medical writing the focus was on the ambient air outdoors, but indoor air was not completely ignored. One of the earliest works entirely on the subject of air quality and health, the 1549 tract *Aerarium Sanitatis,* by Antonio Gazio, warns us that air that is bad for the lungs may include "[a]ir which is wholly bad, northern, smoky, dusty, from an enclosed cavernous space, especially with furnaces in which there are metals or where metalworking is carried out. Charcoal fumes to which there is long or ongoing intermittent exposure. Air exposed to moonbeams. The exhalation of granaries when first opened after being enclosed."[47] Leaving moonbeams aside, many of Gazio's specific indoor-air-quality warnings have since been well established. The commonplace adoption of household carbon monoxide alarms is certainly testament to the dangers of combustion smoke exposure. The more generic suspicion that enclosed air is simply "bad" has also come down to us from Gazio's day.

Relatively more recently, but since Victorian times at least, a central rallying cry of public health has proclaimed the vital need for adequate air in both public and private building spaces. In fact, this concern has often verged on obsession among hygienists. Our current distrust of electronically climate-controlled, air-recirculated spaces pales when compared with standard nineteenth-century invective against the dangers of improper ventilation. Proper home ventilation was considered even more important than proper ventilation in the workplace. For example, one English physician of the time inveighed, "Our houses, like bell glasses, cover and keep in numerous impurities."[48]

In the United States in the nineteenth century, the necessity of good ventilation became, if anything, even more of an idée fixe than it was in England. Lewis Leeds's course of lectures on ventilation, delivered at the Franklin Institute in Philadelphia in the winter of 1866–67, is an excellent example of this school of thought.[49] The lecture texts read as a kind of self-help–popular science hybrid cross between Deepak Chopra and Carl Sagan. The take-home lesson was simple: American buildings, private and public, are overheated, underventilated breeding grounds of ill health, places where disease and disability fester.

Victorian hygienists often invoked the Black Hole of Calcutta as the ultimate example of adequate ventilation denied. For instructive purposes, Captain Holwell and his brave band of British East India Company men, forced to enter an overcrowded cell, constituted ideal witnesses to this danger (at least the few who lived to tell the tale). Indeed, as the very emblems of a fate doomed by the lack of an open window, they served symbolically as something of a "Donner Party of Air Hunger." Suffice it to say, the precise role that lack of ventilation actually played in the demise of the victims of the Black Hole has never really been clear. Much as in current reports of sick buildings, reliable data are scarce.

The Victorian dogma of the dangers of enclosed air was transmitted down to a new generation of public health leaders in the early twentieth century.[50] In this period, the fight for indoor air was also imbued with a touch of the patriotic fervor typical of the times, although it never reached the fevered nationalist pitch of the contemporaneous eugenics movement. Here is the view of the problem of indoor air as sponsored by the American Public Health Association, well articulated in a 1921 self-congratulatory review, "What Fifty Years Have Done for Ventilation": "The lack of ventilation in living quarters is responsible to-day for much of the tuberculosis in the land of our good friend and ally, the French Republic. The American doughboy who sojourned overseas can tell you that good ventilation is an adjunct to health." The same panegyric for pure air goes on, "The mechanical blower and the steam radiator have been a godsend to the factory operative and the girl at the department store counter. Even though located a long distance from the open window, these workers in our immense twentieth century buildings may be supplied with cool, re-vivifying air."[51]

National and international associations of building and safety engineers have long promoted clear-cut guidelines on the amount and type of ventilation needed in public buildings and private residences. There's a hitch, though. However fine these guidelines may be, building codes are largely local matters. Unless specific toxic gases build up indoors to the point of an immediate hazard, which is rarely the nature of sick building problems, corrective interventions are not mandated by federal or even state standards. The concern may be national, but the solutions, at least for the foreseeable future, must be local.

BURNOUT

What about *job burnout*? This occupational illness is prototypically social-environmental in nature rather than produced by either physical or chemical stimuli. Surely the existential condition of job burnout must be a modern problem by its very nature. The alienated, depersonalized worker of the late twentieth century seems to be unique to our time in history. Even when Mrs. Loman, in *Death of a Salesman,* tells us "Attention must be paid," she is obliquely pointing us in the direction of this problem.

In its current meaning, *burnout* implies a profound state of fatigue due to psychic forces rather than physical stress in the workplace. In fact, the lack of substantial physical demands on the job, although not a prerequisite for classic psychic burnout, is stereotypic of the modern occupational scenarios typically associated with this condition. The most extreme form of burnout is manifest in a fatal syndrome known as *karoshi* in Japan. This term has been used to refer to fatalities among young middle managers believed to have literally "worked themselves to death."[52]

A more typically American manifestation of fatal job stress involves externalized lethality.[53] The Japanese may have coined *karoshi,* but the United States has coined "going postal" as a result of this country's experience of an extreme and violent subset of burnout. This particular manifestation of burnout, in which its victim becomes victimizer in a return to the workplace with loaded weapons, is linked to service- and industrial-sector work. Despite the high-profile nature of this type of burnout, highly trained professionals are considered even more prime for work-related burnout, albeit theirs is usually of a nonviolent nature. Such professionals include health care providers, attorneys, and money managers. Even clergy are not felt to be exempt from burnout.

As it turns out, these supposedly "new" professions-at-risk are not so very new to the syndrome after all. Back before *burnout* was a medical term, but melancholy was a distinct and diagnosable condition, similar occupational groups were already the ones identified to be at the greatest risk of mental ill-health because of the nature of their work. The trail of woe for lawyers, students, clerks, and bankers stretches back a long, long way.

As far back as the Renaissance, some of the earliest treatises of the new science of medicine began focusing on the health risks from mental strain in these professions. In 1555, for example, Guglielmo Gratarolo published one of the first books on the subject, translated into English in 1574 as *A Direction for the Health of Magistrates and Studentes.*[54] A hundred years later, the same theme was echoed in a seventeenth-century Latin treatise by Fortunatus Plemp.[55] It best translates as "How to Preserve the Health of Lawyers." In addition to addressing burnout, he also warned about the indoor air hazards to lawyers from the fumes of candles.[56]

In the eighteenth century, medical scientists of the Enlightenment were no less convinced that professional trades carried serious mental risks. By that time enough wisdom on the subject had accumulated to allow a well-known Continental practitioner named Tissot (sometime physician to Voltaire) to write not one but two books on the topic. These were combined in a 1772 English translation, *An Essay on the Disorders of People of Fashion; and a Treatise on the Diseases Incident to Literary and Sedentary Persons.*[57] He cautions against overindulgence (leading to both gout and venereal disease). Yet vocational overuse of one's mental faculties may be no less dangerous; these strains lead, almost inevitably, to melancholy in a direct downward spiral. As another eighteenth-century text notes, "Hence it is often said that the melancholic are talented, but perhaps it would be nearer the mark to say that the talented become melancholic; this is because in mental work the more spirituous part of the blood is used up, whereas the more foul and earthy part is left in the body."[58]

Amazingly, this strain of medical writing did not die out with the ascendance of experimental over empiric medicine in the nineteenth century. S. Weir Mitchell, a leading American physician-writer, published an 1871 best seller entitled *Wear and Tear,* which is essentially a popularized monograph on work burnout, even though that specific term, of course, is never used. Mitchell approaches the problem as a novel and emerging manifestation of post–Civil War American work mores. At particular risk are those persons entering the business world at both too high a level and at too young an age:

> The worst instances to be met with are among young men suddenly cast into business positions involving weighty responsibility. I can recall several cases of men under or just over twenty-one who have lost health while attempting to carry the responsibilities of great manufactories. Excited and stimulated by the pride of such a charge, they have worked with a certain exaltation of brain, and, achieving success, have been stricken down in the moment of triumph.[59]

Like *burnout,* the word *workaholic* had yet to be coined, but the meaning of the comments is clear. S. Weir Mitchell extended his concerns about occupational "neural exhaustion" from the traditional workplace to nonsalaried vocations of all sorts. He goes on to note, "I firmly believe—and I am not alone in this opinion—that as concerns the physical future of women they would do far better if the brain were lightly tasked and the school-hours but three or four a day until they reach the age of seventeen at least."[60]

Mitchell carried this over from formal schooling to intellectual vocations of any sort if attempted by a woman. At the same time, he extended the concept that mental overuse brings on mental disease to mental *underuse* as an effective treatment for spontaneous disease. Not long after Mitchell wrote *Wear and Tear,* he consulted on the case of Charlotte Perkins Gilman (whom he treated for what we recognize today as endogenous depression).[61] His advice to Gilman was to limit herself to a maximum of two hours of intellectual pursuits per day and, by all means, to "never touch pen, brush, or pencil as long as you live." Charlotte Perkins Gilman's early modernist story "The Yellow Wallpaper" frighteningly documents both her own mental breakdown and Dr. S. Weir Mitchell's oppressively proscriptive "rest cure."

THE HUMAN ECOSYSTEM

Even from this brief summary of air and water pollution, asbestos disease, carpal tunnel syndrome, sick buildings, and job burnout, it is abundantly clear that environmentally related illness, in and out of the workplace, is not a modern problem that we have only recently discovered in our own time. We still face old hazards and many new ones too: novel toxic threats that potentially emerge with each technological twist and innovation of human industry, creating ongoing dangers on the job, in the home, and for the wider environment. These are the collective challenges before us. They do not obey artificial divisions between work outside and inside the home, between the environment inside and outside the factory door, among the maker of goods, the supplier of services, and the consumer. In 1962, Rachel Carson wrote, "The most alarming of all man's assaults upon the environment is the contamination of air, earth, rivers, and sea with dangerous and even lethal materials. This pollution is for the most part irrecoverable; the chain of evil it initiates not only in the world that must support life but in living tissues is for the most part irreversible."[62]

The lasting relevance of *Silent Spring* remains the ecological construct that informs it and us, teaching the inescapable interconnectedness among human industry (in the broadest sense), the air we breathe (in which the birds also fly), and the water we drink (in which the fish also swim). We live in an interlocking "environment" of work, home, and community. Changes introduced in one sphere often spill over into another with unexpected effects. Toxic materials seep into the groundwater, migrating out across many miles of aquifer. The same materials spread out by other routes, rippling through waves of human activity, from primary manufacture through commercial distribution.

The human advancements that introduce such risks into our environment need not be sophisticated; it is often a small change in a relatively simple technology that carries great potential for harm, even through the everyday products that surround us. In the coming chapters, I cover the histories of some of these substances. Their stories show how we are all tied together in a single, complex human ecosystem, an environment that, in its fundamentals, is no less delicate than an ocean tide pool or a rain forest grove. Their stories also give shape to critical interrelationships among the past, the present, and the future, compelling us to examine closely a lost environmental history we all would do well to remember.

TWO

The Shadow of Smoke
How to Evade Regulation

RAPID RECOGNITION—SLOW CONTROL

The links between exposure and occupational or environmental disease, even with novel toxins, usually are identified with surprising accuracy and speed. These causal connections, however, seem to require periodic rediscovery over time. In a cyclical pattern, the accumulated knowledge and experience tying toxic risks to adverse health effects are erased with a regular periodicity. The discoveries and then the rediscoveries of new/old environmental hazards, sometimes over many decades or even several centuries, are matched by a repeated pattern of corrective failures when it comes to definitively fixing the problem. In fact, the two are tightly linked in a parody of Newtonian mechanics, reworked so that for every action there appears to be an equal and opposite degree of inaction. This may explain, in part, a relatively short span of collective memory for these events: as public expectations of remediation are slowly dimmed and then eclipsed, time passes and forgetfulness sets in.

The scenarios by which corrective action has so often been thwarted have been staggeringly duplicative over their long history. The same old arguments against the need for protective action, in the workplace and for the wider environment, have been paraded forth time and again, simply reoutfitted in whatever the costume of the day is. Even the revisionists' arguments that environmental concerns are both insubstantial and of recent manufacture do not form a new line of reasoning. Indeed, belittling the problem may be one of the most standard opening gambits when naysayers seek to put off any action.

The scenario for failed protection follows a pattern of responses analogous to the Kubler-Ross four-stage "death and dying process": denial, anger, bargaining, and acceptance. In this instance, in the initial stage, denial, polluters minimize and explain away the purported hazard. Next, they mount angry counterattacks seeking to neutralize those pressing for control of the problem. In the bargaining stage, polluters seek the best deal that can be had by weakening any proposed intervention mechanisms before they are ever put into place. The final stage of the death and dying process has been conceptualized as an acceptance of the true nature of the immutable situation at hand. Unfortunately, in negotiations over occupational and environmental hazards, those who were injured or made ill in the first place are almost always the ones forced into acceptance. Those responsible for the problem most often simply walk away, unscathed.

Thus in practice, the strategies used to block any effective action are:

1. characterizing scientific information as limited, overblown, conflicting, or simply "junk."

2. blaming the victim and simultaneously charging that regulation is overly costly and ineffectual to boot.

3. labeling opponents as unrealistic visionaries or, worse yet, seditionist Luddites standing in the way of inevitable progress.

4. reaching out to the *invisible hand of the marketplace* as the best partner for corrective action, if such action is really needed.

The following pages trace how each of these strategies has been successfully exploited.

MORE DATA ARE NEEDED

Of these four strategies, decrying insufficient information to establish fact may perhaps be the most familiar to us from current debates. Take, for example, the fight over global warming. Its tactical popularity is not surprising, given its rich legal heritage and long track record of success, going back to at least the seventeenth century. In 1700, the Italian physician Bernardino Ramazzini published *Diseases of Workers,* in which he tells the story of a citizen's failed suit against a manufacturer for polluting an entire residential neighborhood with chemical fumes arising from a laboratory situated there (clarifications to text are bracketed):

> A few years ago a violent dispute arose between a citizen of Finale, a town in the dominion of Modena, and a certain business man, a Modenese, who owned a huge laboratory at Finale where he manufactured sublimate [a mercury-containing compound]. The citizen of Finale brought a lawsuit against this manufacturer and demanded that he should move the workshop outside the town or to some other place, on the ground that he poisoned the whole neighborhood whenever his workmen roasted vitriol [a source of sulfuric acid] in the furnace to make sublimate.

Ramazzini goes on to detail the extent of evidence:

> To prove the truth of his accusation he produced the sworn testimony of the doctor of Finale and also the parish register of deaths, from which it appeared that many more persons died annually in that quarter and in the immediate neighborhood of the laboratory than in other localities. Moreover, the doctor gave evidence that the residents of that neighborhood usually died of wasting disease and diseases of the chest; this he ascribed to the fumes given off by the vitriol, which so tainted the air near by that it was rendered unhealthy and dangerous for the lungs.

Ramazzini's story, up to this point, sounds like a slam dunk for the plaintiff. But we have yet to hear from the defense's expert witness. "Dr. Bernardino Corradi, the commissioner of ordinance [overseeing and profiting from munitions manufacture] in the Duchy of Este, defended the manufacturer. . . . Various cleverly worded documents were published by both sides, and this dispute which was literally 'about the shadow of smoke,' as the saying is, was hotly argued. In the end the jury sustained the manufacturer, and vitriol was found not guilty."[1]

One irony in Ramazzini's phrasing is the implication that an inanimate material (the toxin vitriol) was innocent until proven guilty and thus elevated to a level of civil rights protection denied most citizens of the time. Karl Marx was to make the same point in an early and important essay on the priority of rights given to firewood over those of peasants desperate for fuel.[2]

Although Marx did not draw directly on Ramazzini in that particular work, he did cite *Diseases of Workers* in *Das Kapital*. Marx recognized well that the production of illness could represent a hidden cost of industrial manufacture.[3] And Marx was not alone in this realization. Economic arguments have no less venerable a tradition than legal ones in the history of how and why occupational and environmental protections can be blocked. In fact, the presumed ineffectiveness, unfeasibility, and excessive expense of almost any corrective measure have been almost axiomatic as rationales for inaction. On the political front, when any proposed regulation is served up as an absurd recipe for disaster, this is often seasoned with a healthy dash of victim blaming as well.

The lines in these battles do not necessarily fall along a consistently marked out progressive/conservative divide. For example, one of the great nineteenth-century English reformers, Harriet Martineau, despite her elevation to the liberal pantheon as an abolitionist and early feminist, was rabidly reactionary on the subject of workers' health. She was a master of economically driven victim blaming.

Martineau viciously attacked the prospect of even the most rudimentary factory protection proposed at that time in Great Britain. To that end, in 1855 she penned a pamphlet on the subject, titled *The Factory Controversy; A Warning Against Meddling Legislation*. In its pages, Martineau decried what she viewed as a ludicrous regulation that would require protective bars around the moving parts in mills. Martineau felt that such controls would be absurd, given that it was the workers' own failure to follow safety instructions that was the true cause of any equipment-related injury. To make her point, she recounts cold-bloodedly the tale of a worker too foolish to have ever been saved by protective bars:

> James Ashworth, employed by Messrs. Wild and Son, of Heywood, threw away his life by an act which is forbidden in mills so expressly that there is no pretense for saying that he was killed in the course of his occupation. One of the two straps which had slipped from its pulleys became entangled with the other; and Ashworth had the foolhardiness to attempt to disentangle them with his hands. The second strap slipped off, lapped round the shaft, and drew the poor man up to the ceiling, where his brains were dashed out.[4]

Charles Dickens was on the opposite side of this argument, entering into an entertainingly public and acerbic exchange with Martineau. The group that sponsored Martineau's pamphlet was called the National Association of Factory Occupiers. Dickens renames them the National Association for the Protection of the Right to Mangle Operatives.[5] Martineau, in turn, refers to Dickens as "sordid" and "law hating" for his agitation against the mill owners. Then, in an amazing flourish, she compares Dickens to the ineffectual do-gooder Mrs. Jellyby, a character from his novel *Bleak House*. This betrays an impressive degree of psychological projection—as one suspects that Dickens must have modeled Jellyby on Martineau herself or at least on someone very much like her.

That the unfortunate James Ashworth had his brains "dashed out" two days before Christmas in 1854 provides the whole episode with an added Dickensian flourish that seems to have been lost on both sides. The government took Messrs. Wild and Son to court to collect a fine of one thousand pounds. It failed, although the factory owners did eventually settle with Ashworth's survivors to the sum of 150 pounds. This, Ms. Martineau tells us, was an act of "pure benefaction on their part."[6]

Protective safety bars eventually were installed by statute in various workplaces, but they continued to serve as a backdrop for further victim blaming. A classic example can be found in a 1916 U.S. government pamphlet, *How a Miner Can Avoid Some Dangerous Diseases.*[7] Intended to educate the worker in supposedly simple language, it devotes the bulk of its twenty-five pages to personal hygiene around the miner's shack, with subsections such as "Slop Water Causes Nuisances" and "Make the Privy Sanitary."

Only near its conclusion, in the section "Rock Dust," does the pamphlet acknowledge, grudgingly, the real health hazards of the miner's job, "Working in dust, like exposure, is at times unavoidable, but a great deal, if not most of the dust breathing is due to carelessness on the part of the miner himself who does not realize the danger of so doing, or if he does is indifferent to it. *It is another example of failing to keep up the bars around an open place*" (italics added).

THE PRIORITY OF PROGRESS

Victim blaming, as Martineau demonstrates, has a lot of precedent. For at least two hundred years, another tradition has been to dismiss any expressed concern over the adverse health effects of new machinery or other technological innovation as a slackish labor-organizing ploy seeking to avoid the inevitable impact of progress, even if it means a work speedup. Alternatively, some have dismissed this concern as the ravings of Luddite throwbacks seeking to block progress simply because it is progress. Others, as the tactical ideal, lay both charges simultaneously.

We can see this lesson illustrated in one of its earliest forms in an instructive primer called *Tom and Charles, or, the Grinders*.[8] This was a children's book printed in 1824 in Sheffield, England, a manufacturing center long associated with cutlery grinding. Tom Crafty and Charles Lowly are poor orphans, we are told at the outset. Tom, the most popular boy at the charity school, robs a classmate of two shillings. Charles is falsely accused. Eventually, Tom is found out as the real thief and is expelled. After his expulsion, Tom is bound as an apprentice to a grinder. Because he is initially a success (easy charm is one of Tom's several vices), the grinder for whom he works comes back to the school looking for a second boy to apprentice along with him. The grinder picks Charles Lowly, who is thus thrown in with Tom Crafty once again.

The grinders, we learn, are metalworkers who have operated essentially as free agents up to this time. Each has his own "trough" with a water-driven grinding wheel. "When they are employed, they can earn great wages," *The Grinders* instructs us (17). Of course, we also learn that the employment is sporadic, with periods of forced idleness when the water that powers the grinding stones is low (in summer) or frozen (in winter).

Intended as a simple morality tale of Christian virtue, *The Grinders* inadvertently documents a critical turning point in industrial disease. Grinding had always been a dangerous trade, not because of the metals worked, but because of the abrasives used to sharpen and polish them. Grinding stones, in the working of the metal, give off a fine dust of silica. The inhaled silica, in turn, causes a progressive and deadly scarring of the lungs, known as silicosis.

Of all of the many industries in which silica has been a hazard, none was to become as infamous as that of the Sheffield grinders of the generation that followed Charles and Tom. When these two start their apprenticeship in the story, the old water-powered freelance operation is still in place. It is idyllic only by contrast with what is to come. We are told, "In the more open wheels of the country, by the side of rapidly running streams, the strong current of air which is almost always flowing through the room, disperses the dust which is constantly rising under their noses, and which, in a still atmosphere, they imbibe in breathing" (69).

It was exactly during this period in Sheffield that steam power was introduced. This served several purposes. First, it freed the operation of the grinding wheels from any seasonal downtime. Second, it greatly increased the overall pace of production. Third, by controlling the source of power, quite literally, the owners abolished the old freelance system.

Indeed, the central plot line of *The Grinders* revolves around this new mechanization and an unsuccessful strike by the workers opposed to the deterioration in their terms and conditions of employment. To get its message across, the story line invokes a theme echoing the recent Luddite uprising that had taken place in the textile industry a little more than ten years before the time frame of *The Grinders*. Just as the Luddite laborers destroyed mill machinery in an attempt to improve their lot, wicked Tom hatches a plan to physically sabotage the grinding machinery.

His plan is thwarted by Charles. Thus Charles is able to take and hold the moral high ground in *The Grinders,* not only because of his inherent Christian virtues, but also because, inter alia, he is also a strikebreaker. Yet despite his many virtues, Charles Lowly still has a price to pay. "He had found his health considerably affected by constantly working in close rooms in a confined situation. Grinding is at best not a healthy employment; but it has become much more fatal since the introduction of the steam-engines" (68–69).

All the children of Sheffield who first read *The Grinders,* and their children after them as well, had the opportunity to grow up to work and then die young if they were employed in the metal-grinding industry. It was an industry in which silicosis, known also as grinder's asthma, reached the levels of an epidemic disease. By the 1860s, the average life expectancy of a steam-powered Sheffield worker had declined to twenty-nine years for fork grinders, to thirty-two for scissors grinders, and to thirty-five for knife grinders. The lucky saw or sickle worker, in contrast, might expect to live to the ripe age of thirty-eight years. This hierarchy of mortality had a straightforward explanation, as one contemporary report on the working conditions in Sheffield makes clear. "The ascending longevity being in proportion to the amount of water used on the stone, and to the greater amount of adult labor employed; such articles as saws, sickles, and tools are happily too heavy to be manipulated by the children employed, and thus [are] early diseased in the manufacture of the lighter articles."[9]

THE INVISIBLE HAND OF THE MARKETPLACE

The remaining, and debatably most "modern," argument against protective regulation claims that the balance between consumers (or laborers as a special class of consumers) and business acts as an innate and corrective market force. This proposition holds that self-interest on both sides (especially the side on which capital is concentrated) provides the best guarantee of protection. For this recipe to work, even on its own theoretical terms, a symmetric balance of information is a required starting ingredient that is almost never present.

Adam Smith is the spiritual godfather of this line of reasoning, although it took later political theorists of laissez-faire economics to develop these market force arguments in relation to workplace and environmental safety and health. By the latter part of the nineteenth century, the Social Darwinists already had quite a bit to say on the subject. They argued that external regulations for safety and health protection were unwarranted because, simply put, business knows best. Yes, they might allow that child labor is an area in which limited governmental purview may be reasonable. But this sole intervention, if anything, was the exception that proved the rule. This way of thinking was so widespread in the latter half of the nineteenth century that one finds the amazing rationale, explicitly stated, that the protection of adult workers is valid only to the extent that they are like children. "They are supposed, it is true, to be free agents, but, practically, they are little more so than the children Government has so properly taken under its protection."[10]

The most dramatic "proof of concept" experiment for a laissez-faire economic corrective working to the benefit of public safety was supposed to be the case of the modern match industry, an example of an entirely new manufacturing process driven by technological innovation.[11] The modern match was first introduced commercially in the 1830s. This was made possible by the chemical discovery that phosphorous could be used to produce an easily ignitable liquid compound into which wooden sticks could be dipped and then dried. The industry was initially concentrated in Germany and Austria and quickly grew to employ a large number of workers.

Although risk of incendiary mishap due to phosphorous was easily predictable and frequent, another, far more insidious, danger in the match trade also became clear. When chronically inhaled or taken into the mouth, phosphorous, it was discovered, slowly eats away the victim's bones. Because the jawbone was highly exposed through fumes entering the mouth, its degeneration was the most severe. By the mid-1840s (only ten years after the new match was introduced commercially) a new and devastating disease, osteonecrosis of the mandible, was already well documented in the medical literature. The condition became known popularly as phossy jaw.

The new lucifer, or strike-anywhere, matches were wildly popular with consumers, and the highly lucrative industry spread quickly. German and Austrian reports were soon complemented by those from France and England. Then, on 26 January 1852, Dr. H. J. Bigelow presented an unusual surgical case. The minutes of the Boston Society for Medical Improvement duly note:

> In March last, a man with an immensely swollen lower jaw, and highly inflamed tongue and gums, presented himself to Dr. Bigelow for advice; diagnosis difficult. Leeches were ordered. Dr. Bigelow left town soon after for Europe, and in a fortnight after, Dr. Gay saw the patient. The parts affected had now opened, and a probe detected dead bone. The man entered the Massachusetts General Hospital, his health continuing to fail. . . . The patient had been engaged in the fabrication of friction matches, and thus exposed to the fumes of phosphorous, which at last caused the disease.[12]

Dr. Bigelow promised to show a pathologic specimen from the man's autopsy at the next meeting, informing the group that this was the first case in which this condition, already well known in Europe, had been detected in America. It would be far from the last. Phossy jaw spread wherever the match industry took hold. It was so widespread and well recognized a problem that it even became material for contemporary fiction. In Chekhov's late work, "The Steppe: The Story of a Journey," one of its key characters is asked by the protagonist (a child named Yergoruska) why his chin is so swollen, and Vassya replies, "It hurts . . . I used to work at a match factory, young sir. The doctor did say as how that was what made me jaw swell. The air ain't healthy there, and there were three other lads beside me who had swollen jaws, and one of them had it rot right away."[13]

The epidemic need not have continued; there was an easy preventive solution to the problem. As early as 1850, red phosphorous was introduced commercially as the original "safety match" or, because of the original patent, as "Swedish safety matches." It was clearly a safer substitute for the yellow phosphorous used in strike-anywhere matches, and the potential health benefits of this new match were immediately appreciated. The second U.S. medical report on phossy jaw was published by the *Saint Louis Medical and Surgical Journal* in 1854, two years after Bigelow's.[14] The article concludes with a prominent footnote (illustrated with a pointing hand so as to be better noticed) calling the reader's attention to the new red phosphorous alternative formulation for matches that had recently been invented.

Although physicians were in favor of the new red phosphorous, the innovation proved less popular with consumers, because the striking mechanism was more complicated, requiring a special box for ignition. It was even less popular with manufacturers of the strike-anywhere matches; the red phosphorous was more expensive than the yellow, cutting into the profit margin of those who went so far as to substitute the red for the yellow.

In 1874 Denmark wisely banned the production and sale of yellow phosphorous matches, requiring use of the safer substitute. Neighboring Sweden did not follow Denmark's lead; despite its association with the red phosphorous safety match formulation, it was a major exporter of yellow phosphorous matches. In Sweden and in all the other match-manufacturing centers, yellow phosphorous remained in production. Improved workplace hygiene, it was argued, was a more realistic solution to the problem of phossy jaw. As a part of this strategy, specific regulations were passed in a number of countries, beginning with an inspection rule as early as 1846 in Austria, mandating health-screening examinations of workers and other protective steps.

One intervention popular among some employers was to provide the laborers in their factories with turpentine-soaked sponges to wear beneath the chin as a protector against the phosphorous fumes. This was about as effective as the governmental hygiene rules, whose failure was clear from the beginning. In 1863, a British physician named Henry Letheby, who had cared for many patients suffering from phossy jaw, testified to an official commission. "Means might be adopted no doubt to ameliorate the present evils that arise from the manufacture of lucifer matches; but I think that the whole force of the evidence derived from my reading and experience points to the use of red phosphorous as the most likely means of getting rid of the danger to health, which results from the manufacture as it is now conducted."[15]

The British authorities may have listened, but they did not concur with Dr. Letheby that the only viable protective option was to use the red phosphorous substitute. In the following years, Great Britain enacted very detailed and specific factory legislation to prevent phossy jaw while preserving intact the yellow phosphorous manufacturing industry. These factory rules gave particular emphasis to protecting child laborers in the industry, who often bore the brunt of exposure and manifested the worst ravages of the disease. Even these changes, which may have kept some children out of the workhouse, did nothing to diminish another growing yellow phosphorous menace, especially for younger children. Toddlers, it seems, were at particular risk from acute yellow phosphorous poisoning brought about from chewing on the odd match or two. Such cases continued to be commonplace throughout the latter half of the nineteenth century.

By the turn of the century, the new approach of a British firm called Bryant and May's had become the shining example of industrial responsibility in making yellow phosphorous matches. Ironically, Bryant and May's had been the original U.K. patent holder for the Swedish method of producing red phosphorous safety matches, but instead it found that the popular strike-anywhere match was the key to a successful business. Using the old yellow phosphorous method, the firm grew to become one of the largest manufacturers in the industry, admired as its hygienic standard setter. Phossy jaw was supposedly unknown among Bryant and May's lucky employees.

This reputation was finally dispelled as fiction, however, when, on 1 June 1898, Bryant and May's was cited for failing to report phossy jaw cases as required by law.[16] The violation had come to light when the death of one of the Bryant and May's workers, a man named Cornelius Lean, was found at inquest to be due to phosphorous poisoning. Further inquiry revealed seventeen other, similarly unreported cases of disease. Appearing at court for the firm as its managing director, Mr. Gilbert Bartholomew stated that Bryant and May's was extremely sorry. The court inflicted the full penalty allowable, which amounted to a fine of twenty-five pounds, nine shillings. Public outrage was so strongly voiced that a governmental commission was appointed to look into the matter.

At about the same time that Bryant and May's was hauled into court, another new phosphorous derivative was perfected for use in matches. It was as safe to use and easier to strike than red phosphorous, although still more costly than the yellow. This new material was invented in France, where the match industry was a state-run monopoly, facilitating the substitution of the new phosphorous formulation. As individual countries across Europe and around the world, one by one, finally adopted internal national bans on yellow phosphorous matches, the impetus grew for concerted international action. This goal was realized in a 1906 treaty convention. Although Great Britain was not a formal signatory, by 1908 even it agreed to honor the treaty's provisions.[17]

A few holdouts remained. The United States was one of them. Despite examples dating back to Bigelow's Boston report, industry argued that

American cases were rare. Finally, in January 1910, a federal *Bureau of Labor Statistics Bulletin* debunked this argument, documenting hundreds of cases of phossy jaw in multiple U.S. workplaces.[18] Meanwhile, on 16 December 1910, 20 January 1911, and 10 January 1912, the U.S. House Ways and Means Committee held hearings preparatory to legislation meant to control yellow phosphorous.[19] Congressman John J. Esch of Wisconsin, a Republican who was allied with the Progressives, put the legislation forward. Witnesses included Warren B. Hutchinson, president of both the East Jersey Match Company and the Salvation Match Company; F. W. Woods, representing the Ohio Match Company; Fred Fear, of the Fred Fear Match Company; and William A. Fairburn, general superintendent of the Diamond Match Company.

Esch proposed a novel legislative solution to the match hazard. It was believed that on constitutional grounds the United States could not participate in the 1906 treaty because it would dictate to states how they could conduct intrastate commerce. The Esch bill circumvented this problem simply by putting a prohibitive tax on all yellow phosphorous matches sold domestically and simultaneously banning both the export and import of the product. Esch's proposed bill became law in 1913. Business opposition was overcome only after Diamond Match agreed to share with other producers the domestic patent rights it had already locked in for the new safe phosphorous alternative originally developed in France.

This "success story" in controlling the yellow phosphorous menace has been invoked to show the effectiveness of regulation when it works in cooperation with enlightened business interests.[20] In fact, this experience teaches quite the opposite lesson. For over fifty years, halfway regulatory measures that deferred to manufacturing and market priorities could never bring the phosphorous hazard under control. Laissez-faire protection proved to be an utter failure. Only an outright ban, long blocked by business interests, offered an adequate margin of public safety.[21]

THE LEGACY OF SOCIAL DARWINISM

The nineteenth- and early twentieth-century arguments over the role that market forces should play in public protection reverberate to this day. Social Darwinism, with its ambivalent mix of warmed-over paternalism and cold-blooded detachment, continues to cast a long shadow. Herbert Spencer's central 1851 text, *Social Statics,* seems to have had real staying power on the antiregulatory best-seller list, though even Spencer allows that pollution of water or air is not a reasonable sphere of free agency by one citizen, given that it adversely affects others against their will.[22]

In March 2001, John Tierney, a libertarian-oriented *New York Times* columnist, provided a textbook example of how the tired old ideas of laissez-faire protection continue to be recirculated. Under the header "Best Incentive to Make Sure Workers Don't Get Hurt: Money," Tierney writes:

> Here we go again. By rescinding a new set of ergonomic regulations, Congress this week raised an old question: do the workers of the world need politicians and union leaders to write safety rules for them? . . . Workplace safety rules never did much to protect workers. Conditions improved over the last century because safety was profitable: employers wanted to avoid injuries that lessened productivity and drove up costs, notably the bill for workers' compensation insurance.[23]

In his commentary, Tierney reveals his own personal bout of work-related tendonitis brought on by heavy typing, an injury that put him "out of commission" for six months. The *New York Times* eventually invested heavily in work-site ergonomic interventions (the problem was widespread), a scenario of corrective action that he believes is just as likely to be played out for any other employee working anywhere else. He should sort mail at the U.S. Postal Service for a while.

WHEN ACTION IS FINALLY TAKEN

A point comes when the empiric evidence of damage is so overwhelming, the required interventions are so self-evident, and the public's outrage is manifested to such a degree that laws are indeed finally passed, new rules promulgated, or inspectorates expanded or established. In the most egregious cases, imminently hazardous enterprises may even be shut down.

In 1983, exactly such an extreme chain of events transpired near Chicago, Illinois. Paramedics were called to a factory located in a suburban industrial park.[24] A middle-aged worker had fatally collapsed on the job from what, at first, seemed to be an ordinary heart attack. Then the paramedics, attempting to reach the victim, were themselves suddenly overcome with severe symptoms of nausea and light-headedness. They became even more alarmed when several of the dead victim's younger coworkers reported, in broken English, that they, too, were ill with headache, nausea, and dizziness. Such symptoms were frequent in the plant, they readily admitted.

The industrial operations at the facility, which was housed in a converted warehouse, were quite simple. Discarded medical X-ray films were cut into little pieces and placed in large vats of water to which a white powder was added. The liquid resulting from this mix was pumped into a second vat, then processed through a modified electroplating apparatus. In the final step, the electroplating panels were removed, and the metal deposited on them was scraped off by hand. The metal whose extraction was the goal of this entire process was silver, salvaged from the minute quantities present in each chip of spent X-ray photographic film.

The workers in this facility could describe the process up to this initial level of detail but not beyond it. I had the opportunity to interview many of them when I led a team of investigators from Cook County Hospital in documenting the extent to which the former workers continued to experience ill effects even months after cessation of their exposure.

By the time of the interviews, we knew what these workers had not known when they worked at Film Recovery Systems. The white powder, which they took from metal barrels with blacked-out labels and mixed into the tanks many times each day, was cyanide. Cyanide salt was the critical ingredient in the electroplating process that allowed the silver extraction to take place. Cyanide is widely used in the plating industry, but with the mandate of strict precautions. The concentration of cyanide salt in aqueous solution must not be too great, nor can any acid be allowed to interact with the solution, because either situation produces deadly hydrogen cyanide gas. Air levels of cyanide gas in the plant, measured days after active operations ceased, were still at least twice the legal OSHA limit.

Nor is this the only danger from such an operation. Even without being given off as a gas, cyanide salts in solution can be lethal if the solution comes in contact with unprotected skin. The surviving workers described just such exposures. The vats routinely overflowed, leaving large cyanide-laden puddles on the floor. No warnings or specific protective equipment were provided. Since there was no lunchroom, when the concession truck rolled up at lunch break each day, workers often ate and drank in work areas. Altogether, conditions were so hazardous that was it was only a matter of time before a fatality occurred.

The plant was quickly shut down following the death that day in 1983. OSHA levied monetary penalties. But the Cook Country district attorney's office went beyond the closure and the fines. It sought an indictment of murder against the owners of Film Recovery Systems. The shutdown of this factory and the prosecution of its owners for murder represented the strongest possible regulatory and legal response. Although no similar prosecution of industrial murder by poisoning had occurred in the United States, indictments were brought and the case did go to trial. Yet even this set of seemingly definitive actions was eroded over time. Despite an initial conviction, the verdict was later overturned on appeal. Also, one of the key defendants "relocated" to Utah and was never even brought to trial, since that state would not agree to extradition. The OSHA fines, even though they were modest to begin with, were reduced further after negotiations with the owners of Film Recovery Systems.

The worker who died was an immigrant from Poland with no family in the United States. Almost all of the other workers were Mexican immigrants, many of whom spoke little or no English. Although assisted by a local community group, they did not have the resources for lengthy civil tort action. Moreover, despite a variety of ongoing symptoms, the majority of these former employees were too fearful of problems with immigration authorities to allow themselves the luxury of pursuing legal action over any potential long-term health effects from cyanide exposure.

DEFERRED ENFORCEMENT

Extreme examples of ineffective worker protection such as these teach us that even when we eventually take action to control a hazard, those who benefited from an absence of controls may adopt a final course of action geared to negate any possible success. If anything, this strategy is even more cynical than the tactics of dueling expert opinions, blaming the victim, attacking the proponents of control, or invoking market-driven social determinism. This maneuver allows the construction of a rudimentary regulatory apparatus, but what appears to be an effective protective shield is only a simulacrum. Ultimately, should the machinery of protection ever be put into motion, the moving parts of enforcement will not be lubricated, and if they should break, they will go without replacement.

One of the single most publicized occupational disasters in the United States occurred on 25 March 1911. It was on that day that fire swept through the Asch Building in New York City, killing 146 workers of the Triangle Shirtwaist Company. Nineteen-year-old Bessie Gabrilowich's story was not unusual, except that she survived. Bessie was at work on the ninth floor when fire started coming up from the cutting room, one floor below. Many of her coworkers died after leaping from the windows; the firemen's ladders could reach only the seventh floor, and their nets tore, failing from the weight of the employees who jumped simultaneously. Bessie Gabrilowich was one of the lucky ones; instead of jumping she found access to a stairway and made it to the street alive.[25] After the fire, investigators learned that exit doors from the shop had been locked for better control in keeping the women at their sewing machines. The owners of the Triangle Shirtwaist Company were tried for manslaughter but acquitted. In 1914, some of the victims' families won seventy-five dollars each in a civil suit against the owners.[26]

Fire codes are local matters. New York City, in response to the disaster, established the Bureau of Fire Safety. In most other matters, worker safety codes were a state, certainly not a national, prerogative at the time. This remained so until the establishment of the federal OSHA in 1970. OSHA sets national standards for work practices, including requirements for safety exits in case of fire. OSHA enforcement depends on inspections, however, and the agency has always been understaffed. Back in the 1980s, the number of OSHA inspectors then in place was estimated to be sufficient to reach every workplace once for a routine inspection sometime around the year 2050. Under the Reagan administration, new guidelines were developed mandating that only work sites that had reported frequent injuries to OSHA would be prioritized for inspection. In response to this disincentive to accurate reporting, the enforcement gap widened further. It has not been effectively narrowed since.

Bessie Gabrilowich, the Triangle Shirtwaist fire survivor, went on to become Bessie Cohen, raise a family, and live a long and full life. Active in the International Ladies Garment Workers Union, she saw it grow into a major force for worker protection, part of the Union of Needletrades, Industrial, and Textile Employees (UNITE). When Bessie Gabrilowich Cohen passed away at the age of 107, her obituary commented, "For many years after the fire, her son said, she would react fearfully to thunder and lightning, burying her head in her arms and sobbing."[27]

The obituary also noted that Bessie Cohen had lived long enough to see a near replay of the Triangle Shirtwaist fire. In this 1991 incident, the employees, once again mostly women, were trapped in a burning plant that processed chicken parts. The fire occurred in Hamlet, North Carolina. Twenty-five died trying to flee through exit doors, locked just as they had been at the Triangle Shirtwaist site. The authorities, after the fact, were quick to cite the facility's violations, totaling $808,150 in fines. Six months later, its owner was indicted and later convicted of manslaughter. Eventually, the families of the victims received a sixteen-million-dollar cash settlement, a post hoc remediation that contrasts with the aftermath of the Triangle Shirtwaist fire. In both cases, however, the failure in prevention is key. The Hamlet plant had been run by a company called Imperial Food Products. In eleven years of operation until the time of the fire, it had never once been inspected by federal, state, or local safety regulators.

In April 1996, the federal Occupational Safety and Health Administration presented the National Museum of American History with two charred doors left as a record of the Imperial Food Products disaster.[28] As the Hamlet fire makes clear, even if, at long last, regulations are finally on the books, inspection deferred is protection denied. This is no fleeting specter or a mere legal argument about an insubstantial "shadow of smoke," such as Ramazzini described in Modena so many centuries earlier.

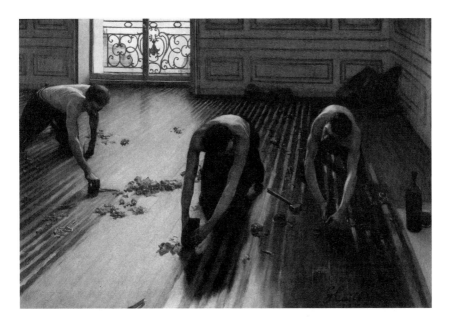

Gustave Caillebotte (1848–1894), *Les roboteurs de parquet* (The Floor Scrapers), 1875. Oil on canvas, 102 cm × 146.6 cm, RF 2718. Photo: Herve Lewandowski. Photo credit: Réunion des musées nationaux/Art Resource, NY, Musee d'Orsay, Paris, France.

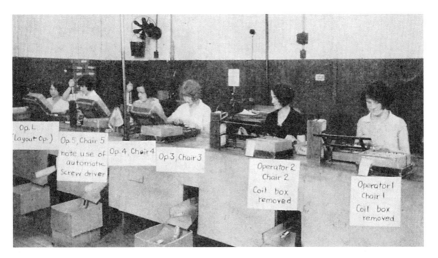

The operatives during the Hawthorne experiment. Photographic illustration reproduced from L. J. Henderson and Elton Mayo, "Effects of the Social Environment," in *The Environment and Its Effect upon Man; Symposium Held at Harvard School of Public Health, August 24–August 29, 1936, as Part of Harvard University Tercentenary Celebration, 1636–1936* (Boston: Harvard School of Public Health, 1937); the image appears on page 3, 9.2 cm × 11.4 cm.

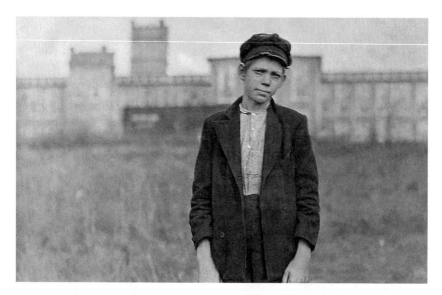

Will Morrill, Wylie Mill; Chester, S.C. Been in the mill 5 years. Photograph by Lewis Hine, 1908. Gelatin silver print in the collection of the author. The image is also held in the records of the National Child Labor Committee, Library of Congress (Lot 7479, vol. 1, no. 0320). Original photograph 12.1 cm × 17.1 cm.

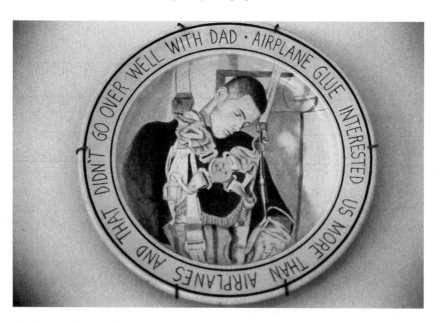

Charles Krafft, *Dead Pilot.* Hand-painted overglaze on production china, 1992. 25.4 cm in diameter. Private collection. Used with permission of the artist.

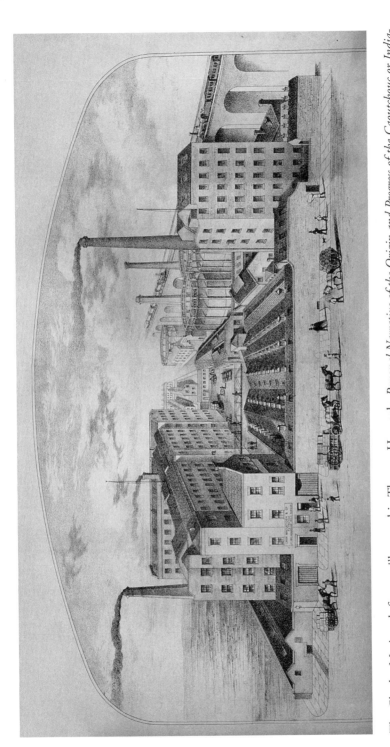

The Charles Macintosh factory, illustrated in Thomas Hancock, *Personal Narrative of the Origin and Progress of the Caoutchouc or India-Rubber Manufacture in England* (London: Longman, Brown, Green, Longman & Roberts, 1857). The printed illustration is an oversized panorama foldout, 22.2 cm × 43 cm, following the title page.

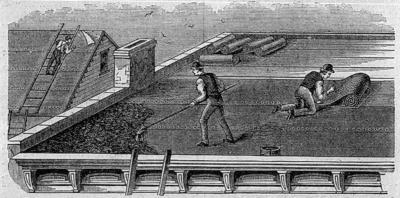
Asbestos advertisement for H. W. Johns, nineteenth century. Original size 11.4 cm × 17.1 cm.

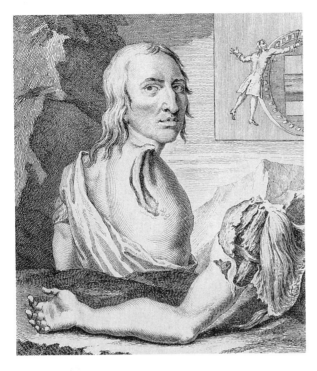

Samuel Wood. Whose Arm with the Shoulder blade was torn off by a Mill y^e: 15th of Aug: 1737. He was brought to S^t. Thomas's Hospital y^e: next day where he was Cured by M^r. Ferne. Etching, plate mark 23.5 cm × 18.6 cm. London: published by Samuel Wood according to an act of Parliament, 1 November 1737. Collection of the author.

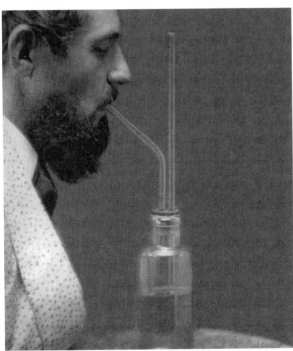

Peter Welling, *James Hyatt Inhaling Chlorine Gas.* Sixth-plate daguerreotype, 1850–1855. This daguerreotype was used as the basis for an engraving illustrating Hyatt's *The Elements of Chemistry.* The Metropolitan Museum of Art, Gilman Collection, Museum Purchase, 2005 (2005.100.386).

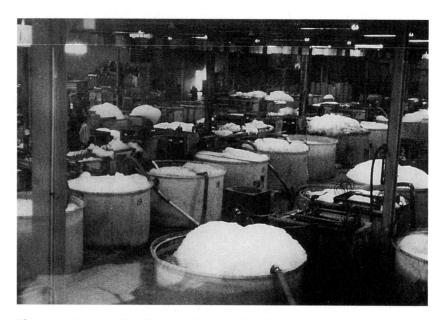

Plant operations at Film Recovery Systems. The image was provided as a photographic transparency slide (2.4 cm × 3.4 cm) to the author in 1985 by the Cook County State's Attorney's Office. See also P. D. Blanc et al., "Cyanide Intoxication among Silver-Reclaiming Workers," *Journal of the American Medical Association* 253 (18 January 1985): 367–371.

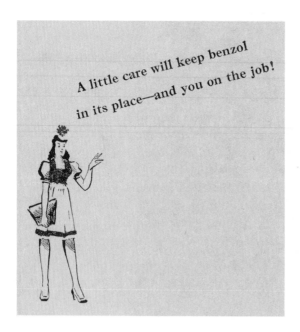

Clara Carelittle, full-page illustration (15 cm × 11.5 cm) in Federal Security Agency, U.S. Public Health Service, *Clara Gives Benzol the Run Around,* Workers' Health Series no. 4 (Washington DC: U.S. Government Printing Office, 1941).

THREE

Good Glue, Better Glue, Superglue

Two contract workers went down into an underground vault to do a one-time job, applying a coating of sealant resin to water pipes. They mixed together two components of the resin product, working quickly to apply the sticky black coating material before it hardened. Essentially, they were spreading a kind of glue onto the pipes. A key ingredient in the substance was a chemical solvent called 2-nitropropane. Its sole purpose in the product was to keep the adhesive runny enough to spread.[1]

Neither man had ever worked with this product before. By the end of three days in the cramped quarters of the vault, both were feeling ill. They had so much nausea and vomiting that they sought care at a nearby hospital emergency department. One of the two was noted to have a chemical smell on his breath; both had a tarlike substance on their hands. They were treated for their symptoms overnight and then discharged home.

In one of the workers the symptoms resolved, but the second worker came back to the hospital three days later. He was already obviously jaundiced. By the time he was transferred to the hospital in which I worked, he was progressing rapidly to complete liver failure, spiraling downhill into a coma and dying ten days after his first exposure to the sealant resin.

We obtained the samples of the patient's and his coworker's blood that had been collected the night they first came into the emergency department. Both samples tested positive for 2-nitropropane. When we extrapolated back from these values, the samples demonstrated a level of exposure equivalent to concentrations that had killed half of the test rats reported in a published paper on nitropropane's toxicity. When we researched the compound further, we found published medical reports of eight other deaths from coatings containing 2-nitropropane. Despite the toxicity of this substance, there were no specific restrictions on its use; it was a totally legal, albeit exceptionally deadly, glue.

And what could be simpler than glue, after all? It is the quintessential everyday item. The tube of glue is in the kitchen drawer, waiting to repair the next broken coffee mug handle. It's in the office supply cabinet, essential for those critical cut-and-paste problems that desktop publishing just won't solve. An extra-large glue container may be up on the shelf above the home hobbyist's worktable. Whether it's used in assembling a model airplane or a do-it-yourself furniture project, the concept involved is not very complicated: stick the materials together and have them stay that way. In industrial manufacturing or commercial construction work, the scale may change, but the basic idea is the same. Glue is the stuff of childhood rhyme ("I'm rubber and you're glue; everything bad you say bounces off me and sticks to you") as well as a tired metaphor (the old swaybacked horse, bound for the glue factory).

Despite this reassuring familiarity, glue is not just glue anymore: it is no longer a simple, homogeneous, all-purpose substance. Glues are composed of many different materials. Glue can be as benign and ordinary as wheat paste or as complex, sophisticated, and potentially poisonous as the deadly sealant the two workers used. Terms such as *sealants, coatings, resins,* and *adhesives,* which refer to materials that are like glue but are not the same as glue, have all come to be so interrelated as to apply to a single family of potential hazards. Concepts involving polymers, catalysts, solvents, latex, and plasticizers, which were once the purview of only chemical engineers, have come to be so intertwined with the technology of modern glues that the language of these products cannot be understood without fluency in the terminology of chemical engineering.

This has not always been so. Glue was once just a simple and fairly standard material. Indeed, even to refer to the "history of glue" may sound, on the face of it, absurdly grandiose. And yet, glue has traveled a long and complicated path of small innovations, each one building on the last, many of them taking advantage of some of the most significant technological breakthroughs in the wider world of chemical discovery.

Along the way, strewn beside that trail of technological advancement, are the unmarked memorials of the women and men who have paid dearly for the cost of this "ever-improving" product. They labored in turn-of-the-century factory workrooms filled with the toxic fumes of solvent-soaked glues acting as slow poisons to their bone marrow. They still toil around the world today as cottage-industry pieceworkers exposed to any number of insidious chemical toxins that are present in many modern adhesives. Sometimes, like the unfortunate workers exposed to the nitropropane-laced sealant, they are working with the latest product on the market. Highly reactive chemical components that would have been curiosities of research chemists fifty years ago are now freely available for unwitting consumers in the hardware aisle of every supermarket in the country. Surgeons can exploit remarkably effective adhesive cements in life-saving procedures, while their colleagues in the emergency department struggle to extract similar high-tech chemical adhesives from eyelids sealed shut through misuse of instant glues. Glue does have a history, and with it comes the story of its hidden human costs.

GOOD GLUE

Making old-fashioned *good* glue is pretty simple. This kind of glue has been around for a very long time and hasn't changed much over the years. The affected naïveté of the term *gluon,* which physicists have coined with ironic humor as the name for the theoretical subatomic construct holding quarks together, underscores the point—glue is basic.

In its fundamentals, traditional glue making is a kind of antitechnology. Indeed, the voluminous *History of Technology* has only one entry for glue in its more than three thousand pages, and that is in reference to ancient Egyptian furniture making.[2] One has to go to erudite sub-subspecialty references to learn more about the earliest glues. For example, *Ancient Egyptian Materials and Industries,* whose first chapter devotes itself to adhesives, teaches us that plaster and glue mixed together (gesso) dates to the Third Dynasty, whereas actual furniture glue emerged only later in the Twelfth Dynasty, four thousand years ago.[3] That's still a fair time back.

Glue making was so basic, neither elegant nor proprietary, that the ancients didn't even bother to document much about it. The earliest detailed account we have dates from as recently as around 1100, when a medieval monk named Rugerus, also known as Theophilus, compiled an instruction manual for artisans. We have little reason to think the process had changed much since the time of the pyramids' construction, though. Rugerus's preferred glue recipe reads:

> Of glue of skins and stag-horns. The above being carefully dried, take cuttings of the same skins, dried in the same manner, and carefully cut them up into small pieces, and taking the stag-horns, broken very small with a smith's hammer upon an anvil, place them together in a new pot, until it is half full, and fill it with water, and so apply the fire until a third part of this water be evaporated, so, however, that it may not boil. And you will thus try it; moisten your fingers with this water, and if, when they have become cool, they adhere together, the glue is good; but if not, cook it until they do adhere together. Then pour this glue into a clean vessel and again fill the pot with water, and simmer as before; and do this four times.[4]

Rugerus also provides an alternative recipe for glue using vellum, eel skin, and the head of a wolf-fish. The operative principle is the same: take animal products and cook them down until sticky. For the next thousand years or so, as it had been for several millennia of human craftsmanship before Rugerus, not much was to change.

True, by the nineteenth century glue making had become industrialized, but the underlying concept remained the same. As an early Victorian occupational health text noted,

> Glue and size boilers are exposed to strong putrid and ammoniacal exhalations from the decomposition of animal refuse. The stench of the boiling and drying rooms is indeed well known to be highly offensive, even to the neighborhood. . . . Yet the men [who work with glue] declare it agrees well with them—nay, many assert that on entering this employ, they experience a great increase in appetite and health. All the glue and size makers we saw, were remarkably fresh-looking and robust.[5]

This kind of glue is still available, and it is preferred for use in any application that requires the simplest and most conservative agent, for example, in the repair of fine antiques. A leading conservator of French-period furniture told me that his atelier hosts a resident house cat on whom he depends to detect "imposters" on the basis of glue traces. When, for example, a Louis XIV escritoire, purported to be pristine and original, arrives in the shop, the atelier closely scrutinizes the cat. Should the cat display great interest in the object, smelling the remnants of old fish glue, the piece of furniture passes the test. Feline disregard signals a telltale synthetic glue, a sure mark of later modifications decreasing the piece's value.

Although infectious agents can be spread through working with hides and meat by-products or even fish by-products, once these parts are rendered for glue, the cooking process sterilizes the materials, effectively removing this risk. The general public, who were the ultimate consumers of animal-derived glues, may have found the factories a nuisance because of the smells emitted, but they used the products without incident. For most of history, old-fashioned *good* glue has been synonymous with animal-derived materials extracted by slow cooking, without too much attention to other details. For this very reason, through all those many generations of glue making, glue has been an exceedingly safe material.

The nontoxic common denominator of animal glues is a natural material called collagen. This is the basic ingredient of gelatin, too. Leaving matters of taste aside, the use of traditional glue is about as hazardous as encountering a tomato aspic. Through its innate binding qualities, collagen is a natural substance that provides the principal building matrix framework for bones, cartilage, sinew, and skin. Collagen is also present in other body parts as well. For example, the liver has special threads of collagen that help to preserve the architecture and the function of that vital organ. An overabundance of collagen can be a problem, although it might be theoretically advantageous from a glue maker's perspective by providing more starting material. Too much collagen in the liver is what happens in alcoholic cirrhosis: the body lays down excessive collagen in response to injury, scarring the liver and disrupting its function.

Collagen molecules are made up of very long repeated chemical sequences. Such long, sequenced molecules are called polymers. This is what gives collagen its strength and flexibility and, ultimately, what makes it sticky when converted into glue. Collagen is a protein polymer, a specific category of molecules in which the structural backbone is made up of repeating sequences of amino acids.

Although plants do not make collagen, they do produce their own long molecular polymers that, like collagen, help them hold themselves together. These polymers, too, can be exploited for their adhesive qualities. In contrast to collagen, however, gluey plant polymers are made up of repeated sequences of sugars, not amino acids. Very long polymer strings of sugar occurring in nature are called cellulose. Somewhat shorter strings of sugar also occur in nature. They are not as stiff as cellulose, but they too can be usefully sticky.

Wheat paste is the most familiar example of a shorter sugar polymer glue (microwaved instant oatmeal may be a close runner-up). A variety of different plant-derived, sugar-based polymers are exploited commercially for their gluelike qualities. Despite their pedestrian applications as fillers, sizing agents, and binders, these materials have exotic names such as gum tragacanth, gum arabic, and gum karaya. At best, none is a very strong glue (one tends not to make furniture out of papier-mâché, after all), but just as with protein collagen, none is particularly toxic, either.

The animal glues and the vegetable gums may differ in their strength and utility, but they have one very important thing in common: both are water soluble. Even in the eleventh century, Rugerus understood that glue-stuff dissolves in water, even if he didn't know that it was collagen that he was extracting by so patiently simmering his fish heads and stag horns.

Collagen and starch are water soluble because, fundamentally, the world of a living cell is water bound. All its vital connections interface with an aqueous environment. The water solubility of the plant and animal glues has critical importance for evaluating any adverse health effects these glues might have. Moreover, water solubility is a key to understanding the later changes in glue technology and the risks that have come about with those changes. Animal glues may be smelly to make and wheat paste may be messy to apply, but when the work is all done, they can be cleaned up with water. No toxic chemical solvents are needed to mix vegetable or animal glue, to ease their application, or to remove any excess or unwanted amounts.

Water solubility is not automatic just because a material is naturally derived. In fact, a number of plants (particularly trees), in addition to containing water-soluble gums, produce a wholly different type of polymer known as resins, which are made up of repeating units of acid or alcohol molecules instead of long chains of sugars. Like plant gums, resins are sticky, but far more so. Unlike gums, resins have the peculiar property of not being very soluble in water. These poorly soluble plant resins provide the first inkling of a dangerous turn that glue making, in its first technological advance, was about to take. The initial incremental change in this direction occurred when artisans, using very simple materials, first figured out how to adapt the insoluble plant resins for other purposes, paving the way for a technological revolution in glue making that would eventually follow this same path.

On the face of it, the insolubility that resins display seems to go against the fundamental living requirement of water compatibility. If vegetable gum and animal collagen both have to play by these rules, why not resins? And if plant resins are so sticky, how is it that sap flows so well? Part of the answer is that a resin is not a sap; both serve different functions. Sugar-rich saps carry the internal nutrient flow of trees and are, in fact, highly soluble in water. That is why maple syrup doesn't glue our pancakes together. In contrast, precisely by reason of their incompatibility with normal living functions, true plant resins (as opposed to saps) are not for internal consumption at all. They are produced and then excreted onto the plant's outside surface. Small amounts may be exuded under normal conditions, but following injury to the bark of a tree (for example, by an attacking insect), resin flow increases dramatically.

The sticky, viscous resin excreted by an injured tree plugs the damaged area and hardens as it dries, trapping along with it any pests that didn't get out of the way (fossilized tree resin is familiar to us as amber). One obvious challenge to trees making such a substance is how to prevent the viscous and water-insoluble resin from clogging up the very mechanisms needed to make and excrete it. Trees solve this problem by producing their own specialized solvents to make the resin flow. Turpentine, for example, is the natural solvent that pine trees produce to enable the flow of resin out to the bark's surface. In the air, the turpentine solvent evaporates, and the resin efficiently hardens.

RUBBER CEMENT

Some plants have come up with an entirely different way of taking poorly soluble polymers and "packaging" them for export. This mechanism also has critical implications for glue making, because it provides an important clue for a possible way to engineer an alternative to toxic chemical solvents. By suspending otherwise insoluble polymers as microscopic droplets, certain specialized plants can turn them into water-based solutions. Like resins, these water-suspended polymers also reach the plant's surface when needed, particularly after injury. Once there, the water evaporates and an adhesive layer of protection forms. Because of their milky appearance (as opposed to the see-through quality of solvent-based resins), the generic term for these suspended polymer droplets is *latex*.[6]

Rubber is the most important but not the only source of a natural latex substance. It can be harvested by repeatedly wounding the bark of latex-producing trees and collecting the exuded liquid. Very early in the processing of natural rubber, the tiny suspended droplets of polymer are condensed from the liquid (*coagulated* is the technical term). From that point on, just as with resins, chemical solvents must be used if the rubber polymer is to be made malleable enough to spread or flow at room temperature.

Chemical solvents are a key component of non-water-soluble sealants or adhesive glues, because to be usable they have to be spreadable. Natural plant resins have long been used as coating materials, although not directly as glues until much more recently. One example of an early use of a non-water-soluble resin is traditional Chinese lacquering. This craft, which goes back at least to the sixth century, employs the resin of a variety of sumac tree. In Europe, medieval artisans prized recipes for resin-containing varnishes that could protect paintings without discoloring them (Theophilus recommends the use of sandarac, a North African resin). Because none of these resins is water soluble, they could be used only when mixed with turpentine or oil.

It was natural rubber latex that was destined to become the first commercial plant glue. Even as late as the 1850s, however, this future role for rubber was impossible to foresee. In contrast to most resins, rubber was far more difficult to render into a spreadable state. Turpentine, if added as a solvent for rubber, utterly failed in this regard. Vulcanization, the chemical process using sulfur to make rubber stable for a myriad of other uses, was the opposite of what was needed to create a rubber-based glue. A variety of different solvents, including the highly flammable anesthetic ether, could be employed to make small-scale samples of "rubber cement" in the laboratory, but none was commercially applicable. The technology to make rubber glue for mass marketing simply was not there.

Finally, in the mid-nineteenth century a technical breakthrough in dye making, an industry entirely unrelated to rubber and even more remote from glue, provided the ideal solvent that was to impact the production of both. This solvent, benzene, permanently changed the technology of glue making and, through it, was responsible for an epidemic of deadly illness that lasted for nearly a century thereafter. The industrial origins of benzene can be directly traced back to the tremendous financial successes of the synthetic dyestuffs industry.[7] This was the engine of profit that drove benzene manufacturing, transforming what was once a costly and exotic chemical into a material so cheap and plentiful that it could find its way into other niches in the commercial marketplace, especially in glue making.

The roots of the benzene problem go back to 1856, when a young English student of chemistry, William Henry Perkin, created *mauve*, the first aniline dye. Perkin synthesized mauve dye from coal tar, a by-product residue of coal gas manufacturing.[8] Gas for illuminating and heating, derived from coal, had been introduced only recently on a large scale. England set the pace for illuminating gas. Its initial economic appeal lay in a demand created by shortages in the existing alternative resources. In the second decade of the nineteenth century, the American whale oil trade was down because of the War of 1812, and Russian sources for candle tallow were disrupted by Napoleon. Moreover, illuminating gas proved to be a godsend for mill and factory owners, who suddenly could light their premises well into the night, maintaining production with less risk of fire and, as a consequence, with lower insurance payments, too. Demand was so great that illuminating gas could not be produced fast enough.

Such large-scale use of coal gas was the prerequisite to making its by-product, coal tar, abundant and cheap.[9] At first, the coal tar residue left over from gas production was of little or no value except as a plaything for curious chemists. Perkin's discovery of mauve and the other synthetic dyes that soon followed transformed coal tar from a useless by-product to a commercially valuable raw material. Moreover, aniline dyes constituted only one of a number of different groups of carbon-based chemicals that could be synthesized from the starting materials present in coal tar residues. To derive those starting materials, the coal tar had to be broken down by heat and its components distilled off. The technology needed to accomplish that initial processing was well established by the laboratory chemists of the mid-nineteenth century. Thus, once Perkin and his contemporaries began to apply existing techniques to the search for dyes, related advances were rapid.

The money to be made was staggering. The biggest challenge seemed to be coming up with marketable names for the new colors being synthesized. Some of these are now completely obscure, such as the brilliant golden yellow shade *chrysaniline*. Others garnered synonyms that have survived the original dye designation. *Rosaniline*, although obsolete now, also became popularly known as *fuschine* and then even more widely referred to as *magenta*, named after an 1859 battle site in Italy where the blood flowed, if you will, magenta.

Many of the chemicals being derived from coal tar shared one critical common feature: the carbon atoms present in them were linked together in tight, circular chains. One of the simplest and most abundant of the cyclic molecules extractable through coal tar distillation is benzene. Thus benzene was the pivotal starting point for aniline dye synthesis.

Benzene is made up of a six-carbon atomic chain closed in on itself to form a hexagonal ring, like a charm bracelet with half a dozen tokens. This chain is particularly strong because its carbon links are high in the form of energy that holds atoms together rather than letting them drift apart easily or be broken by interactions with heat, light, or other molecules. A number of other coal tar derivatives are chemically related to benzene and, like it, have similar ring structures with high-energy bonds. These ring-shaped carbon molecules, as a group, tend to have a pungent, somewhat sweet odor. For this reason they are called *aromatic* molecules. Benzene is the prototypical aromatic chemical, the chief progenitor of the clan. From benzene, many others substances, including aniline, can be chemically synthesized through various chemical reactions.

Benzene's usefulness as a starting material for dyes and other products was not its only potentially valuable application. All the aromatics, as a class, can act as useful chemical solvents. Although many aromatic chemicals were being isolated at the time, such as xylene and toluene, benzene still seemed to be one of the most effective solvents of the group. Nonetheless, despite its solvent potency, benzene was too precious to use for that purpose in the early years following its first isolation.

All of the benzene available from coal tar extraction was required for aniline manufacture. There was none to spare; the seemingly insatiable appetite for benzene was driven by the huge new market for aniline dyes. The commercial explosion of the nineteenth-century dyestuffs industry is a powerful example of an industrial innovation rapidly impacting consumer product sales on a global scale. It belies the notion that such technological "shocks" are solely a phenomenon of the latter half of the twentieth century.

Queen Victoria is said to have worn a mauve dress in public not long after the technology first became available. By the time the queen was dressing solely in mourning colors after the prince consort's death in 1861, the synthetic dye industry was already fast at work perfecting a more brilliant black than had ever been possible to achieve with natural dyes. In the interim William Henry Perkin, all of twenty-three years old at that point, had become spectacularly wealthy, a technologically empowered wunderkind who was the Bill Gates of his time and place.

Following Perkin's initial success in the Mauve Decade, named after his discovery and the years thereafter, intense industrial competition for the discovery, synthesis, and control of other new chemical dyes continued unabated. At first, benzene production remained a key priority within the rapidly growing coal tar distillation industry. But this was the case only insofar as benzene continued to be a necessary starting material for synthetic dyes, which held true only as long as aniline derivatives dominated the industry.

Dye technology, like any other, is not static. The first-generation aniline dyes were brilliant and relatively inexpensive, but sadly, they were not durable. As their brilliance faded, so too did their market attractiveness. Chemists, some like Perkin experimenting in England while others worked aggressively on the Continent (especially in Germany), soon discovered that a multiringed aromatic coal tar distillation by-product called anthracene was the new alternative to aniline. The important factor was that anthracene, even though obtained from coal tar and chemically related to benzene, was not derived from it.

Anthracene yielded dyes that were unquestionably superior to the benzene-dependent anilines, in particular synthetic substitutes for the natural red of the plant-derived dye madder and the blue of indigo. For this reason it was the anthracene dyes, far more than the anilines, that spelled economic ruin for the farmers who raised natural dyestuffs. It also meant that coal tar distillation, at the ever higher production levels needed to yield sufficient anthracene, produced far more benzene than was needed as a derivative for the shrinking aniline market. Benzene, at first so indispensable, had come to be little more than a hard-to-market by-product from the coal distillation needed to purify anthracene.

BETTER GLUE

This shifting economic reality illustrates a pattern that is often repeated: a technological change (in this instance synthetic dye manufacturing) transformed a by-product that previously was of little value (here, coal tar) into a lucrative commodity. At aniline's apogee, benzene was riding high; when it fell, benzene's fortunes followed suit. Benzene became one of the many stepchildren that any technological innovation produces: a by-product looking for a viable end-use market.

Benzene did not have to wait long for adoption, given its potential utility as a cheap industrial and commercial solvent. Benzene, it turned out, could fill a new market niche by surmounting the long-standing challenge of dissolving rubber and converting it into an effective adhesive. As the nineteenth century turned into the twentieth, the first major technological change in more than three thousand years of glue making had finally arrived, resulting in rubber cement. And when the new rubber cement hit the marketplace, with it came a novel and deadly threat to health.

In the summer of 1909, within only a few years of this technological breakthrough in making rubber cement, a physician in Baltimore was called in to treat a woman with pneumonia. The pneumonia case was unremarkable, but the patient's daughter caught the doctor's attention. She was a fourteen-year-old girl who, despite claiming to be in good health, appeared remarkably pale. More than that, she exhibited ominous tiny purple blotches indicating small hemorrhages under the surface of her skin.

Four weeks later, on 28 June 1909, the girl was admitted to Johns Hopkins Hospital with bleeding from her gums, nose, and throat. She was anemic, had a low white blood cell count as well, and virtually no blood platelets. Because she was so ill, on 3 July a blood transfusion was performed, at that time a risky and aggressive maneuver. The girl rallied briefly but then, on the 6th, deteriorated again. Her physician noted tersely, "She became steadily weaker until the exitus which occurred on that day."[10] That very same day, two other girls, both aged fourteen as well, were also admitted to Johns Hopkins Hospital with similar skin hemorrhages and low platelet counts. One of the girls died within the week; the second, who did not have concomitant anemia and a low white count, survived.

All three had worked as laborers in the same canning factory, none longer than five months altogether. Although the facility employed more than three hundred workers, the three stricken all worked in the same small room, part of a group of fourteen girls, aged fourteen to sixteen, operating special coating machines. The coating machines sealed the cans rather than soldering them. The sealant was a mixture of rubber, natural resin, and benzene. Coated caps dried on open racks, evaporating off the benzene.

This was the first medical report in the United States of benzene-caused, toxic aplastic anemia, a disease wherein the bone marrow fails to produce enough of any of the critical blood cells needed by the body. Two separate benzene incidents had already been documented in foreign reports that appeared within weeks of each other in 1897.[11] One was a very similar cluster of poisonings in a bicycle tire factory in Uppsala, Sweden. In that outbreak four workers, all young women as well, also died of bone marrow failure.

These early cases of benzene poisoning, occurring so soon after the introduction of the "new" technology of rubber cement, highlight how quickly a distinct pattern in an unusual disease process can be recognized.

In the case of aplastic anemia caused by benzene, this recognition occurred even though the primary diagnosis of the disease process required considerable diagnostic and pathological acumen, aside from connecting this disease, usually of unknown etiology, to a novel toxic mechanism. Still further sophistication is evident in the comments on benzene that the author of the Johns Hopkins report makes near the end of his paper. "Experiments with chemically pure benzene yielded results identical with benzol (e.g., industrial benzene), that is leucopaenia and aplasia of the bone marrow, and we have thus in benzene an intense poison for the white cells of the blood." This statement is footnoted by the author with the following ominous addendum: "Exposure to Roentgen Rays is likewise able to produce an enormous destruction of white cells."[12]

The year was 1910. It had taken less than twenty years from their near simultaneous technological introduction to the scientific recognition that two new toxins, X-rays and benzene, seemed to share a similar profile of toxic action.[13] These first U.S. cases of benzene poisoning were not to be the last. The industrial rubber cement trade relied almost exclusively on young boys and girls who worked at hand-filling cans or running equipment that mechanically filled metal tubes with the profitable, benzene-rich glue. The early warnings of the initial cases went unheeded. In fact, the benzene–rubber cement industry expanded considerably as the adhesive began to be marketed for home and commercial use.[14]

WAR MATÉRIEL

The growing rubber cement industry was limited by the nature of its feedstock. Benzene, as noted previously, was a by-product of coal tar distillation carried out for the chemical dye industry. That industry, from its very inception, was a very high-stakes international enterprise in which the United States was not a major player. England and France had important economic roles, but in the early twentieth-century organic chemical industry, Germany was king of the hill. The "aniline" in Badische Anilin-und-Soda Fabrik (BASF) underscores the national preeminence in the organic chemical industry that Germany achieved in this period. American supplies of benzene were imported and, largely for that reason, relatively limited and expensive.

On the eve of World War I, the petroleum industry was still callow, whereas the international coal-based chemical industry was full grown. The war changed the geopolitical equation for both of these manufacturing sectors. The control of dyestuffs did not carry much strategic weight per se, and the rubber cement trade was marginally important at best. But when World War I interrupted the German flow of benzene to the United States, raw military power hung in the balance. Although munitions manufacturing was not directly related to glue making, benzene was crucial for the manufacture of trinitrotoluene (TNT) and related explosives, which meant that a trade flow of the solvent had to be assured. The American munitions industry required massive amounts of this feedstock to supply TNT to the war effort. In response, a homegrown industry of coal tar distillation took off in the United States. The stockpiling of benzene would later be crucial in the way that glue and related coatings were formulated.

In the short term, while the flow of benzene was diverted into munitions manufacturing, another war-related industry exploited the new technology of polymer sealants, an innovation closely linked to glues and adhesives. These early man-modified polymers were engineered using cellulose as their key starting point. Chemical modification of this natural plant substance causes different polymer links to form, yielding substances with new resinous properties. In the chemical transformation of cellulose into a resin, the water solubility of the original material is unavoidably lost, which is why synthetic resins, like natural plant resins, are unusable unless solvents are added.

Nitrocellulose was the first of these new resinous materials to be invented, the earliest industrial plastic. In the 1860s an American, John Wesley Hyatt, developed it commercially as a substitute for ivory in the manufacture of billiard balls. Nitrocellulose could be formed into a variety of hard shapes. Furthermore, when dissolved in the appropriate solvent and spread very thinly, nitrocellulose could be transformed into a transparent film. In 1889, George Eastman pioneered this application of nitrocellulose, making possible the first motion picture film, known more commonly by an alternative name for nitrocellulose, *celluloid.*

Celluloid, however, is highly inflammable. Early in the twentieth century a related synthetic, cellulose acetate, was also introduced commercially. By 1908, Kodak had patented a cellulose acetate–based fire safety film, but this alternative product found a limited market for film use in its early years. The big industrial application that established cellulose acetate as a real moneymaker was the new business of making planes, specifically, fighter aircraft. The earlier technology of producing airplanes had utilized linen, canvas, and other cloth, which were coated for durability and water repellence. In the trade, this kind of coating was known as *dope,* a term that was originally used for the coating applied to the underside of snowshoes. Nitrocellulose, which could be spread when mixed with one of a variety of solvents, had served as an acceptable dope for standard civilian airplane construction, but it was considered unacceptable for fighter craft because of the fire hazard of warfare.

Cellulose acetate fit the bill as a substitute, but not without a hitch. It was less inflammable, but it was also less soluble than nitrocellulose. Different chemical solvents were tried for its application, but to make the new airplane coating, cellulose acetate dope required a new kind of solvent. The solvent called for was one so special that it could not be found even among the myriad natural molecules extractable from coal tar. This solvent, tetrachloroethane, had been synthesized for the first time only in the latter part of the nineteenth century. Because it is chemically related to chloroform, being a hydrocarbon to which one or more chlorine atoms are linked (a "chloroderivative of hydrocarbon," in the terminology of the time), initial studies focused almost exclusively on its anesthetic-like effects. In 1910, a British researcher studying the anesthetic properties of tetrachloroethane on frog muscle introduced his paper by stating, "Within the last few years chloroderivatives of the aliphatic hydrocarbons, other than the familiar chloroform, have been used for various purposes, occasionally with fatal results."[15]

The investigator concluded that tetrachloroethane was approximately four times as toxic in the frog tests as chloroform was. A year later, a 1911 German research study in cats confirmed tetrachloroethane's toxicity.[16] A key finding in those experiments was that liver damage could be readily induced by the chemical. The makers and distributors of Cellon, the trade name for cellulose acetate dissolved in tetrachloroethane, saw to it that the animal experimental findings could be reproduced in humans. In 1914, a German physician reported a new industrial disease in the form of a toxic jaundice attacking four out of eight men in a workforce he investigated. In one case the liver damage was so severe it proved to be fatal.

Despite the German scientific publication on Cellon, which may well have received notice in Britain, airplane production was a high priority there, just as in Germany, with the coming of the war. And the British could also obtain Cellon as a doping agent. The makers of Cellon, being under Swiss licensure, were not taking sides. The day after Christmas in 1914, the *Lancet* published the results of a newsworthy coroner's inquest:

On Saturday last, December 19th, Mr. Luxmore Drew and a jury resumed an inquiry into the cause of death of an employee at an aeroplane factory, when highly interesting scientific information was given in accordance with which the verdict was returned. . . . Evidence was given by the Aircraft Manufacturing Company, the proprietors of the factory, describing the procedure of applying "dope," this being the work which was presumed to have led to the condition. From the evidence it was obvious that there had been a considerable number of cases of sickness, in some of which jaundice was present.[17]

Age thirty-six, Mr. Gilbert Moody had begun work as an airplane doper in early August. By late October he was ill; in November he was admitted to the hospital; twelve days later he was dead. The factory in which he was employed operated out of a converted omnibus shed, with intermittently operative ventilating fans. When the fans did work, they served only to distribute the toxic fumes rather than remove them. In concluding its report, the *Lancet* noted that the coroner's jury "hoped the investigation would be the means of preventing further deaths."[18]

They were to be disappointed. The very day after the *Lancet* publication, a female worker at another doping plant became acutely ill, lapsed into a coma from liver failure, and died within the week. She was nineteen years old. All told, it took another two years for the British to eliminate tetrachloroethane from airplane dope. At least a dozen fatalities were documented, and far more workers became ill without succumbing fatally to the effects of the poison.

At this time, America was only just gearing up its manufacture of aircraft. Attention had already been given to the potential dangers of tetrachloroethane, including notice in the *Journal of the American Medical Association*.[19] In the United States, the chemical was not banned outright, but other solvents were promoted in its place. Scattered cases of illness did indeed occur, but no fatalities were reported. Ironically, one of the principal solvent substitutes favored for use in doping was benzene.

NEW MARKET OPPORTUNITIES

The post–World War I period presented economic challenges to the nascent American coal tar distilling industry. With munitions manufacturing winding down fast, the industry faced a huge capacity for benzene production with no obvious market for its key product. The economic imperative was the same as it had been when benzene changed from a valuable dye feedstock to a useless by-product on the way to making anthracene. The solution was the same. Benzene was put forward more strongly than ever as a cheap and efficacious industrial chemical, especially for the manufacture of rubber cement and natural and synthetic coatings requiring the need of a potent solvent.

Similar post–World War I economic pressures were at work in Europe. In response to benzene's availability and low cost, its industrial uses multiplied. Medical notice of a spreading epidemic of blood disease soon followed. Throughout the 1920s, numerous scientific reports reconfirmed the terrible link between benzene exposure and aplastic anemia, which had first been reported more than a decade before. Researchers were even able to show the same relationship between benzene and human bone marrow toxicity and benzene and blood-forming cells in controlled animal studies, displaying a methodological sophistication that remains impressive to this day.

Further medical interest was briefly generated when a Hungarian scientist suggested that benzene might be capable of acting as a therapeutic agent as well as a toxin. It was already well recognized that benzene was capable of suppressing the bone marrow's production of white blood cell precursors. Since leukemia is a cancer manifest in the overproduction of white blood cells, might not benzene, the Hungarian scientist postulated, be a potential therapy for that disease?

This scientist might have done well to pay more heed to the key earlier observation made in the first American report of aplastic anemia in Baltimore, wherein the author pointed out that X-ray radiation and benzene shared a predilection for acting on blood cells in a similar way. It was known by this time that radiation could have a twofold effect: an initial suppression of bone marrow's capacity to form blood cells, followed only later by a loss of normal controls over cell production. Leukemia is the end-stage, cancerous manifestation of cell proliferation caused by radiation exposure.

Documenting the same dual effect of benzene took only a matter of time. In 1928, a French medical journal reported the first case of leukemia developing because of workplace exposure to benzene. The forty-one-year-old patient had been heavily exposed to benzene over a number of years while working in a chemical manufacturing plant. Admitted to the hospital on Bastille Day in 1927, he died only three days later. In an erudite discussion of the case, the reporting physicians went so far as to comment on the theoretical risks of benzene were it to be used as a therapy (as had been proposed by the Hungarian scientist, for example). The authors speculated on benzene's potential to transform chronic leukemia to an acute form of the disease, since "this possibility is well recognized from radiation therapy."[20] After this case, there was little rationale for further discussion of benzene use as a possibly curative chemotherapy drug.

In 1932 and 1933, two additional reports of benzene-induced leukemia appeared, including the first to come from the United States.[21] Then, in October 1939, an entire issue of the U.S. *Journal of Industrial Hygiene and Toxicology* was devoted exclusively to benzene poisoning.[22] The journal cited fifty-four different scientific articles that had accumulated by then on benzene's effects on the bone marrow.

The 1939 publication also contained new reports, including data on eighty-nine additional exposure cases, twenty-six of whom had worked directly with rubber cement. Of the ten deaths involved, one was attributed to leukemia, the others to aplastic anemia. After this publication, one would have difficulty arguing that the failure to control benzene might be attributable to a lack of sufficient hard scientific data.

W. M., the unfortunate man with leukemia whose case was documented in the *Journal of Industrial Hygiene and Toxicology*, was twenty-eight when he died in March 1939. He had started working at age eighteen in a factory that made "artificial leather," using large amounts of benzene in the process. In 1937, two years before his death, the plant had stopped using the toxic solvent, but even by that time, W. M.'s blood had already begun to demonstrate subtle abnormalities. When his leukemia erupted full force, the final illness was rapidly progressive. Most of the people whose cases appeared in the 1939 report had worked in one of several different factories using benzene as a solvent for artificial leather, which was manufactured by coating natural textile fabric with nitrocellulose. It was another version of the doping story all over again.

At the same time as these leukemia cases were incubating in the glue trades and related artificial leather industry, cellulose acetate was hunting for its own new markets after the falloff in warplane demand following the armistice. The makers of Cellon came up with a new process, also solvent intensive, converting cellulose acetate into spun fibers. These could be woven into a sheeny, albeit somewhat stiff, fabric known as acetate silk, which for a time became quite the rage. This is the industry, as a paradigm of modernity, that Aldous Huxley singled out to include among the deadening jobs suitable for Epsilon laborers in his fictional dystopia of the future. "Hot tunnels alternated with cool tunnels. Coolness was wedded to discomfort in the form of hard X-rays. By the time they were decanted the embryos had a horror of cold. They were predestined to emigrate to the tropics, to be miners and acetate silk spinners and steel workers."[23]

Far from symbols of a brave new world, the emerging industries of artificial leather and spun acetate were actually indicative of the technological limits of the time. These were not wholly synthetic alternatives to natural materials that were represented by leather or by both animal and natural rubber glues. Nitrocellulose and cellulose acetate were not truly man-made materials; they were merely the human modifications of a common natural polymer, cellulose.

PLASTIC

The goal of making an entirely new polymer of any kind from scratch was proving far more challenging than any modification of cellulose, no matter how elegant. Above all else, elasticity and flexibility seemed the most difficult properties to engineer in a polymer. In 1909, Leo Baekeland synthesized the first wholly "new" polymer, a material that came to be known as Bakelite. When first formulated, Bakelite can be formed into a hard shell-like material initially capable of conforming with great versatility to virtually any molded shape. It is there that the versatility stops. Its flexibility is temporary. Once Bakelite plastic has become set in a fixed form, it is what it is, which is certainly not elastic.

To make a polymer de novo, elastic or otherwise, one must begin with individual separate units, or monomers, and then link them together into polymer chains. Nature carries out this daunting task quite cleverly. Of course it has the advantage of time, employing, as it does, biosynthetic strategies learned through millions of years of evolutionary trial and error. One of nature's basic tricks of the trade is to construct polymers in a consistent spatial orientation. In practice, this means that the molecules serving as monomer subunits are attached together, taking into account a kind of left- or right-"handedness." This left/right duality occurs because many carbon-based molecules can exist in two forms, mirror images of each other with exactly the same chemical structure but different spatial symmetry. They are matched, left and right, like a pair of gloves.

Natural rubber provides a perfect example of this. All of the monomer subunits of rubber, each an identical chemical molecule called isoprene on its own, are aligned in an identical orientation. This alignment, in large part, is what allows rubber to be rubbery, especially with the boost provided by vulcanization. Another natural polymer is a close relative of rubber. It, too, is made entirely of isoprene chemical subunits, or monomers, also linked up like a chain in a consistent orientation, as if left- or right-handed. It just happens to be the opposite orientation to that of rubber. This mirror polymer is called *gutta-percha*.

Although latex rubber is originally a product of the New World, gutta-percha is derived from an Asian plant native to Malaya, where it had limited traditional use for fashioning small, solid objects.[24] There is good reason for the limited use of this mirror-image rubber; although gutta-percha has excellent properties for being molded into a shape, it has none of the elasticity of its fraternal twin. Gutta-percha is the equivalent of a natural analogue of Bakelite. The European commercial discovery of gutta-percha in 1843 was followed in short order by two significant milestones in Western civilization: the gutta-percha golf ball (replacing a leather ball stuffed with feathers) and gutta-percha-insulated telegraph wire, suitable for undersea cables.

The *trans*-polyisoprene structure of gutta-percha, the chemical designation for its precise spatial configuration, is no match for the elastic performance characteristics of *cis*-polyisoprene, that is, rubber. Gutta-percha never achieved broad economic success, because without elasticity its commercial applications were far more restricted than those of rubber. Nonetheless, the repeated *trans*-polymer configuration still allows for structural consistency. The proof is in the sticky pudding of naturally mixed *cis*- and *trans*-polyisoprene: chicle, the raw material of chewing gum, echoed in the trade name Chiclets.

If such subtleties of structure are all that critical to essential polymer qualities such as elasticity and plasticity of form, then a successful yield is likely to be problematic when one crudely cooks together a pot of monomer subunits meant to combine haphazardly. Brother Rugerus had the know-how and equipment to brew glue from natural preformed polymers, but he could not have synthesized polymers from scratch.

The young plastics industry of the first part of the twentieth century made slow progress, yielding a handful of early synthetic materials that could be "set" into shapes. In addition to Bakelite, another leading brand of plastic was called Galalith, a polymer with vaguely biblical connotations derived from a combination of formaldehyde and milk protein. Milk protein (casein) had already found its way into modified glues that needed to be less water soluble, especially compared with wheat paste. For example, such casein glues are still de rigueur for the labels on champagne bottles, since they have to stay on the bottle despite its submersion in a bucket of ice.

The early inflexible plastics such as Bakelite and Galalith have been reincarnated into a second existence as popular and lucrative eBay collectibles,[25] but in their art deco heyday the hard, inflexible plastics served a utilitarian purpose. Elasticity is not always advantageous—one does not want a hair comb with the consistency of a rubber band. But elasticity or flexibility is critical at other times. The forward progress of the plastic industry seemed to hit a wall when it came to engineering synthetic elasticity.

A flexible plastic in general and an artificial rubber in particular became the technological Holy Grail of polymer chemists working in the 1920s and '30s. At the time that the first benzene leukemia cases were reported in Europe and the United States, no large-scale commercial synthetic rubber manufacturing existed yet anywhere in the world. Especially in Germany, but in the United States as well, the first synthetic substitute elastic polymers were just coming on line. In the 1930s, *synthetic rubber cement* would have been a household item only in a science fiction story.

SYNTHETIC RUBBER CEMENT

Just as World War I led to a dramatic shift in the coal tar distillation industry that ultimately came to impact glue making in fundamental ways, the matériel demands of World War II spurred the technological evolution of the polymer industry, including the fabrication of glue and other sealants. Glue making was to join the ranks of other synthetic chemical industries, magnifying old hazards and raising entirely new toxic threats. The key factor in the ultimate transformation of glue was the disrupted access to most of the world's supplies of natural rubber, brought about by the advent of World War II.

The disruption of the rubber supply greatly escalated the demand for synthetic substitutes. Several major successes had already occurred in the race for artificial rubber substitutes in the years leading up to the war. The chemical monomer *butadiene* was polymerized to butadiene rubber, or Buna in Germany. *Styrene,* a close chemical relative of benzene, was combined with butadiene. In Germany this copolymer was trademarked as Buna-S, and the Allies referred to it as GR-S (government rubber-styrene). Yet another artificial rubber was named *neoprene.* Neoprene was formed as a polymer of the chlorinated version of isoprene. Making synthetic rubber became a mainstay of war production for the Allies and the Axis powers alike.

In Germany, Buna had been developed by the former BASF in its later embodiment as part of the megachemical concern Interessengemeinschaft Farbenindustrie Aktiengesellschaft (IG Farben). The chemist and writer Primo Levi was one of the survivors of IG Farben's Buna manufacturing. Levi worked in the synthetic rubber facility as part of the slave labor serving from Auschwitz. His writings bear testimony to the priority given to the polymer as a key war matériel.[26] The synthetic rubbers were of great use because they could do just about anything that natural rubber could do, including act as a pretty effective adhesive cement if dissolved in the right solvent, like benzene.

By this point, benzene was such a common solvent that the Federal Security Agency of the U.S. Public Health Service highlighted it for its 1941 Workers' Health Series education campaign. The ten-page pamphlet *Clara Gives Benzol the Run Around* tells the story of Clara Carelittle, an assembly-line worker who is not compliant with her scheduled medical exam for benzene surveillance. "I've got a date with Jim tonight. I won't have time for my hair-do if I go to the doctor for that examination. I'll skip it. Once won't make a difference."[27] Clara was being dangerously short-sighted, we quickly learn:

Clara was on her first job, cementing crepe rubber soles in a shoe factory. Every 2 weeks, the factory doctor and Miss Fairly, the nurse, examined the girls in Clara's room.

This seemed foolish to Clara. With her good health and high spirits, she couldn't imagine what it was like to be sick.

About a week later, Clara had a nosebleed at work. Not a bad one—but the foreman sent her right up to Miss Fairly.

"He sure is fussy about a nosebleed," Clara said.

The foreman, the pamphlet makes clear, is the one who sets Clara straight. "'He's right, Clara. A nosebleed *may* mean you've been breathing too much benzol which is used to make the rubber cement. Benzol vapor can make you sick. That's why we insist on regular examinations for workers who use materials containing benzol. You missed your last one. Now let's get busy on that check-up.'"

The pamphlet never tells us exactly what happens to Clara after her nosebleed. A drawing of her appears on the back cover with the message

"A little care will keep benzol in its place—and you on the job," and a final paragraph emphasizes that benzene is good for business. "Clara is one of about 30,000 American workers whose jobs call for the use of benzol in some form. Thousands more are employed to manufacture this valuable solvent. A lot of people would be out of work if there were no benzol."

Natural rubber stockpiles were being exploited strategically. Butadiene polymers and neoprene were useful and important supplements. Yet, even together, these natural and synthetic materials could not meet all of the polymer needs of war production.

POLYVINYL CHLORIDE

Once again, as had been the case in World War I, aviation production set the pace for novel materials and applications. In particular, the complicated and vulnerable electrical wiring systems of fighter planes had a desperate key need for a flexible, stable, synthetic insulation of relatively low flammability.

B. F. Goodrich had just the polymer for the job. Actually, this polymer had been around for quite some time, becoming a bit of the spinster sister as each of a series of younger debutantes emerged from industrial laboratories and was married off to a new application. It was synthesized from a simple monomer subunit that could be mass-produced from a common, small carbon molecule into which chlorine had been chemically introduced. No complex ring structures were needed, nor were sophisticated synthetic steps involved. The basic two-member carbon starting point could be obtained from coal or even more easily from petroleum.

The original Goodrich trade name for the product was Koroseal. Soon it was known more widely by its technical designation, *polyvinyl chloride,* and later predominantly by its initials, *PVC,* almost as if it were a familiar political leader. Ultimately, it just went generic: it was simply *vinyl.*

Vinyl chloride monomer can trace its pedigree back to the first generation of industrially oriented organic chemists. It had been synthesized initially in 1835 by a French researcher, Henri Victor Regnault. Regnault was a multitalented scientist who authored one of the leading chemistry texts of the nineteenth century.[28] He became the director of the royal porcelain manufacture at Sévres, where his acumen in chemistry was highly relevant to glazing and other technical aspects of the industry. In his spare time he also applied his skills to the relatively new technique of photography. His surviving photographs, quite rare and sought after by collectors today, include images of the workshops at Sévres and the chemical equipment of his laboratory.

Regnault quickly noted that vinyl chloride had some unusual qualities. At room temperature, it was a gas, possessing a sweet odor. Most of the other new substances that were chemically synthesized with chlorine formed volatile liquids, not gases. Being a gas, of course, vinyl chloride could not be used as a possible solvent. This substance had another strange and important property. When it was sealed in a glass, especially if exposed to the action of sunlight, a viscous deposit would develop on the sides of the container. Regnault had observed the first spontaneous polymerization of PVC, indeed, the first synthetic polymerization of any sort.

This attribute of vinyl chloride, its ability to react easily with itself to auto-polymerize, makes the promotion of its chemical reaction fairly straightforward. As early as 1916, a time when almost no synthetic polymers were around other than Bakelite and celluloid, the controlled polymerization of vinyl chloride was perfected by a Russian scientist named Ostrumuislenskii. But, despite its easy polymerization, the material had little use because it was not much good to work with. In its pure form, it was stiff and brittle and inflexible. The original PVC just wasn't very plastic at all.

Ostrumuislenskii was a staunch tsarist who left Russia in 1921.[29] For a time, he carried on his polymer research for the United States Rubber Company. It was not Dr. O.'s, however, but an industrial competitor's research that made PVC's future. A B. F. Goodrich chemical engineer with an only slightly less tongue-tripping name, Waldo Lonsbury Semon, came up with a way to make PVC usable, applying an approach that has been generalized since then to a wide variety of polymers.

The first step in making PVC on a large scale was easy, because it so readily polymerized. For this reason, the early years of industrial PVC polymerization involved little more than pumping vinyl chloride into sealed "reaction vessels," adding a little pressure or heat, and letting the chemistry take off by itself. Semon's contribution was to devise a technique of adding secondary chemicals, known generally as *plasticizers,* to make a finished polymer that was more malleable.[30] The amount and type of plasticizer help to determine the ultimate use of the product, without changing its basic polymer formula. PVC of a proper consistency for coating electrical wire that could be used in fighter planes was only one of any number of options made possible by Semon's key technical innovation.

As additional new polymer plastics followed in the tracks of artificial rubber and PVC, each required its own set of chemical additives. Plasticizers guaranteed the desired flexibility, stabilizers defended the polymer against degradation, and colorants provided aesthetic appeal and even practical advantages (especially in color-coded wiring insulation). For certain applications, especially when a polymer served as the basis of a synthetic coating, sealant, or bonding agent, the key additive would take the form of a solvent in an exact amount and of a specific kind. The kind of solvent called for was often benzene.

BENZENE RUBBER CEMENT HANGS ON

By 1945, the first fully synthetic glues had arrived as part of a wholly new plastics manufacturing sector, an industry that had never existed before. Yet in terms of the new sector's solvent use, its approach was mostly business as usual. In practice, this meant benzene and then more benzene. Despite the fatal anemia cases linked to benzene for over forty years and the growing certainty that benzene was also linked to leukemia, it became the glue solvent of choice for synthetic rubber cement, just as it had been for its natural rubber predecessor.

And then benzene suddenly got even cheaper. Shortly after World War II, the petrochemical industry discovered an effective way of "cracking" gasoline to yield a number of by-products, including benzene. This had never been technically achievable on a large scale before. The coal tar industry was history; petrochemicals were the future. As postwar refining for automobile gasoline expanded exponentially, benzene was ever more abundant. In fact, there was an awful lot on the market to be unloaded. The production of rubber cement, using both natural rubber and artificial rubber substitutes, was able to absorb a healthy portion of this excess by-product. It was good for business all the way around.

A heavy cost was hidden in the profitable sale of benzene-laced rubber and synthetic polymer cements. Shoemakers, more than any other working group, paid the price: people such as Clara Carelittle, representing a sizable cadre of U.S. workers, and her cousins across the Atlantic, especially in Italy, where shoe manufacturing had become particularly prominent.

In October 1964, the *New England Journal of Medicine* carried a report entitled "Benzene and Leukemia," cowritten by Dr. Enrico Vigliani. Based in Milan, Dr. Vigliani had a long and painful familiarity with the link between benzene used as a glue solvent and cancer in those who applied it. His first paper on the subject had been published more than a quarter of a century before, in 1938. His 1964 report, however, was far from historical.

Of the forty-two cases it described, the most recent had died of leukemia less than a year before the article was published. Vigliani recognized that many still discounted benzene's leukemia link, despite many years of accumulated evidence to the contrary. Vigliani writes near the conclusion of his paper:

> We are fully aware of the fact that no final statement about the existence of a true "benzene leukemia" can be made, without a statistical analysis of the incidence of leukemia among workers exposed to benzene as compared with that among a control group of the same age, sex and living habits. Unfortunately, this analysis is particularly difficult in our cases because of the large number of shoe and other factories handling benzene, the artisan work carried out at home by many factory-employed workers and the frequent and unexpected changes in [the] benzene content of glues and solvents used by the workers.[31]

Benzene poisoning was on the rise, but there was next to no effort to bring it under control because industry had little incentive to embrace Vigliani's findings. The Italian shoe industry behaved as if the deaths were an unavoidable industrial by-product of the economic engine driving *la dolce vita*. Just like Americans, the Italians, too, could state that many people would be out of a job without benzene.

Epidemiological study, as Vigliani emphasized, is a slow and arduous process, all the more so when those at greatest risk are scattered among small and poorly regulated job sites. Nonetheless, by 1964, there was ample precedent for a link between cancer and on-the-job exposure to benzene or closely related chemicals.

In 1895, for example, an outbreak of occupational chemically caused cancer of the bladder had been scientifically documented among workers in the dyestuff industry.[32] Despite this outbreak and several others that had been reported by researchers in the first part of the twentieth century, Vigliani was realistic in his expectation of skepticism. In the 1960s, little credence was given to the possibility that cancer in the workplace might be anything more than an isolated event.

There was one relevant exception to this. Radiation exposure was very well accepted as the environmental and occupational cancer-causing agent par excellence. For radiation, the link to several types of cancer, especially leukemia, could not be disputed. This established association went back as far as case reports among the first researchers in the field, scientists and physicians who were victims of their own early experiments. Anecdotal data based on such individual cases may have suffered from the same weaknesses that Vigliani highlighted in the benzene data, but the meticulous epidemiological follow-up studies of survivors of atomic weapon blasts put any question of cause and effect beyond doubt.

CANCER IN THE PLASTICS INDUSTRY

Another ten years passed after Vigliani's report. More benzene-related deaths accumulated, but still no concerted action was taken to curtail benzene's use substantially, either industrially in factories or in the final commercial products they produced. It proved to be a different chemical in the polymer industry that finally put work-related cancer on the agenda. In 1973, John Creech, a physician employed by B. F. Goodrich, in Louisville, Kentucky, noticed a strange and alarming coincidence at one of the company's main polyvinyl chloride polymerization factories, for which he served as plant physician.

Three years before, in 1970, a patient under Creech's care, a thirty-six-year-old who had worked at the Goodrich facility for fourteen years, was diagnosed with an exceptionally rare liver tumor. The cancer was typed as *angiosarcoma,* a malignancy that arises from cells associated with blood vessels. It is hard to diagnose, both because it is so uncommon and because attempts at biopsy can easily lead to copious bleeding. Furthermore, treatment options are no impetus for early diagnosis. Angiosarcoma, at any stage, carries a very poor prognosis.

Creech's first patient died of the disease in 1971, fourteen months after his diagnosis. Even if Creech had a suspicion that the vinyl chloride played a role in the cancer, he would have had nothing solid to go on. A single animal study implicating vinyl chloride as a cancer-causing agent had only just been published in 1971; the cancers identified were not of the same cell type as angiosarcoma. Nevertheless, it was presumed that vinyl chloride could cause liver damage, if not cancer. In the early 1960s, Dow Chemical cut by tenfold the exposures it allowed to vinyl chloride in its own factories. This action was based on company-sponsored animal studies that indicated liver injury.

Creech himself had particular expertise with another peculiar toxic manifestation of vinyl chloride. In 1967, he had been one of the first to publish a description of a new disease, peculiar to vinyl chloride polymerization workers and given the rarified label of *occupational acro-osteolysis.* This is a condition in which the ends of the finger bones gradually disintegrate, a dis-

GOOD GLUE, BETTER GLUE, SUPERGLUE   71

abling process that leaves the afflicted hands crippled with painful blunted digits. Those at risk were the workers assigned to climb into the plastic reaction vats after completion of the polymerization. Using simple hand tools, they were assigned the task of manually scraping off any residual PVC. In the process, they were exposed to the exceptionally high levels of unreacted vinyl chloride gas that typically remained sealed in the tanks.

The death of the single 1971 angiosarcoma victim seemed to be an isolated event at first. Then, in 1973, Creech became aware of a second and then a third additional death from angiosarcoma of the liver. All were among employees of the same plant. This might have been unusual for even a more common type of cancer. The odds against this as a chance occurrence for angiosarcoma were staggering. Up until that time, the annual reported incidence of angiosarcoma of the liver was only twenty-five cases in the entire United States.

The third case died on 19 December 1973. The final angiosarcoma-specific diagnosis was revealed only at autopsy. On 22 January 1974, B. F. Goodrich officially notified governmental health agencies and the general public about the outbreak of the disease. In the interim, records of another case of the disease in a plant employee dating back to 1968 had also been uncovered. In the case of vinyl chloride, the otherwise slow pace of epidemiological investigation was fairly rapid. Less than a month after the public announcement by Goodrich, the *Morbidity and Mortality Weekly Report* prominently featured a summary of the CDC's initial outbreak assessment. Still, its editorial comment was guarded. "Four cases, therefore, among a small number of workers at a single plant is a most unusual event, and one which raises the possibility of some work-related carcinogen, conceivably vinyl chloride itself."[33]

An initial case report by Dr. Creech, coauthored with the Goodrich corporate medical director, was already in press as a brief "special communication" to the *Journal of Occupational Medicine,* with a summary header acknowledging "the probability that this condition, in some instances, may be causally related to . . . polyvinyl chloride resins."[34]

The special communication also included an accompanying editor's note, which was equally significant. Dated 21 February 1974, it highlighted a presentation given one week before by Professor Cesare Maltoni.[35] Maltoni, an Italian toxicologist, had exposed laboratory animals to low levels of vinyl chloride and produced the very same rare angiosarcomas that Creech had seen in his cases. Needless to say, animal experiments take time; Maltoni's experiments had not been set up following the news of the

Louisville cases. In fact, the results of the animal studies showing that vinyl chloride causes angiosarcoma had been in the hopper for months, but earlier dissemination of the findings had been actively blocked by chemical manufacturers on both sides of the Atlantic.

By early October 1974, the *JAMA* carried a full-length paper on the outbreak, which had now climbed to seven confirmed cases, including two diagnosed in February, within weeks or even days of the delayed release of Maltoni's data.[36] The *JAMA* report referred to "a direct causal relationship between exposure to vinyl chloride monomer and pathologic findings," leaving little room for equivocation. Underscoring this, in a highly unusual step, the senior author of the paper was then the director of the National Institute for Occupational Safety and Health, Dr. Marcus Key, the highest ranking occupational health scientist in the U.S. government.

Eight months had elapsed between February's equivocation ("possible"; "conceivable") and October's certainty ("direct"; "causal"). This is a blink of the eye in epidemiological time, but it is glacially slow compared with the lay public's exposure to the news coming out of Louisville. It rapidly became unequivocally clear to any reader of the *New York Times* (and other major newspapers) that vinyl chloride was a cause of cancer in the workplace. Furthermore, evidence indicated that this might be only the tip of the iceberg of vinyl chloride's danger. The litany of news articles published in the weeks following the first announcement of the deaths linked to vinyl chloride in early 1974 document the broader concern that this event had awakened, a concern that spiraled out from the core group of the production workers to outer circles of PVC users and even consumers more peripherally exposed:

27 January. "Job Link to Deaths Studied"

15 February. "Liver Cancer Alert Declared to Protect Plastics Workers"

20 February. "Rare Liver Cancer Discovered in Two More at a Chemical Plant"

13 March. "Plastic Workers Screened for Ill Effects of Vinyl Chloride"

23 March. "Discovery of Rare Cancer Spurs Concern About Environment"

4 April. "Clairol Recalls Aerosol Sprays"

18 April. "Aerosol Sprays Recalled by FDA"

19 April. "Twenty Sprays Listed in Drive by EPA"

30 April. Consumer Product Safety Commission announces investigation . . .

11 May. "Vinyl Chloride Parley Told of Dangers to Workers"

1 June. "New Cancer Cases Widen Fears on Vinyl Chloride"

14 June. "New Cases Linked to Chemical"

26 June. "Vinyl Chloride Exposure Limit is Opposed by Plastics Industry"

2 October. "Vinyl Chloride Rules Seek to Guard Workers' Health"

6 October. "Carcinogens: Unchecked, They Threaten an Epidemic"[37]

BENZENE AND LEUKEMIA REVISITED

Because vinyl chloride was relatively cheap and easy to manufacture, it turned out that it had many applications beyond polymer chemistry. One of the most alarming of these applications was as a spray-can propellant in consumer goods.

Beyond that, the public legitimately asked itself, if a product as common as vinyl holds such hidden hazards, what other carcinogens are waiting to be discovered? The clear-cut identification of vinyl chloride as a cancer-causing agent and the strict regulatory controls that followed (despite vocal industry opposition) gave a new impetus to the researchers who were trying to establish benzene's role in causing leukemia.

The issue of determining benzene's cancer-causing potential fell to the International Agency for Research on Cancer (IARC). Based in Lyon, France, IARC is the key arbiter in a formal process of officially determining whether a chemical agent does indeed cause cancer. In June 1974, in the immediate wake of the deaths caused by vinyl chloride that were reported early that year, a group of IARC experts met in Lyon to discuss benzene.[38] They reviewed Vigliani's Italian cases reported in 1964, along with another fifty cases of leukemia among benzene-exposed workers occurring over a fifteen-year period and reported from France in 1967. Six of the victims whose cases were documented in the French series had been exposed while using benzene-contaminated rubber cement in raincoat manufacturing, an industry that in all of France employed only one thousand workers. Six cases of leukemia among one thousand persons over fifteen years is many times the expected rate in the general population.

The IARC committee did not find these cases compelling. They gave heavier weighting to a Japanese study they felt was more rigorous in its epidemiological methods. Ironically, that study used the Atomic Bomb Casualty Commission Leukemia Registry to track down cases and determine the occupations of the individuals involved. The risk of the disease among those with jobs likely to involve benzene exposure was double that of those who did not have such jobs. In the end, the experts would conclude only that a relationship between benzene exposure and leukemia was *suggested* by the scientific data at hand, not conclusively established.

In the years that followed, new epidemiological studies linking benzene to leukemia continued to appear. By 1978, the U.S. Occupational Safety and Health Administration was sufficiently convinced of the cancer link to propose a new workplace limit for benzene exposure. The new OSHA regulation, which was meant to cover over two hundred thousand U.S. workers regularly exposed to the toxin, would have tightened the limits on air contamination by a factor of ten. The standard would also have banned outright any direct skin contact with benzene.

The American Petroleum Institute, which was not convinced by the benzene body count, had its day in court. On 2 July 1980, the U.S. Supreme Court voided the benzene limit on the grounds that OSHA had not sufficiently quantified its claims of benzene's dangers. It was an anniversary of sorts. On a July day exactly seventy-one years earlier, in a Baltimore hospital less than fifty miles away from the Supreme Court building where the decision was handed down, the fourteen-year-old glue worker had lain dying from benzene-caused anemia.

In the dissenting Supreme Court opinion, Justice Thurgood Marshall cogently warned, "In recent years there has been increasing recognition that the products of technological development may have harmful effects whose incidence and severity cannot be predicted with certainty. . . . Risks of harm are often uncertain, but inaction has considerable costs of its own."[39]

Overexposure to benzene continued unabated. One year later, in October 1981, another meeting on benzene was convened by IARC in Lyon. This time the experts came down from the fence, finally concluding, "There is *sufficient* evidence that benzene is carcinogenic to man" (italics in original).[40]

It took OSHA another seven years to redo the quantification math sufficiently that it might pass court muster. The new OSHA standard finally took effect in 1988, the same year that the first actual visual image of the benzene molecule was achieved through a sophisticated technology called scanning tunneling microscopy. In 1989, even the U.S. Environmental Protection Agency finally took on benzene as a toxic air pollutant that might be in need of regulation.

A decade later, bottled mineral water's appeal was tainted by the possibility that minute amounts of benzene had contaminated Perrier. A worst-case scenario of exposure by this route was thousands of times lower than the levels to which so many had been so long subjected with so little control. By this time, pure benzene had finally been removed as an intentional solvent additive from almost all industrial and consumer glues, although it continues to be introduced into commerce as a trace contaminant of other solvents.

None of this abrogated the industrial demand for solvents: benzene was not the only chemical on the shelf. Hexane, for example, proved to be a prime alternative solvent for both natural and synthetic rubber cements. Hexane began to gain in commercial popularity as benzene's regulatory fortunes waned. Just like benzene, hexane is a molecule made up of exactly six carbon atoms joined together. Hexane is a straight chain molecule rather than a closed ring linked end to end, like benzene. From the American Petroleum Institute's perspective, hexane was still an attractive commodity to market, since it too is an abundant by-product of petrochemical refining.

Hexane, at first, was considered a rather innocuous solvent. Like most hydrocarbons, at higher levels of exposure it has an alcohol-like effect, inducing lightheadedness, giddiness, or even drunkenness. Limits on workplace exposure were based on this effect alone, allowing inhalation at levels fifty times as concentrated as the old benzene standard, even as lax as that was.

Indications that something might be wrong appeared not long after hexane's commercial applications became more widespread. In fact, a series of medical notices published in Japan in the late 1960s made it clear that something was terribly amiss, even though hexane did not seem to have the same propensity as benzene for attacking the blood system. The Japanese reports described an unusual outbreak of a new neurological illness. The victims in this small epidemic suffered from loss of both sensation and muscle strength, which was particularly marked in the arms but sometimes progressed to full quadriplegia. The common link in all the cases was exposure to hexane. The largest outbreak claimed ninety-three victims, the youngest only ten years old; the oldest, seventy-five. All of them lived in a small region dominated by a single cottage industry that had recently gone through a technological upgrade:

> Typical of inhabitants of this area, it had been their conventional means of livelihood to make sandals or slippers. In recent years, utilization of synthetic resins to this household industry has occurred and many kinds of organic solvents have been used as a rubber paste base. . . . They have engaged in the work more than 8 hours a day in narrow badly ventilated dwellings where vapor of the volatile solvent filled the rooms.[41]

Soon additional reports began to come in from other countries, too. By the 1970s the illness had a name: *shoemaker's polyneuropathy*. Although Italy was the country to coin this name in its medical reports, the United States was not free of the "new" disease.[42] In 1971, a series of cases were identified at the largest public hospital in the Bronx. The afflicted women who came in to be treated all worked as furniture strippers, using hexane from an open fifty-gallon drum. These cases were clinically identical to the syndrome that had been originally described in Japan.

The most renowned victim of shoemaker's polyneuropathy is undoubtedly Bill Bowerman, coach, inventor, and Nike cofounder. Working in a small closet in his home as he developed the prototype of the shoes that were to make him a multimillionaire, he so poisoned himself with hexane-laced glue that he was initially misdiagnosed as suffering from Lou Gehrig's disease (amyotrophic lateral sclerosis, or ALS).[43]

As other U.S. case reports began to accumulate, not all involved hexane use on the job. A novel and alarmingly different public health threat was arising from hexane-laced glue. Rather than shoemaker's polyneuropathy, *glue sniffer's neuropathy* was becoming a prime diagnostic consideration. An early case from Philadelphia was typical. By age nineteen, when the patient sought medical care, he had already been abusing glue for five years.[44] He got high either by sniffing the solvent vapors generated by heating up glue in a pan or by inhaling glue vapors from a plastic bag placed over his nose and mouth. This latter practice is known as *bagging;* solvents can also be abused by placing a chemical-soaked rag over the nose and mouth, known as *huffing,* but this is impractical with glue for obvious reasons. Despite the years of glue sniffing, the young man had remained in relatively good health. Then he switched from glue containing a mixed, petroleum distillate solvent to a new, hexane-based rubber cement. Over two months, he lost forty pounds and developed pain, tingling, and weakness in his legs. As his unnamed syndrome advanced, he was unable to stand or even sit without assistance.

In response to the rising frequency of hexane abuse, a German glue manufacturer attempted to discourage the practice by adding a second, mildly irritating solvent, methyl ethyl ketone, to its product. The abuse continued unabated. Unfortunately, it turned out that methyl ethyl ketone, relatively benign on its own, actually magnifies the toxicity of hexane. Although this was later confirmed in laboratory animal studies, such testing with combined industrial toxins is almost never done before marketing.

Toluene was another substitute for benzene in glue. This solvent is structurally similar to benzene but lacks its bone marrow toxicity and is not believed to be a carcinogen unless contaminated with benzene (which it often is, at least in trace amounts). Like toxicity from hexane alone or hexane combined with methyl ethyl ketone, however, toluene-related problems also began to show up in glue sniffers. Instead of damage to the distant nerve endings supplying sensation and power to the limbs, the effect manifest with toluene was subtler. Very high levels of toluene exposure appeared to lead to impaired cognitive function, marked by memory loss and an inability to process new information.

At first the association between toluene exposure and long-term mental deficits was discounted, but the significant risk that toluene carries slowly came to be accepted. Magnetic resonance imaging (MRI), a technology that was not clinically available when toluene-related nervous system toxicity was first reported, has since shown that parts of the brain simply wither away in chronic toluene-laced glue sniffers. Occupational groups heavily exposed to toluene, especially shoemakers and printers, might be at risk of nervous system injury as well.

SUPERGLUE

Many brands of glue still contain toluene or even hexane, but they no longer dominate the market. A stroll through any hardware store will quickly demonstrate that rubber cement has lost shelf space. Rubber cement glues were *better* in their day, but the chemical industry had plans for really *super*adhesives. A new technology of glue making came into being.

The consumer would no longer need to buy a polymer product; the polymer could be synthesized in the privacy of his or her own home.

PVC's Semon and the chemical engineers of his generation had successfully overcome the challenge of turning monomers into any number of different, novel polymers. Needless to say, this was all accomplished within the controlled setting of the manufacturing factory. Because of their inherent structure, all of the polymers used in glues manifest excellent bonding characteristics as their solvents vaporize. In this they are essentially no different from animal or vegetable glues that adhere as the water they contain evaporates. Put in plain terms, the way good glue and even better glue works is to simply *dry.*

Beginning in the 1950s, polymer chemists began to develop a fundamentally different concept of glue. Suppose a new kind of glue could be created that was applied as monomer subunits that polymerized on the spot? This would not be an improved glue that simply dried more quickly than the competition, but rather a glue that *catalyzed.* Materials wouldn't just adhere to one another; they'd be bonded by a seam of cross-linking molecules forming a solid polymer weld.

Going from concept to execution was no mean feat: it meant creating glues that would polymerize on command. For this, the monomer starting material must be in a form that will remain stable until the right time comes; otherwise the tube of would-be glue will have turned itself into a hard lump of plastic long before it can be used. A chemical stabilizer is usually required to impede such a process, and just the opposite, a catalyst, may be needed when rapid polymerization is required.

The glue catalyst may consist of an added chemical, or the glue reaction may be catalyzed by its exposure to heat or water or air or even by preventing its exposure to air (glues of this last type are called anaerobic and are sometimes used to hold threaded screws in place). If the polymer is made from a combination of two different monomers (in which the end product is a copolymer) or is cross-linked by a hardening agent, then two separate starting materials may have to be combined to make the glue polymerize itself on-site. Chemical solvents often need to be included too, ensuring spreadability before the reaction takes hold.

If you have ever followed the step-by-step instructions for using an epoxy glue ("Squeeze out equal parts of tube A and tube B . . ."), then you have performed this complicated chemical choreography. Epoxy polymerizes when its principal chemical constituents, a monomer and a cross-linking hardener, are combined with a catalyst that cures the reaction.

Other reactive adhesives and surface coatings that polymerize as they are being used are not fundamentally different. These include cyanoacrylates, methacrylates, and polyurethanes.

One big problem occurs with the chemical intermediates that make up these Generation X glues. They are all, perforce, reactive chemical intermediates. If they can't bond to one thing, they will bond to another. In the living organism, if inhaled or absorbed through the skin, such reactive chemicals can quickly cross-link to the body's own proteins. This gets them out of circulation, but, unfortunately, it also transforms the chemicals into a form ideal for stimulating an allergic response. Each of the reactive glues and sealants, to a greater or lesser extent, can cause allergic skin rashes, nasal symptoms resembling hay fever, new and often disabling bronchial asthma, and, in rare instances, even more serious immune responses.

Cyanoacrylate is a good example of a material that causes such complications. Cyanoacrylate glues were first introduced commercially in the late 1950s. By the 1970s, allergic skin rashes were established as a clear health risk arising from its use. In 1985, the first case of asthma in the United States from a cyanoacrylate *instant glue* was published in a medical journal.[45] The person affected was a thirty-two-year-old accountant whose exposure was not on the job but rather through his hobby of model airplane building. He had been wheezing and short of breath for about a year. The pattern was always the same: about an hour after he'd use the glue, his eyes would become puffy and his nose would run profusely. Three to five hours later, usually waking him from sleep, he would experience wheezing and couldn't catch his breath. He'd never had asthma before.

Because *instant-glue asthma* had never previously been reported, the physicians investigating the case went so far as to have the patient re-create his home gluing activity under laboratory conditions. They then watched him closely over twenty-four hours. His lung function fell by almost 25 percent, which greatly impressed his doctors, although the patient himself described it as only a "mild" attack relative to some others he had experienced.

The same year, a British medical report detailed seven similar cases of asthma, five from cyanoacrylates and two from methyl methacrylate. It was around this same time that these materials were just gaining popularity in medical applications as high-tech surgical cements. They are well suited for that purpose precisely because they harden quickly and, once polymerized, have fewer complications, such as allergic responses, than occur with alternative materials. The main problem arises not among patients but among medical personnel who have to work repeatedly with the reactive monomer. By 1986, the first case of methyl methacrylate asthma in an orthopedic operating room nurse was verified. Dental technicians, who also use methyl methacrylate cements, have been identified as another group at risk of asthma from these products.[46]

As much as polymerizing glues have been a health problem, even greater hazards have resulted from the use of these materials in sprayed-on coating or painting applications, especially if the final step involves baking or heat-curing. Polyurethane is the most important polymer associated with this type of hazard. Polyurethane paints and sealants, because of their durability and finish, are now nearly ubiquitous in both industrial and home applications. By the 1980s, the designer Issey Miyake had even introduced a line of dresses created by applying polyurethane to cloth that was molded over mannequins. One need not look to the haute couture atelier for sources of urethane exposure, however. Virtually no auto body repair shop in the developed world does touch-up without using urethane paints, often with few or no employee protections at all in place.

The critical active monomer ingredient in urethane polymers is called an isocyanate. Depending on the urethane product involved, varying amounts of residual isocyanate remain in the end product as it is actually being applied. Some urethanes come as partly prepolymerized one-part products with only a modest amount of pure residual monomer left to react. Other urethanes are packaged just like epoxy glues, with two separate components that must be mixed and used immediately afterward.

Spray painting constitutes an especially popular application of urethane. It also happens to be a particularly effective means of generating high levels of a fine isocyanate mist that can penetrate deeply and efficiently into the lungs. According to current estimates from industrialized countries, about one in every ten cases of asthma with onset in adulthood has a link to workplace exposures. Isocyanate-induced asthma has become the leading single cause of this occupationally related disease.

Moreover, new uses for urethanes continue to be introduced, further expanding possible sources of exposure. Methylene diphenyl diisocyanate (MDI) has become particularly popular as a glue and adhesive sealant (e.g., Gorilla Glue), because it can be formulated so that moisture in the air catalyzes its final polymer cross-linking. This characteristic also accounts for the widespread use of MDI-based, lightweight casts that have all but replaced less efficient, old-fashioned plaster casts. With the change, asthma has become a new "orthopedic" problem.[47]

When used as sprayed-on coatings, epoxy resins can also act as potent asthma-inducing agents similar to the urethanes. Epoxies used in this way can also cause other allergic responses leading to even more devastating damage. For instance, some epoxy-spray workers develop inflammation deep in the lung, causing scarring that, if left unchecked, can leave the lungs permanently stiff and dysfunctional. Other epoxy sprayers contract an even more unusual condition. This syndrome is marked by profuse bleeding deep in the air sacs of the lungs, taking away much of the body's ability to capture oxygen. This rare and life-threatening disorder has occurred almost exclusively when epoxy has been sprayed onto hot metal, a work practice that generates very high levels of toxic fumes.

As a matter of fact, overheating any of these polymers, not just the epoxy resins, is generally a bad idea. One of the latest related incidents occurred among a group of fax machine repair technicians who developed an unusual illness characterized by eye and respiratory irritation and, in at least one case, lymph gland swelling. The illness was traced to the fax machines, because they released butyl methacrylate fume as the top coating of the electrosensitive paper was vaporized in the transmission process. New high-temperature *hot-melt* urethane glues also release breakdown fumes that can cause illness. Yet another new technology that intentionally heats polymers is the introduction of *susceptors* in food packaging for microwave cooking. Susceptors are used to generate localized areas of very high temperature for browning. Unfortunately, microwaved pizzas using epoxy-containing susceptors were found to be laced with epoxy monomer. Luckily, this particular product was reformulated prior to any documented outbreak of human illness.[48]

NEW GLUES AND GLUE REMOVERS

Asthma, chemical irritation, and allergies make up only one group of health risks from the new glues and related polymers. The rapidity with which the glues set and the strength of their bonds can also lead to an entirely different set of problems. Almost a thousand years ago, Rugerus instructed us to test glue with our fingers, and if "they adhere together, the glue is good." With superglue technology, such a finger test often means a trip to the emergency department. Indeed, every year in the United States, there are thousands of such visits for body parts instantly glued together. These emergencies include many cases in which an inadvertent glue splash or wipe to the eye has occurred. Even more serious, direct installation into the eye has taken place when visually impaired individuals mistake an instant glue container for their prescription eyedrops. The packaging of both, it should be noted, is often remarkably similar. One medical paper on the subject noted, "Despite 10 years of published reports attributing such accidents to similar packaging of cyanoacrylate and ophthalmic medicines and preparations, glue manufacturers have yet to answer the professional pleas to change their package."[49]

Even more disturbing, deliberate installation to the eyes of children has been reported as a particularly cruel form of physical abuse.[50] In cases of direct installation, the glue may virtually seal the eyelids together, requiring prolonged softening until the skin can work itself free. In especially severe cases in which there is rapid need to remove residual polymer because of risk of long-term complications, sedation or even general anesthesia may be needed.

Yet another set of problems exists. The new, more sophisticated polymers require ever more aggressive solvents if they must be de-adhered. Common sense dictates that a person should have more reason to glue things together in the first place than to unglue them later on. Fashion, of course, is not ruled by common sense. Artificial nails are a case in point. Artificial nails, or *sculptured* nails as the preferred term in salon parlance would have it, are glued (sculpted) onto the natural nail through polymerization, often with methacrylate. To remove the polymer, a variety of potent solvents are widely sold that might not otherwise have become available to the unwary consumer. One of the most unfortunate marketing choices for a nail remover was the solvent acetonitrile, which was otherwise intended for industrial use only.

Acetonitrile's use in the home was promoted as an effective methacrylate or cyanoacrylate instant glue remover. Initially sold in non–child resistant packaging, each two-ounce screw-top bottle contained enough acetonitrile to kill one or two toddlers. Acetonitrile is not highly toxic to start with, but over several hours the body's own metabolism converts it into the potent poison cyanide. The first acetonitrile artificial nail remover death was reported in the *JAMA* in 1988.[51] A sixteen-month-old had taken a few sips of the product. The parents did telephone a poison control center, but in the call the product was misidentified as a far less toxic acetone nail *polish* remover. The parents were reassured, and the child was put to bed. He was found dead in his crib the next morning. Autopsy testing verified lethal cyanide levels.

Other reports soon followed of additional cases of profound toxicity after ingestion of even tiny amounts of the nail remover by small children. Poison control centers, having been alerted to the danger, acted quickly to recommend antidote therapy, and the exposed children survived. After public pressure from the medical community, beginning in 1990 manufacturers were required to market acetonitrile in child-resistant packaging.

This success with nail remover was short lived. In 1994, a new threat was uncovered in the form of an alternative artificial nail solvent (sold under the brand name Remove) made from a different but no less potent industrial solvent, nitroethane. Nitroethane does not act as a poison through the same mechanism as acetonitrile. Acetonitrile breaks down to cyanide and blocks the body's ability to use oxygen, thus stopping critical life functions. Nitroethane, acting more rapidly, simply blocks the blood's ability to transport oxygen in the first place. For example, in the case of a nitroethane-poisoned twenty-month-old who arrived at the hospital emergency room blue and short of breath, almost half of the blood's capacity to carry oxygen had been blocked. Fortunately, a chemical antidote was available and the infant survived.[52] Certain artificial nail "primers" have a similar toxic effect on the blood.[53]

JURISDICTIONAL SQUABBLES

To date, no regulations have formally banned or recalled the nitroethane nail remover. The Food and Drug Administration (FDA) has jurisdiction over cosmetics and has had some experience with regulating artificial nails, although with mixed success. Because of growing numbers of reported adverse reactions, in 1974 the FDA took action against methyl methacrylate nails. Although some cosmetic ingredients have been banned by specific regulations, this action is rarely taken (the FDA's action to limit vinyl chloride, independent of OSHA, is one of the few examples of such a step).

In the case of methyl methacrylate, the FDA sought a court injunction for a single manufacturer and limited sales by seizing materials from several others. Some states followed up with local bans on methyl methacrylate, but despite these restrictions, the product has continued to be widely used even in states where it is supposedly prohibited. A safer substitute, *ethyl* methacrylate, is more expensive.

Acetonitrile and nitroethane fall into an even grayer regulatory zone. When those chemicals are used in a factory or construction site, they clearly come under strict OSHA regulations. Even when off-gassed into the atmosphere or dumped down the sewer, they fall under the purview of the EPA. Potentially toxic chemicals used around the house, including glues, are another matter. The default regulatory body for household hazards—and *default* is the operative word—is called the Consumer Product Safety Commission (CPSC).

The CPSC, which has taken no action whatsoever on nitroethane, at least mandated protective packaging for acetonitrile in 1990 (two years after the initial deaths were publicized). In an unusual swipe at another federal agency, the FDA has gone so far as to be openly critical that this packaging restriction was insufficient, noting on its Web site, "The fact that a product is in 'child-resistant packaging' does not mean that a child could not possibly open it."[54]

Even to people who have heard of OSHA, the FDA, and the EPA, the CPSC does not exactly come trippingly on the tongue. Its obscurity may simply mirror its ineffectiveness. The CPSC was created in 1973 with the goal of closing regulatory loopholes for common household products. One of its first regulatory challenges was vinyl chloride in spray cans. After OSHA, the EPA, and the FDA had all promulgated concrete regulatory measures for products under their jurisdictions, the CPSC announced it was "investigating" the problem of vinyl chloride.[55]

In 1978, the CPSC finally decided to do something about benzene, trailing the other agencies in regard to this substance as well. In April of that year, it proposed a ban on benzene for all household products, including rubber cement, whether the benzene was added intentionally or was introduced as a contaminant that constituted 0.1 percent or more of the product. According to the CPSC press release, of fifty-two rubber cement makers it had contacted, only one still intentionally added benzene.[56] Two years later, in 1980, the CPSC had still not put the proposed ban into force. Instead, it issued a press release announcing that it would require all U.S. corporations to inform the commission of any benzene intentionally added to current products.[57]

In January 1981, the CPSC announced its intention to withdraw the proposed ban, which had never come into force anyway. This time the commission did not issue a press release to trumpet the nonachievement, but it did produce a lengthy justification published in the *Federal Register.*[58] The CPSC could no longer identify products to which benzene was added intentionally, but it did acknowledge in its *Federal Register* apologia that one out of ten products tested still contained the solvent at 0.1 percent or more. This was the trigger level for action named in its originally proposed ban.

Even by the CPSC's own calculations, the use of sixteen ounces or more of a product containing this much contaminant in an enclosed room would yield benzene levels as high as the old OSHA limit. One highlighted example was contact cement applied to a large surface area. Rubber cement used in smaller quantities might be less risky, although the CPSC noted the highest contamination (0.23 percent) in one such product it sampled. The CPSC admitted that benzene-contaminated rubber cement "may reflect a risk for certain hobbyists and artists."[59]

Instead of banning benzene, the CPSC fell back to a standard position requiring warning labels on glues containing solvents. Its current regulations detail that the designation *danger*, along with the warning *Harmful or fatal if swallowed*, must be present when solvents such as toluene make up 10 percent or more of a product by weight.

Benzene is a special case for the CPSC. For example, on a bottle of glue composed of 5 percent or more of benzene (granted, half the level for toluene warnings, but *fifty times* the level of the ban that was never instituted), the label must state *danger* and include the words *Vapor harmful* and *poison,* along with a skull and crossbones. Although the specific cautions of "leukemia" or "cancer" might be warranted, they are not mandated as warnings.

Back in 1978, one of the early chairmen of the CPSC, S. John Byington, was widely criticized for his flamboyantly poor leadership. One of his most publicized acts was an attempt to formally place his daughters as exhibits to support his congressional testimony asserting that carcinogen-treated sleepwear posed no real danger. By the CPSC's ten-year anniversary in 1983, the *Washington Post* documented that little had changed, noting, "The CPSC is on a downhill cycle, in part because of the Reagan administration's emphasis on deregulation. . . . One sign of decline is the criticism of Chairman Nancy Harvey Steorts and her style of leadership."[60]

Steorts was followed by Chairman Terrence Scanlon, who successfully promoted the concept that, in place of unequivocal regulatory controls, the CPSC should rely on vague "voluntary safety actions" by industry. He left the CPSC in 1988 to join the conservative Heritage Foundation.

The CPSC continues on a bumpy ride. In 2001, the Senate Commerce Committee rejected President George W. Bush's initial nominee for chair of the CPSC, Mary Gall.[61] At an earlier time, as a seated member of the three-person commission but not its chair, Gall had made a name for herself by blocking an investigation into a reportedly faulty design of baby bath seats. Later, she voted against a requirement that bunk bed manufacturers rectify a problem with faulty rails that injured children (she felt manufacturers should be encouraged to take voluntary action).

The CPSC has been consistently reluctant to take on politically controversial or high-stakes economic issues. As established by legislation, the watchdog agency may have teeth, but it is effectively muzzled. The petrochemical industry has had little to fear from the CPSC. Hexane and toluene, two principal solvent replacements for benzene, are still widely marketed in over-the-counter glues and adhesives, despite their toxicity to the nervous system.

Even on its own terms, the labeling policy that is the mainstay of CPSC action on toxic materials is inadequate. In 1991, the Public Interest Research Group called on the CPSC to crack down on improper labeling of arts and crafts supplies, including glues, when it found that 44 percent of the products it surveyed carried insufficient warnings. "'Our compliance people will take a look at it,' replied a CPSC spokesperson."[62]

In 2001, the CPSC did announce the voluntary recall of ninety thousand packages of "super contact adhesive" containing toluene for failing to have the required cautionary labels, one of its few recent actions in this area. In the last two decades, the CPSC has called for stricter labeling in the case of only a single solvent, methylene chloride. It is widely used in furniture strippers but is not a major component of glues. The CPSC took action on methylene chloride at the same 1978 meeting in which it decided to officially warn against using a handheld hair dryer while in the bathtub.

FALLING BEHIND

Regulatory inaction in an arena where new problems are constantly coming to the fore means falling ever further behind in effective control measures. This is true not only for the CPSC but also on a larger national and even an international level. New and potentially toxic materials are routinely introduced or combined with other processes to create novel risks; at the same time, old established hazards are recirculated into the workplace or the marketplace, their past histories conveniently forgotten. For synthetic glues, sealants, and related products, there are no shortages of examples of new hazards with familiar dangers.

Dimethylformamide (DMF) is one such material. An industrial solvent of relatively recent popularity used primarily in gluelike coatings, DMF is a potent cause of liver injury. It can bring on chemical hepatitis after as little as a few weeks of heavy workplace contact. Less extreme DMF exposure can lead to fatty infiltration of the liver, a condition usually associated with long-term alcohol abuse. One industry in which DMF has been a particular problem has been the application of polymer coatings in the manufacture of artificial leather, the same process in which benzene made an early name for itself as a cause of leukemia.

Nitromethane, a chemical closely related to nitroethane, has also been introduced as a solvent for acrylates. For the nail sculptor, this use may involve the product D-Zolve Tip Blender. "One drop on the line of demarcation cuts filing time to a minimum with no hard, heat producing file strokes."[63]

Industrial settings can involve a heavier use of nitromethane as a solvent for glue or sealant removal. One well-documented example comes from a headlight subassembly shop, where excess residues of a combination cyanoacrylate-methacrylate glue were removed by spraying them with nitromethane, then wiping them off with a rag. Two of the headlight assemblers who used the product began to have symptoms of numbness and weakness in their arms and legs. Although their illness was remarkably similar to hexane-related disease, at first they were misdiagnosed as suffering from Guillain-Barré syndrome, a no-fault neurological illness presumed to be triggered by a viral infection. Later, an investigation carried out by the National Institute for Occupational Safety and Health finally identified nitromethane as the cause.[64]

With increasing amounts of nitromethane in the marketplace, other health effects from overexposure are also beginning to be documented. One of the popular non-glue-related uses of nitromethane is as a fuel additive to give an extra kick in small motors. Model engine makers, especially model airplane racers, often use it. One reported overdose occurred in a two-year-old child who ingested some model aviation fuel while on a family outing in a park. Although the child did not appear ill, testing seemed to indicate severe kidney dysfunction. This chemical, however, specifically interferes with the most commonly used laboratory assay for creatinine, a primary blood test for kidney status. Luckily, this testing error didn't result in a drastic intervention for presumed kidney failure, such as dialysis.[65]

Another nail care solvent is also turning out to pose a health threat—this time through misuse in a scenario reminiscent of classic glue sniffing. The solvent, gamma butyrolactone, can be used to make the "party drug" gamma hydroxybutyrate (GHB) and can be converted on an industrial

scale in any makeshift home laboratory. One common means of this manufacture had been to mix the solvent with a strong alkali (a caustic), but if
this mixture is not neutralized, the resulting GHB can lead to severe throat
injury similar to that of swallowed drain cleaner.[66] Of course, GHB is, in
and of itself, a dangerous substance that easily induces coma in those taking it to get high. Unfortunately, the laboratory of the human body,
through its own metabolism, can also produce GHB from ingested gamma
butyrolactone. The Drug Enforcement Administration restricts sale of the
solvent for drug manufacture or ingestion, but this does not ban its use
for "valid" commercial purposes, one of which is as a key component of
"acetone-free" nail polish removers. Additional chemical additives may or
may not deter recreational use of the acetone-free products, but childhood
ingestions of nail polish remover have led to more than one case of coma
from GHB.[67]

Amid all these new threats, old hazards remain as well. As a solvent for rubber cement, benzene has not been entirely removed from commerce either
in the United States or in Europe. Not surprisingly, in developing economies benzene is often minimally regulated, if at all. Hexane use is even
more widespread worldwide as a glue solvent, and outbreaks of shoemaker's polyneuropathy continue to occur.[68] Hexane has even gained new
popularity as a solvent for general uses, as documented by a report of progressive neuropathy affecting a California man who had repaired cars for
twenty-four years.[69] He used up to nine spray cans a day of an aerosol
brake cleaner that turned out to be more than 50 percent hexane.

Even the old doping toxin tetrachloroethane, which should have seen its
last use in 1918, is an old soldier that has not completely faded away. As late
as the 1960s, an outbreak of tetrachloroethane-related illness was reported
in Bombay.[70] At least twenty-three small factories were using the solvent to
make wrist bangles from recycled cellulose acetate film. Other holdover uses
of the solvent have occurred as well. In the early 1980s, the U.S. National
Cancer Institute undertook a follow-up study of more than a thousand veterans who had been exposed to tetrachloroethane during World War II.[71]
Incredibly, the chemical had been used to impregnate uniforms against
chemical warfare agents. The veterans studied had been assigned to field
units processing the uniforms. The later concern was over possible long-
term effects, because laboratory studies had shown that tetrachloroethane

exhibited cancer potential in test animals. Although a modest elevation in cancer risk was apparent among the exposed veterans who were studied, no definitive conclusions based on the research were ever reached.

For a truly effective shield to be formed between the public and the myriad of old and new potential toxins such as those associated with modern glues and sealants, a number of regulatory agencies must be involved. The CPSC, the FDA, the EPA, and OSHA need to work together proactively for the effective control of these hazards. Some materials should be removed from general commerce altogether. For instance, there is no compelling reason to continue to market nitroethane for removal of artificial nails or hexane- or toluene-based rubber cements for household use or benzene-contaminated glues for any purpose.

Other products need not be removed from the marketplace but could be restricted through different regulatory controls. For example, instant glues provide bonds far stronger than actually needed for most applications. Is the world really better off with a coffee mug whose reglued handle has a more powerful seam than the original ceramic? If tested by force, the mug may disintegrate into a hundred pieces while the handle holds—and the unlucky repairer may have self-induced allergic asthma. With sufficient data, a better-informed public could theoretically adjust its demand for the supply of potentially hazardous consumer products in the first place, short of absolute restrictions. Yet in the face of a greater public need for information, product labels and other manufacturers' safety data that could provide a key source of consumer information are often out-of-date and inadequate.

Even those involved in industrial use of potentially hazardous products suffer from inadequate protection. Current OSHA limits regarding isocyanates, for example, take into account identification of only the isolated monomer isocyanate component, even though most products on the market today are partly polymerized, a form in which isocyanates are still reactive but fall through a regulatory loophole for OSHA limits on air exposure to them.

We must also think on a global scale. Beyond our own borders, U.S. regulatory restrictions have little direct impact. An editorial in the influential *British Medical Journal* was on point in stating, "Industrial risk in poor countries is vast: exposure ranges from dangerous glues used to make shoes in shanty huts to unsafe steel smelting plants."[72] The American industrialist Peter Cooper made his fortune early in the nineteenth century from glue, a market over which he held a virtual monopoly for decades. Cooper acknowledged glue manufacturing as the source of his wealth in a once famous aphorism, "If you would succeed, stick."

Cooper was a staunch supporter of an ethos of corporate responsibility. He died in 1883 at ninety-two years of age, just as benzene was about to make rubber cement a possibility.[73] Perhaps he was blessed in not living to see the advances that glue making underwent after his death. The survival of his ethos would be a good thing, however. It dictated that corporations should independently take responsibility for product modifications, thus reducing hazards at their source.

For one example of a basic chemical engineering solution that would fit this practice, we can take a lesson from the rubber tree's natural product and its manufactured facsimiles. Many polymers can be modified to make artificial latex, turning insoluble materials into droplets suspended in a water-based emulsion. The familiar white nontoxic glue in the squeeze bottle is a good example of a modern product for an old need. Despite Elmer, the friendly bull on the label, the glue does not contain natural collagen but rather a man-made polymer. This polymer, however, is engineered to be benign and water soluble, eliminating the need for potentially toxic solvents.

On a classic episode of the television comedy series *Seinfeld,* George, one of the main characters, is rescued from an ill-suited engagement. His fiancée succumbs to glue toxicity from licking the seals of too many cut-rate envelopes for their wedding invitations.[74] The plot device is devilishly absurd. But such a product might indeed fall between the cracks of effective regulatory control in an all too plausible way.

We have progressed from good glue through better glue and on to superglue, with a recurring set of problems with each cycle of technological change. We can enjoy the reruns of the *Seinfeld* television satire, but it is high time we stop revisiting the same repeated episodes of failed public protection.

FOUR

Under a Green Sea

The Rising Tide of Chlorine

A SILENT EPIDEMIC

A bottle of household bleach sitting peacefully on the laundry room shelf is not a ticking time bomb. It is merely a small tactical weapon in our never-ending war against dirt, germs, and stains. Bleach is not benign, however, because the chlorine that is trapped inside it, if released, can be a potent toxin. Chlorine is one of the most common causes, worldwide, of chemical gas poisonings. The most dramatic chlorine gas inhalation scenario is played out when a derailed gas tanker leads to mass evacuations and large-scale injuries. Far more common, however, are the everyday small-scale chlorine gassings that take place in the quiet comfort of the home: in laundry rooms, kitchens, and bathrooms.

This silent epidemic of intoxications went wholly unnoticed in the United States until the initial establishment of poison control centers in the late 1950s, such as Boston's Poison Information Center. Set up to advise both medical providers and the general public on the hazards of childhood ingestions, Boston's Poison Information Center also, from the beginning, fielded calls on adult cases. During each winter, almost one in ten of these adult consultations involved exposures of a disturbingly similar kind. Mrs. B. was typical of the cases. She "cleaned her kitchen floor just prior to meal-time with a mixture of 5 per cent solution of sodium hypochlorite, an anionic detergent-hydrocarbon combination, a commercial bleach mixture and vinegar."[1]

Shortly afterward, the entire family became ill. Mrs. B., described as a "36-year-old housewife," was still sick the next day when she finally called the Poison Information Center. The report, published in the *New England Journal of Medicine* in 1964, begins with the following time-encapsulated introduction: "Mixing household cleaners is a common practice among American housewives. Experimenting and unconscious of the fumes that some of these mixtures release, they hope that their own formulation will clean better than a single commercial product will."

Not every homemaker was as lucky as Mrs. B. A few years after that first report, *JAMA* published the case of an eighty-three-year-old woman who nearly died after developing an injury-related buildup of fluid in the lungs following a bleach mishap. She, too, fell victim as a soldier in the war against stains. "Provoked by a stubborn stain unresponsive to soap, she had emptied about half a gallon of Clorox (an aqueous solution of 5.25% sodium hypochlorite) and thereupon added most of a can of Sani-Flush. . . . Almost immediately she experienced intense burning of the eyes, mouth, throat and began to cough."[2]

Over the last thirty years, Ozzie and Harriet's classic kitchen and bathroom may have been replaced by a trendy work-live-eat loft space, but just the same, each year's tally of poison control center calls around the country shows that chlorine is still one of the most frequent sources of chemical injury in the home. When I speak to general medical audiences on occupational and environmental toxins, I often ask how many physicians in the room have ever treated a patient with breathing problems following a household bleach mishap. Typically, about 15–20 percent of the audience raise their hands. When I ask in follow-up how many in the room have actually had to treat themselves for this same exposure, several hands always stay aloft.

It would be easy to assume that these overzealous bleach attacks are a peculiarly American problem. For example, in her book *Chasing Dirt: The American Pursuit of Cleanliness,* Suellen Hoy argues that the American obsession with cleanliness is peculiarly local and rooted firmly in an endemic culture of Puritan compulsiveness. This, she proposes, has combined historically with the commercial marketing of hygiene products to a melting pot of immigrants eager to fit in.[3]

Yet the data on bleach suggest that the United States is far from the leader in use of this product. By the early 1990s, Spain, not the United

States, had the greatest average use of household bleach per capita per year, at more than twelve liters for every citizen. Portugal outstripped the United States too, coming in at more than eight liters per capita. The United States trailed behind at 6.4 liters.

Household bleach exposures account for 6 percent of all poison control center calls across Europe.[4] Deaths from household mixing exposures have been reported in Germany, the Netherlands, Turkey, and Japan. The Japanese scientific literature has contributed the longest-titled study on the subject (with eight coauthors), "Dangerous Mixture of Household Detergents in an Old-style Toilet: A Case Report with Simulation Experiments of the Working Environment and Warning of Potential Hazard Relevant to the General Environment."[5] Household bleach has even been found a health threat in the former Yugoslavia. A scientific report on eighty-seven patients treated in Skopje, Macedonia, over a two-year period alone concluded, in somewhat Byzantine prose, "Housewives are usually unaware of danger from their own mixtures while cleaning at home in poor ventilated spaces with no protection devices and acute inhalatory poisoning remains an actual and frequent problem in our clinic work needing continuous scientific and therapeutic enterprise."[6]

The household manufacture of chlorine gas is typically, although not always, unintended. Indeed, creating chlorine gas is an altogether simple operation. It occurs when hypochlorite bleach is mixed with any acid substance. This can be plain vinegar or any one of a number of widely marketed tile or toilet bowl cleaners containing acid. Some of these cleaners are little more than dilute hydrochloric acid; others contain phosphoric or oxalic acid. Direct mixing of these products immediately produces a plume of noxious gas. Concentrated hypochlorite and hydrochloric acid are intentionally mixed at times to generate fumes, which are thought to be better for thorough cleaning. A sufficiently dangerous, but somewhat more insidious, mixture of hypochlorite and acid can also occur by unwittingly combining the products through their separate sequential use without sufficiently rinsing between their applications.

THE DISCOVERY OF CHLORINE

Home-based toxic gas release is all too consistent with the entire history of chlorine. Chlorine's story is not a saga of high technology. Household hypochlorite bleach did not come to us through a series of coordinated breakthroughs, proceeding step by step with ever more sophisticated applications, eventually leading to the widespread marketing of a final product. In short, chlorine's discovery and manufacture were not on a par with rocket science. The history of chlorine rests with a happenstance series of a few simple innovations.[7] It was these small discoveries that led to rapid and mass repercussions.

The "splitting" of salt was, in its way, as much a scientific turning point in 1774 as true fission would be more than 150 years later. Even though salt had been a basic commodity throughout time, up until then its key component, the chlorine of sodium chloride, could never be pulled apart and isolated in a pure form. When this was achieved, salt's properties were jarring to some of the fundamental principles accepted by the scientists of the time. Simple salt seemed to have locked within it a powerful substance that did not follow the rules. Chlorine could penetrate other substances usually impervious to attack. In fact, it was capable of killing nearby plants or animals or even the unlucky experimental bystander.

The chemical breakdown of sea salt was first reported by a modest Swedish druggist, Carl Scheele, who went on to become recognized as one of the great research chemists of his age. Scheele performed a series of experiments to try to understand better the behavior of "marine," or "muriatic," acid. *Muriatic acid* is still a common term for hydrochloric acid. In another form, the acid was known by an even older name, *aqua regia (regis)*, or, literally, "royal water." Aqua regia is a mixture of hydrochloric and nitric acids, which alchemists valued highly. It was known as one of the few substances that can dissolve pure gold.

Those in Scheele's time already appreciated that muriatic acid can be derived from brine (salt solution). A powerful acid, it reacts with other materials to break them down. This reactive capacity was understood only to the extent that it could be made to fit with an accepted and basic experimental characteristic known to the chemists of the day as *phlogiston*. Phlogiston theory is one of the great false principles in the history of scientific discovery, a primary tenet of the new church of chemistry in the mid-eighteenth century.

Phlogiston theory was a useful construct because it seemed to explain so much. It was the explanation for why wood burns and iron rusts. Phlogiston was held to be the innate, albeit theoretical, part of each material that was capable of being carried away by air in a reaction such as combustion or acid dissolution. When Scheele mixed marine (muriatic) acid with manganese, the metal appeared to react in just this way. The manganese dissolved in the acid and gave off a pungent smell, "like warm aqua regis," as he described it.[8]

Scheele wasn't exactly sure how this acid contained phlogiston, but he believed it must to act in the way it did. When Scheele applied external heat to the mix, he was further surprised by an even greater reaction. This time, a yellow-colored air appeared. Scheele reported that it had "a quite characteristically suffocating smell, which was most oppressive to the lungs" (7).

Scheele had just recorded the first case of chlorine gas inhalation. He called his discovery *dephlogisticated marine acid*, because, like a piece of wood burned to ash, the acid had reacted with a metal, giving up its phlogiston. Scheele set about producing more of this curious yellow-colored air. With some effort, he was able to collect it in small glass bottles. Even in his earliest experiments he noted an unusual property of the gas. When exposed to it, "all vegetable flowers—red, blue, and yellow—became white in a short time; the same thing also occurred with green plants. . . . The former colours of these flowers, as well as those of green plants, could not be restored either by alkalis or by acids" (9).

In his crude but tantalizing experiments with chlorine, Scheele was onto something very, very big. The odd whitening of vegetable colors that he observed was the harbinger of an entire industry that was to follow. But before that could happen, the new chemistry, born at the beginning of the eighteenth century, needed to mature. And to do that, phlogiston needed to be left behind. Chlorine was just the tonic to help chemistry grow up.

Scheele's fellow scientists, especially a new generation of French chemists beginning to question the underlying validity of phlogiston, saw in his observations of dephlogisticated marine acid a critical piece of evidence they needed to prove the theory's central fallacy. A list of the researchers who directly pursued Scheele's initial findings in their own laboratories reads like a who's who of French chemistry of the eighteenth century, including Berthollet, Guyton de Morveau, and Gay-Lussac. Others followed the reports closely, incorporating them into a growing body of experimental data from a variety of chemical reactions.

The most important of all of the scientists marshaling the evidence against the phlogiston theory was Lavoisier. By the 1780s it had become clear to him that experimental evidence could not support the presence of an innate physical-chemical force corresponding to phlogiston. Instead, a ubiquitous elemental substance, composing approximately one-fifth the volume of Earth's ambient air, accounted on its own for nearly all of phlogiston's supposed properties. That element, recently named by Lavoisier, was oxygen. Oxygen, it turned out, not phlogiston, was the explanation for both the combustion of wood and the rusting of iron.

In 1788, Lavoisier seized an opportunity to utterly demolish phlogiston. An Irish chemist, Richard Kirwin, had just published *An Essay on Phlogiston,* a fairly pedestrian recapitulation and defense of the theory. Lavoisier's wife translated the text into French. Then Lavoisier and his colleagues— Berthollet, Guyton de Morveau, and other prominent French chemists— set to work, adding scathingly critical commentary to the end of each of Kirwin's original chapters.[9] It is important to note that *An Essay on Phlogiston* includes a chapter that Kirwin specifically devoted to marine acid and the potent gas it gives off, a phenomenon that phlogiston could not successfully explain. Lavoisier's critique had a decisive effect on the scientific community on both sides of the English Channel. Phlogiston was dead—long live oxidation.

Even though these French scientists had used muriatic acid as a prime example to help disprove phlogiston theory, they still could not explain what exactly was going on in the manganese–muriatic acid reaction. Acids seemed to behave like other chemicals whose actions occur in the presence of oxygen. On that basis, they mistakenly assumed that the gas of muriatic acid contains oxygen. This certainly seemed to be true of nitric acid, muriatic acid's old alchemical partner in aqua regis and a substance far better understood at the time. Lavoisier and other chemists argued that muriatic acid must be acting through oxygen, since phlogiston was a fiction. On the basis of this reasoning, they believed the yellow-green gas produced from muriatic acid had to have oxygen attached to it. Thus, they rechristened dephlogisticated marine acid with an equally unwieldy name, *oxygenated marine acid.*

Lavoisier remained firm in the belief that all acids, including marine acid, work in concert with oxygen. It was a rare but important example of Lavoisier making a critical scientific error. Lavoisier had done more than any other scientist to unmask the sophistry of phlogiston masquerading as a scientific theory, but his misstep on how acids act could have set back the new chemistry he had pioneered had it persisted as a general principle. With sufficient time Lavoisier likely would have gained further insights into how marine acid acts and modified his views. Unfortunately for him, he was not only a brilliant chemist but also an official of the French state's tax collection apparatus. He was guillotined at age fifty.

It took a young British chemist named Humphry Davy to decisively overthrow the late Lavoisier's view on the composition of acid. In so doing, he raised the first serious British challenge to French chemical hegemony and led the way past the last remaining obstacle standing before the new chemistry as it strove to abandon the last vestiges of phlogiston. Through a series of elegant experiments, Davy showed that the gas liberated from marine acid is not an oxygen-containing compound after all. By 1810, Davy could argue that it was not rational to persist in using the name *oxygenated marine acid* for this oxygen-free gas. Davy suggested an entirely new name for the substance, *chlorine,* derived from the Greek and based on its yellow-green color.[10] The acid from which the gas is liberated became *hydrochloric acid.* Popularly, Davy is known best for his invention of the coal miners' Davy safety lamp. Yet Davy's work on chlorine (and on a derivative, chlorine dioxide, a bleaching gas that he later discovered as well) has had a far more lasting social, economic, and environmental impact.

The birthright claimed by chlorine, almost from the moment of its discovery, was its status as the once and future king of all bleaching agents. Scheele had first commented on the strange whitening property of the gas. In 1785, nine years after Scheele's initial discovery, Claude-Louis Berthollet once again noted that this new substance, yet to be named chlorine, acted as a potent bleaching agent.[11] Like so many of the top-notch chemists of his generation, Berthollet, then early in his career, was linked closely to Lavoisier. Berthollet, though, seemed better able to land on his feet than his colleague had.

After 1790, Berthollet, an active "committee man" in the Revolution, did not fall under the shadow of the Terror. Rather, he was appointed a commissioner of the National Mint. Later, under the empire, he became Napoleon's adviser on all matters chemical. He died *Comte* Berthollet at age seventy-two, in 1822. Maybe Berthollet was always looking for an angle or he was just farsighted, but he was the first to suggest that oxygenated muriatic acid might have a commercial application as a bleaching agent. Even so, he recognized a drawback to the gas, its "suffocating odor . . . which is extremely disagreeable, and would even be dangerous if workmen were long exposed to it at one time."[12]

Indeed, "commercial application" is far too modest a way of putting it. What Scheele and Berthollet had stumbled on was, in fact, no less than the equivalent of the Northwest Passage of textile processing.

It is hard to comprehend the implications of chlorine gas bleaching without understanding what bleaching entailed prior to 1800, in labor and, as important, in time.[13] Bleaching is an ancient activity, dating back to the earliest history of woven fabrics. For much of antiquity, the task of bleaching was linked so closely to laundering in a more general sense that the origins of the two are inseparable. At some point in prerecorded history, someone figured out that the ashes of burned plants (some more than others) were capable of a caustic action that could be used in cleansing. This ash, mixed in large pots, supplies the English derivation *potash* and, through it, the etymological source of *potassium*.

The Middle East, as it turned out, was quite a center for this sort of thing, in part through botanical and in part through geologic chance. A number of plants and minerals in the region are particularly rich sources of potassium or sodium alkalis that can be used in cleaning. In more than one place, the Bible has something to say on the subject. One of the relevant verses, mixing metaphor with practical advice, occurs in Jeremiah 2:22. "For though thou wash thee with nitre, and take thee much soap, yet thine iniquity is marked before me, saith the Lord God."[14]

In the literal Hebrew text, nobody is actually doing anything with soap in any modern sense of the word. The technological leap from potash to soap requires the addition of fat to the pot and to the ash. Although soap making was known to a limited extent in the classical period, it later died out. True soap was reintroduced into Europe only in the late Middle Ages. In the ancient world, washing with a cleanser, by and large, meant washing with an alkali substance. The alkali could be vegetable (usually meaning potassium carbonate), mineral (soda, derived from plant or mineral), or animal. Animal alkali equated with ammonia, the best source of which was urine, the most reliable donors being humans.

The Romans perfected the cleaning of cloth, with and without urine, to an art. This was the trade of the fuller. Being a plebeian of the Collegium Aquae, or in other words, a rank-and-file fuller, accounted for something, despite its smellier aspects. And it was, undeniably, a good business. This fact was not lost on the state, which placed a special tax on the urine that was collected at public lavatories to be sold to fullers. The emperor Vespasian took some political heat for this tax. In response to derision from no less than Titus on the subject, Vespasian is reported to have held a coin under his critic's nose and said, "Yet, it's made from urine *(Atqui e lotio est*)." This was later boiled down to the sound bite "It doesn't stink *(non olet)*." Soaking cloth in an alkaline solution was a critical step in whitening it in Roman times. Whitening was a long and tedious process, requiring multiple alternating alkaline washes and clear-water rinses and rubbing with special clays ("fuller's earth"). As valued as the dyes of the ancients were, even the royal Tyrian purple, pure white cloth was the rarer commodity. The Roman Pliny the Elder tells us, "For all these paintings and rich dyes, yet, when all is done, the white linen held the pre-eminence still, and was highly esteemed above all colors."[15]

Little changed over the next fifteen hundred years, except for the addition of soap. When Ramazzini described the fuller's trade at the close of the Italian Renaissance in 1700, it was still a laborious and repugnant process that would have been easily understandable to his Roman forefathers:

> In the workshops of the cloth-weavers where they comb the wool and weave broad woolen cloth, one sees small barrels into which all the workmen urinate, and they keep the urine in these till it actually putrefies, and only then do they use it. When I happened to go see such workers I perceived a horrible smell that assailed the nostrils, and when I asked the reason for it they showed me a barrel full of urine in which all were required to urinate by a rule of the trade.[16]

The further details that Ramazzini provides later in the same passage underscore the tedious nature of whitening cloth and its effects on the health of fullers:

> After the cloth or other woolen fabrics have been woven, to cleanse them of oil and dirt they put into a wooden vessel urine that has been stored in this way, with an equal part of tepid water and a certain quantity of Venice soap; in this they immerse the cloth, and to make the liquid soak in deeper and completely saturate the cloth, they stamp on it with their feet and repeat this two or three times, always throwing out the liquid left from the previous washing and pouring into the vessel a fresh supply of the mixture. When this process is finished they squeeze out the liquid with a press and finally wash the cloth in clean water with Venice soap. This is how the cloth-makers bleach cloth white so that it may more readily absorb any color. (111)

A few lines later, Ramazzini also notes, "It follows that fullers and cloth-makers who spend their time with these bad smells from stinking urine and oil in a hot room, at times half-naked, are almost all cachectic [wasted away], wan, short of breath, and subject to coughs and nausea" (111).

Over the centuries, the fuller's profession may have made for reliable employment, but it was thoroughly unpleasant and unhealthy work. Certainly nothing in it was quaintly redeeming or humorous; it was not like some scatological version of Lucille Ball pantomiming a peasant pressing grapes, as she did in a classic episode of her television situation comedy. But despite all its drawbacks, the small-scale fuller's craft persisted largely unchanged for a very long period of time. Then, as the Renaissance faded into the baroque period, the winds of change finally began to blow through the trade. The smell of urine became less pungent, only to be replaced by a burning spray of lye.

Large-scale textile processing began to replace the fuller's workshop early on, a century or more *before* the Industrial Revolution. During this time, bleaching was first differentiated as a separate craft distinct from washing and cleaning per se. For linen in particular, which was especially difficult to whiten, bleaching evolved into a pivotal, multistage process. Steeping or even boiling in an alkaline bath (lye rather than urine), called *bucking,* became a mainstay of bleaching. To this process, two other critical steps were added. One was called *souring,* involving an acid immersion in soured milk. Second, and the most important step, was bleaching in the sun, called *crofting.* We like to think of sunlight as a metaphorical bleaching instrument, but even Shakespeare is being quite concrete, given the practices of his day, when he invokes an image of spring with the phrase "the white sheet bleaching on the hedge."[17]

By the early 1700s, the lowlands of Holland had become the bleaching capital of the Continent, the place where the *whitening grounds of Haarlem* were renowned.[18] Linen and cotton cloth that needed to be bleached was shipped to Holland from all over Europe. The first steps in the process would typically begin in March, but it took so long to complete that the bleaching did not end until September. This timetable optimistically assumed that the material would be put out on the grass to bleach by midsummer. Often, cloth had to be held over to complete its crofting the following spring.

The first real "modern" breakthrough in bleaching occurred in the mid-1700s, when it was found that dilute sulfuric acid could be substituted for sour milk. Even though the chemical action of the acid was not fully understood at that time, this single change in the process cut the souring time down from six weeks to twenty-four hours. There was still no substitute for crofting, however, dependent as it was on the action of time and sunny skies.

The use of sulfuric acid as a chemical aid to bleaching had another important impact beyond the time it saved: it set the stage for chlorine's introduction only a few decades later. The use of sulfuric acid, in and of itself, was not an entirely novel process. Rather, it reflected an adaptation of a long-standing trick of the old fuller's trade. Sulfur fumes, from burning brimstone, had been used to bleach woolens since antiquity. Indeed, Apuleius's *Golden Ass* tells the tale of a fuller's wife whose indiscretion is discovered when her paramour is forced by sulfur fumes to give himself away:

> She could find no better hiding-place for her lover than a high wicker cage, with cloths hung over it to bleach in the fumes of the sulfur fire inside. It seemed a safe enough place, so she came and sat down to supper with us. But the lover was forced to breathe in the suffocating sulfur fumes, and you know how it is with sulfur: the smell is so acrid and penetrating that it makes one sneeze and sneeze. The laundryman, who was on his couch at the other side of the table from his wife, heard the first sneeze from immediately behind her. "Bless you, my dear!" he said, and "bless you, bless you!" at the second and third sneeze. But the noise went on and on, and at last he began to take notice and suspect that something was wrong. He pushed the table aside, got up, turned the cage over, and there he found his rival panting for breath, nearly at his last gasp.[19]

Brimstone bleaching was used for wool, but the damage that the fumes caused to cotton and linen made it unsuitable for those types of cloth. For that reason, there was an initial reluctance to adopt sulfuric acid. When it was found that cotton and linen tolerated the new treatment, this objection was overcome fairly quickly. The sulfuric acid baths proved extremely advantageous in time saving, and time was money. Perhaps cautiously at first, but then more widely and more rapidly, the use of sulfuric acid souring spread throughout the industry.[20]

THE INTRODUCTION OF CHLORINE BLEACHING

When the change to chlorine bleaching arrived, it came about quickly. It is an arrogance born of faxes, cellular phones, and e-mail communications that makes us assume that technical innovation must have diffused at little more than a snail's pace prior to our own time. Even if we overcome this modern bias, however, the rapidity with which chlorine bleaching spread from a laboratory curiosity to a mass industrial process is startling.

Berthollet first presented his observations on chlorine in 1785. Early in 1787, a Professor Copland from Scotland and his patron, the Duke of Gordon, were traveling on the Continent. While in Geneva, they visited a Professor de Saussure, who demonstrated for them the method of producing chlorine gas that he had gleaned from Berthollet's scientific papers. Professor de Saussure showed them, firsthand, chlorine's bleaching power. At this time Scotland was already an industrial textile center, second only to Manchester. By the end of July 1787, Professor Copland returned home. Immediately, he had a chlorine-based bleaching operation up and running at an Aberdeen factory. Copland had gone to Switzerland to learn indirectly of Berthollet's work. James Watt, whose steam engine had not yet been widely adopted by the textile mills, went straight to Paris. There, Berthollet himself impressed on Watt the potential advantages of chlorine bleaching. As it turned out, Watt's father-in-law, James McGrigor, was a bleacher (by the old nonchlorine methods) in Glasgow. There, Watt also introduced commercial chlorine bleaching in 1787; Manchester and other English textile centers were not far behind.[21]

By 1790, less than five years after the initial scientific report that chlorine might serve as bleaching agent, its commercial adoption in Great Britain was widespread. An English translation of Berthollet's *Essay on the New Method of Bleaching*, published that year, sold out its run in just four months. By 1807, *The Edinburgh Medical and Physical Dictionary* had the following entry: "Oxygenated muriatic acid gas has a yellow transparent color, and possesses a peculiar and suffocating smell. It . . . is the most noxious to the lungs of all the gases with which we are acquainted. This acid is not employed in medicine, but very extensively in the arts, particularly for bleaching."[22]

The gas was not only suffocating; it was also inefficient to use:

The articles having been suspended within large wooden boxes, each of which had a close bottom capable of holding water, the gas was conveyed into these receptacles; and, to prevent any injury by the immediate application of the gas, the goods were, by means of a frame and pulley, let down occasionally, and indeed frequently, into the water beneath. But by this method there was great difficulty in exposing all the surfaces of the goods equally, without which no perfect bleaching can ever be effected.[23]

The potential *injury* of concern, to be sure, was to the goods, not to the laborers. For the early bleaching entrepreneurs, the noxious quality of chlorine presented an inconvenience because chlorine gas was difficult to work with technically, not because it was hazardous to workers.

Another alternative to working with the pure gas released in air was to bubble it through water and then use the chlorine-saturated water as a bleaching agent. But this option had its difficulties, too. Chlorine water didn't travel well, because the gas diluted in it came out of solution rather easily. As you might imagine, if you were the unlucky operative working with chlorine water, this characteristic made bleaching with it a noxious occupation; stomping on rancid urine-soaked cloth would have been pleasant by comparison. One writer later in the nineteenth century summarized the situation succinctly, "Owing to chlorine-water being practically incapable of transport, each bleacher had to manufacture his own chlorine; and owing to its tendency to give off its dissolved gas, its use was all but intolerable to workers."[24]

The French claimed to have a remedy for the problem. It was called Liquor de Javelle, named for the town outside Paris where it was first manufactured. This was no aperitif; it was a solution of chlorine gas dissolved in a potash alkali solution. The Liquor de Javelle business did not flourish in France, so its proprietors moved to Liverpool. Then they even went so far as to apply for a twenty-eight-year British patent. This would have had the effect of securing under their business control any and all rights to all chlorine-based bleaching, even by other methods not employing Liquor de Javelle.

A meeting of manufacturers and merchants in Manchester was hastily called to address this looming economic threat. Mr. Cooper, Mr. Baker, and Mr. Taylor produced a large piece of cloth bleached with Liquor de Javelle. Mr. Henry produced a much smaller piece of cotton bleached by chlorine gas, the "old" new method. The latter was considered superior in whiteness. But could the same be said to hold true for linen? Mr. Henry then produced and read a letter from none other than James Watt himself, stating that *at that very moment* he had fifteen hundred yards of linen bleaching by means of chlorine gas (presumably under the auspices of his father-in-law, the Scottish bleaching baron). Needless to say, chlorine gas won the day over the Liverpool-transplanted Liquor de Javelle. A petition was dispatched to Parliament to block the patent.

As if this wasn't bad enough for the hapless French, on the very day their patent was considered in Parliament, one of the original chlorine gas bleachers from Scotland happened to be in the visitors' gallery at the House of Commons. He fancied, little more than the group of Manchester manufacturers did, the prospect of suddenly paying someone else royalties for chlorine bleaching. He made certain that a number of well-placed MPs were aware of his concerns.

The French hung on briefly in Liverpool, but without a patent they soon gave up. Shortly thereafter, a Monsieur Foy put himself at the service of the Manchester textile manufacturers. Formerly in the employ of the French, M. Foy was willing to share the technology of manufacturing Liquor de Javelle, for a price (or, as it was more genteelly described, for a *considerable premium*). The supposed advantages of chlorine gas quickly evaporated; the easier-to-work-with solution, now off-patent and home-brewed, was adopted generally. A subsequent advancement came about when chloride of lime, in place of chloride of potash, was introduced in 1798, further ensuring the standard use of a chlorine-based bleaching liquid rather than gas. The same contemporary observer who had described the cumbersome chlorine gas method of bleaching in a box commented on the new innovation:

The peculiar advantages of combining the chlorine gas with lime or potash, consists in this circumstance, that the saline solution gives out the gas gradually to the goods which require bleaching, but does not give it out with facility to the atmosphere. In consequence of this, the operation of bleaching is now not injurious, nor even very disagreeable, to the workmen; whereas in the former process, when the gas was merely received into water, it was given out again so freely that no man could long endure to work with it, or even for any considerable time to superintend the operation.[25]

Transportation remained a problem. The chloride solutions, even by the modified process, were still bulky and relatively unstable. This required each large-scale textile bleaching establishment to erect a small chlorine gas manufacturing facility on-site.

By 1799, the invention of a *dry* bleaching powder by a Scottish chemical manufacturer, James Tenant, solved this outstanding problem, too. Dry bleaching powder was technically easy to manufacture, transport, and use. But it was not necessarily cheap. Its price would have to depend on both supply and demand. Demand for chlorine was certainly growing and could easily have outstripped supply, driving up price. This might have proved a major economic stumbling block. The ultimate market supremacy of chlorine bleach, however, was guaranteed by a parallel breakthrough in chemical technology that took place just when the need was greatest.

SODA MANUFACTURING

The key to this chlorine problem, once again, was to be found in table salt. Separating the chlorine from sodium chloride was a critical turning point in applied chemistry. So, too, was the development of a process for taking the sodium out of common salt. The process for freeing chlorine gas from marine acid did not free sodium in a form that could be used. Indeed, pure sodium was still unknown when oxymuriatic gas bleaching was already in use commercially.

The chemical properties of sodium and closely related potassium salts were elucidated by the same generation of chemists who first produced oxygenated muriatic gas from sodium chloride. Studying the chemical makeup of vegetable alkali (potash) and mineral alkali (soda ash), it was Humphry Davy who finally settled matters on the elements trapped within them, writing in 1808, "Potassium and Sodium are the names by which I have ventured to call the two new substances."[26]

Of the two, sodium-containing soda ash was by the far the most valuable commercially, with important applications in the growing glass, porcelain, and soap industries of the time. Stimulated by a prize offered by the Académie des sciences, France pioneered several different large-scale methods of soda manufacturing in the 1780s. The most successful was developed by a chemist, Leblanc, whose name was given to this process. Leblanc was awarded a patent in 1791, and the same year, underwritten by the duc d'Orleans, the first Leblanc process soda ash factory was erected near Paris at St. Denis.

Leblanc's timing was poor. His patron, the duc d'Orleans, was executed; the factory, confiscated; and, to add insult to injury, the postrevolutionary Académie des sciences (about to be reorganized by the ever-present Berthollet) denied Leblanc his rightful prize. Although he was later rehabilitated under Napoleon, Leblanc was never commercially successful. He eventually killed himself.[27]

Once again, Britain reaped the harvest from the seeds of innovation planted by France. The Leblanc process was simple to replicate. It merely required common salt to be broken down by sulfuric acid, yielding sodium sulfate as one of the key products of the reaction. When the sodium sulfate was mixed with chalk and charcoal and then heated, copious amounts of soda ash could be cheaply produced.

There was a catch, nonetheless. For every atom of sodium retrieved from common salt, an atom of chlorine is also liberated. The soda ash manufacturers, led by Mr. James Muspratt, had a simple way of disposing of this by-product: they sent it up their smokestacks. The name Muspratt suggests a character in a Sheridan comedy rather than a capitalist overseer who was a principal in an early Victorian morality tale. Muspratt's neighbors, living next to the first Leblanc soda ash factory in England, needless to say found nothing amusing in his crude smokestack eructations.

The massive amounts of hydrochloric acid vapors released by Muspratt's works caused widespread destruction of vegetation, livestock, and other property belonging to those living nearby. Muspratt was arraigned in this matter *for the first time* in 1828. Muspratt's solution was to move his business outside town, building a large facility in a village called St. Helens. Nonetheless, his first facility in Liverpool was never, in fact, shut down by legal action. Finally, eight years later, one of the earliest industrial smokestack scrubbing devices was patented, capturing pollutants as they went up the chimney and before they could be released. This innovation, introduced in soda ash manufacturing in order to reduce acid discharges, is still the basis of much modern smokestack pollution control.

Hydrochloric acid had a potential value that had been going up the smokestacks and now was being retrieved by the scrubber. This was clearest to Charles Tennant in Scotland, Muspratt's main competitor, who was already manufacturing both soda ash and bleaching powder. The thrifty Tennant realized the by-product of one chemical process (soda manufacturing) could provide cheap feedstock for another (chlorine bleach manufacturing). Muspratt soon followed Tennant's innovative lead and also put to use the smokestack by-product in bleach making.

The early legal suits against soda ash pollution have been cited as a precedent-setting example of economic accommodation with environmental protection, because, in the end, manufacturers ameliorated the situation by recapturing at least part of the hydrochloric acid to use in the expanding bleaching powder market. This rosy interpretation of history, which invokes the existence of a protorecycling ethos, ignores the darker reality. Even after the institution of the smokestack modifications, which provided a modest reduction of the extreme levels of the industry's first years, environmental contamination from the soda ash industry remained rampant. As late as the first decade of the twentieth century, one observer could still write, "It is only necessary to be in a town like St. Helens on a moist evening to realize the fact that from these various chemical works large quantities of hydrochloric acid and other gases are evidently escaping."[28]

It was not only air contamination that was associated with soda ash and related bleach production. Other routes of pollution also remained. An important source was the voluminous sulfuric acid runoff at these plants. As one industrial chemist described it, "A product more unfit to go into an inland river would be difficult to conceive."[29]

Chlorine gas also escaped by routes other than the chimneys—routes that put the soda industry workers directly in harm's way. Half a century after the first pollution suit against Muspratt, on 12 October 1876 the Royal Commission on Noxious Vapours took the testimony of Mr. John Gallimore, a laborer:

Q: Did you formerly work for the Widnes Alkali Company,—for Messrs. Pilkington at Widnes?

A: Yes.

Q: As a labourer?

A: Yes.

Q: What did you do at Messrs. Pilkington's?

A: I was mixing for the revolvers,—charge mixing.

Q: Did you work there at night?

A: Yes.

Q: In the morning, what did you do, about half-past five?

A: We used to go out sometimes into the yard; it depends upon the wind, on account of the gas.

Q: Will you just explain that?

A: They used to knock the door down every morning at half-past five,—the man that looks after the chambers,—and he used to give us warning.

Q: To let the gas out?

A: Yes.

Q: Instead of letting it go up the chimney?

A: Yes, of course.

Q: What was his object?

A: I do not know; but he used to knock the door down, and the gas used to come out, in the open air.

Q: Who told him to do it?

A: It was the master's orders, of course.

Q: Were you obliged to give up work on account of your health suffering?

A: Yes, and to put cloths over our mouths.

Q: What effect had it upon you?

A: It used to make us cough, and we got a proper dose of it. We used to be bad after it—that still gas.[30]

Making soda ash was inarguably a dirty job. However much of the hydrochloric acid fume may have been carried off, up the chimney or out the hatch, much remained. "In order to protect himself to a certain extent from hydrochloric acid, the workman either wears a flannel muffler tied over his face, or he bites a piece of flannel between his teeth and breathes through it. The fumes of acid quickly cause the teeth to rot away."[31]

The next step in the process, making bleaching powder from chlorine gas, added yet another new scenario for further exposure to irritating fumes. In a series of lectures, "Occupation in Relation to Disease," delivered in Manchester in 1886–87, a chemist named Arthur Vacher described the methods for manufacturing bleaching powder that had, by then, been in place for more than fifty years. "As illustrating the slowness of manufacturers to adopt improved processes, I may state that chloride of lime (bleaching powder) is now commonly made in the old way, by spreading lime on the floor of a large room into which chlorine is delivered. When the lime has taken up as much chlorine as it will, the doors of the room are opened and volumes of chlorine suffered to escape."[32]

Bleach packers had to enter these rooms to shovel the powder immediately after the doors were opened, as was detailed by an observer in the same period (who earlier described hydrochloric acid workers protecting themselves from hazards with pieces of flannel cloth):

> The bleach packer wraps his face in roll upon roll of flannel, the flannel being drawn over his mouth and leaving his nostrils free. These layers of flannel stand out some three inches beyond his face, and have to be of just the right dampness to prevent the gas from reaching his lungs. He then puts on leather goggles to protect his eyes, and ties a piece of paper round his trousers to keep the bleach from attacking them.

Under the running head "Bleach packing extremely disagreeable," the same writer goes on,

> The chlorine rises from the bleach as it is disturbed, and it would be impossible for anyone to remain for a few seconds in a bleach chamber unless he was protected from breathing the gas in the way I have described. On the other hand, such wrappings make breathing very difficult. In fact a man who has not got accustomed to the bleach packer's flannel would imagine that he was going to die of suffocation, and could not bear it round his face for more that a few seconds.[33]

The duo of the Leblanc soda process and bleach powder manufacturing dominated the industry for many decades. There was little impetus for change. The economic impact of chlorine bleach during this period cannot be overstated. By the 1870s, Great Britain's bleach industry produced two-thirds of the world's supply of chlorine, valued at one million pounds sterling annually (more than one hundred million current U.S. dollars). Perhaps Walter Weldon, who had developed a key process linking hydrochloric acid derived from soda ash to bleach powder manufacturing (the "Weldon process"), waxed a bit grandiloquent in an 1874 oration when he stated, "Not even the steam-engine, the carding-machine, the spinning-jenny, and the power-loom could have produced our modern Manchester, and all that it represents, without the aid of that discovery in pure science . . . that operation of bleaching."[34]

Despite Weldon's boosterism for bleach, "modern" Manchester was not an Eden or demiparadise. Yet Weldon does put forward a reasonable argument for chlorine's importance, at least in raw economic terms. James Watt, inventor of the steam engine to which Weldon alluded, died a wealthy man in 1819. James Muspratt, the baron of bleach who reaped the most profit from the Leblanc process, was only twenty-six the year Watt died. Muspratt went on to amass a far greater fortune than Watt's, in both relative and absolute terms, before he shuffled off this mortal coil at age ninety-three in 1886.[35]

CHLORINE AS A MEDICAL TREATMENT

After bleaching directly with gas was eliminated in the textile industry, relatively few, other than those who made bleaching powders, accidentally inhaled chlorine on the job. Although those who packed chlorine bleach powder were exposed heavily and suffered greatly, their cohort was relatively small in number, and users of the powders were not heavily exposed. Experimental chemists constituted one of the only other groups of workers at significant risk for gas inhalation during this period.[36]

Thus, by the middle decades of the nineteenth century, it seems that chlorine's deleterious effects began to be ignored or were forgotten altogether. Moreover, a curious belief that breathing in chlorine might actually be good for you began to take hold. By 1832, Dr. Charles Thackrah, usually a thorough and cautious recorder of occupational hazards, was somewhat cavalier about bleach. "Bleachers are exposed to chlorine both in inhalation, and by often standing for the whole day in water strongly impregnated with this gas. . . . They are healthy and strong. . . . They live to a good age."[37]

It was still a stretch to go from an absence of harm to a presumption of benefit. The origin of a specific belief in the medicinal benefits of chlorine gas inhalation is obscure but likely owes a debt to the *pneumatic school of medicine* (led by Thomas Beddoes and Erasmus Darwin), which several decades before had promoted the healing value of inhaled oxygen.[38] This was around the same time that Guyton de Morveau first published a treatise (which went through several editions) promoting chlorine gas as an ideal decontaminating fumigant.[39] These fumigations, it was admitted, did produce "violent irritation in the pulmonary passages; an intense heat, a feeling of oppression, and soon after, a sharp fit of coughing."[40]

Despite this cautionary note, medical practitioners began to promote intentional chlorine exposure as a treatment. Thackrah, among the promoters, noted:

> The inhalation of chlorine gas we have tried rather extensively among the workers in flax, suffering from chronic bronchitis. Sixteen of these men I

induced to come every evening, after the day's work, to an apartment, the atmosphere of which we impregnated with chlorine, by pouring muriatic acid on manganese. Here they remained at first for a quarter of an hour, and afterwards for about an hour. One individual declared the second evening, that he had not slept so soundly for several years as he did the night after inhaling; and on the fifth evening, all the men declared their breathing freer, and the cough considerably reduced.[41]

One of the strangest works of the chlorine-gas-is-good-for-you genre is *Researches Respecting the Medical Powers of Chlorine Gas Particularly in Diseases of the Liver.* Its author recommends construction of a tight box into which the patient can be sealed, excluding the head of course, so that he may absorb, through the skin, the beneficial chlorine gas atmosphere within the therapeutic cabinet. At least this chlorine-quack warns of the danger of leakage. "It is scarcely necessary to remark, that if the apparatus be not perfectly constructed, there will be a great loss of the material. Indeed, with a bad apparatus, it cannot be applied in a state of sufficient concentration, without its escaping into the apartment, and instantly producing such distress of respiration, as renders it impossible to continue the operation."[42]

The obvious irritant dangers of chlorine did not seem to dissuade those eager to treat. In 1830, an Englishman translated the work of a Mr. Gannal entitled *Two Memoirs Read Before L'Academie Royale des Sciences, at Paris, on the Successful Inhalation of Dilute Chlorine, in the Early Stages of Pulmonary Consumption.* In the memoirs, Gannal shared his experiences of the clear benefits of chlorine gas treatment for consumption or phthisis, the terms then used for tuberculosis. "Being in the year 1817, attached to the manufactory of printed calicoes at St. Denis, I observed that those workmen who happened to be affected with phthisical symptoms experienced relief, and greatly recovered their health while exposed to the exhalations of chlorine disengaged in the various processes."[43]

The book provides additional practical information for the reader, including information about where an apparatus for the home manufacture and inhalation of chlorine might be obtained. One of the distributors was Perrins, Lea & Perrins, 68 Broad Street, Worcester, at the time dabbling in quasi-medical equipment before its owners later concentrated their business acumen on steak sauce.[44]

Intentional chlorine inhalation remained a popular therapy for consumption and other lung problems for many years, including in the

United States.[45] It was consumption that likely prompted Thackrah's original interest, for both professional and personal reasons. By 1832, when he published the second edition of his landmark text, *The Effects of Arts, Trades, and Professions on Health and Longevity* (the book that included his medical experiments with chlorine gas), Thackrah's tuberculosis was already advanced. Most likely he acquired the disease occupationally, like many of his fellow physicians. Thackrah never lived to publish a third edition of his text. Like his medical school classmate John Keats, who predeceased him, Thackrah succumbed to tuberculosis in 1833.[46]

BLEACHING PAPER

By the close of the nineteenth century, chlorine therapy, never a big market anyway, dissipated. Textile bleaching was still important but was not expanding. The chlorine industry might have stagnated, but it was about to expand into what would become its greatest market—papermaking. Coming to rely on chlorine gas rather than dry bleaching powder, this was the industry that eventually enabled a far more deadly application of gas technology.[47]

Early on, makers of rag paper realized chlorine's potential. Rag paper, derived from recycled linen or cotton, was the form of paper predominantly used in Europe for centuries. It had been introduced in the Middle Ages by the more advanced Arab civilization, which had learned the technique of rag paper making from the Chinese, with whom it originated.[48] Rag paper was relatively expensive and time consuming to produce because of the need to whiten the rags for high-quality paper. For this reason, cheap and efficient chemical treatment with chlorine bleaching powder was a boon for the rag paper industry, much as it had been for textiles. But as demand for printing paper expanded, rag scarcity, rather than bleaching capacity, became the rate-limiting factor in paper manufacturing.

Various substitutes for rag were tried, the most successful of which was paper from a desert grass called esparto, introduced in Great Britain in 1856. This was not the ultimate answer either, however. The solution for the paper shortage lay not in the esparto grass fields of the Mediterranean but rather in the immense softwood forests of North America and Scandinavia.

Rag paper making was brought from China to the West early on. Wood pulp paper also had been developed in China many centuries before. Ts'ai Lun is attributed with the introduction of this practice, using mulberry trees as the starting material, in the year A.D. 105. But Europeans required an additional millennium to understand the technique of using wood pulp for paper.

The change to wood pulp had a technical drawback. The industrial-scale manufacture of this type of paper was far more chemically intensive than the manufacture of rag paper had ever been. The first major method of making wood pulp paper, introduced in Europe in the middle of the nineteenth century, used soda ash (more business for Muspratt!) as its major additive; a second method, called the sulfite process, evolved soon after. In either of these two processes, dry chlorine bleaching powder is used as the pulp whitening agent and is sufficiently effective when added to the liquid mix during its processing.

Then, in 1884, a German chemist introduced an important innovation in pulp paper manufacturing that came to be called the Kraft process. This process substituted sodium sulfate for soda ash. This technical advance allowed pulp paper to be made from a greater variety of poorer-quality, lower-cost trees, thus dramatically increasing profitability. So advantageous in its expansion of the menu of cheap raw materials, the new technology of Kraft pulp paper brought with it a serious disadvantage, too. Bleaching Kraft pulp presented a particularly tough technical challenge: powdered chlorine bleach was not up to the test; it was simply too weak to bleach the pulp effectively.

There was a remedy for this problem, albeit a dangerous one. Chlorine *gas,* even though it had proved too potent and too unpredictable for textile fabric bleaching, had the very strength needed to bleach Kraft process wood pulp paper. Thus pure chlorine gas, all but abandoned for use as an industrial bleaching agent fifty years earlier, was rapidly reintroduced into commerce.

Soon after chlorine gas was once again bubbling through factory bleaching vats—on a major scale at that—reports describing respiratory distress in paper workers surfaced. In Germany, where the Kraft process was invented, the specific name *Bleichererkrankung* (bleach worker's disease) was coined to describe the phenomenon.[49] In Scandinavia, where some of the earliest plants were put into operation, pulp paper gassings from chlorine also became a routine part of operations.

Two other technological developments at the close of the nineteenth century and the beginning of the twentieth were also pivotal in the industrialization of chlorine gas. First, new electrolytic processes allowed large quantities of chlorine to be produced without the need of coal, mineral lime, or manganese, materials on which chlorine's manufacture had previously depended. This was important because these resources were in demand for other purposes, especially high-quality steelmaking, thus driving up the cost of chlorine manufacture. Second, the capability of storing gases under pressure in sealed metal cylinders finally made transportation of chlorine gas over long distances feasible, although far from foolproof. This new transportation option allowed the site of chlorine manufacture to be far removed from the site of its eventual use.

TOXICOLOGY OF CHLORINE

At the same time that these changes occurred, a new science of toxicology and industrial hygiene—German-dominated for the most part—began to quantify the exact levels of chlorine gas that might be encountered in any given workplace atmosphere and to correlate this with a precise set of symptoms that were anticipated at each increment of exposure. Then, with exacting experimental rigor, scientists could compare these field observations with detailed laboratory animal studies documenting the precise chlorine concentrations that induced injury or death on a test-by-test basis.[50]

Although he was not active in the bleach industry per se, Professor Fritz Haber, appointed director of the Kaiser Wilhelm Institute in 1912, was well aware that chlorine represented a critical intersection between synthetic industrial chemistry and the exploit of raw materials. Haber, after all, had made his reputation in the years prior to his institute appointment by developing the Haber-Bosch process for the industrial synthesis of ammonia from nitrogen and hydrogen.[51] This key discovery later freed Germany from dependence on the importation of ammonia feedstock, which was the lifeblood of both domestic fertilizer and munitions manufacture.

Fritz Haber came to chlorine as an applied chemist, not as a technician narrowly focused on the problem of bleaching. With the outbreak of hostilities in 1914, Haber led a huge team of the institute's scientists working for the war effort. At the peak of the project he spearheaded, an estimated staff of two thousand was devoted to it.

Early on, a decision seems to have been made to proceed with chlorine gas as a prototype weapon, and this was certainly a logical approach. It could be mass produced without depleting strategic matériel, and it could be transported to the point of delivery. Just as critically important, the acrid green-yellow gas was also heavier than air. Although this physical property was never particularly advantageous in its earlier industrial applications in textile or paper bleaching, it made chlorine ideal as a gas that might keep low to the ground and so pour into trenches and dugouts.

Dr. Haber, whose work won him promotion to the rank of captain, spent many days at the front directly overseeing the effort. Spring had come, and the weather was not cooperating. Then, on the afternoon of 22 April 1915, the winds were favorable at last. The German forces released 1,600 steel cylinders and 4,160 smaller canisters totaling 146 tons of chlorine gas. The first chemical weapon of modern warfare had been implemented.

In a bitter foreshadowing of the marginalized being the first ones gassed, that initial attack fell mainly on the dark-skinned Algerian forces under French command. In the following days, Canadian and British troops were also hit. No respirators were available, although makeshift protective gear was improvised by soaking handkerchiefs in urine. The first soldier to propose this ad hoc respirator for self-protection from the initial gas attacks has never been documented. It may have been a field officer who, by some remote chance, had enough chemistry training to guess at a neutralizing reaction. Given the long record of exposure in the British bleaching industry, a far more likely scenario is that some infantryman serving in the trenches had been a former bleach packer. His own personal experience in earlier civilian life would have well placed such a soldier to instruct his mates in self-protection from chlorine gas.

The gas attacks came as a complete surprise to the Allies. They were not even certain that chlorine was the substance that had been used. There was no technology in the field to collect the gas for later analysis, although chloride deposits on the buttons of the most heavily gassed soldiers seemed to confirm the suspicion that chlorine was indeed the toxin. Lewis Freeman, a Canadian soldier gassed in one of the first attacks, later described the experience:

> I shall never forget the horrible agony of surprise in the eyes of the men who got that first dose. It was the look of a dog being suddenly beaten for something it hadn't done. They looked at each other with questioning eyes—I only remember hearing one man start cursing—then they began gulping and coughing, and then fell down with their faces in their hands. . . . My first sensation was of a smarting away up inside of my nose; this quickly extended to my throat, and then as my lungs suddenly seemed filled with red-hot needles, I was seized with a spasm of coughing. . . . I had rolled and writhed, in the agony of the pain of the gas in my lungs, in a pool of slush in the bottom of the trench, and it must have been the lying with my face buried in the shoulder of my wet woolen tunic that saved my life.[52]

Freeman's narrative is echoed in Wilfred Owen's "Dulce et Decorum Est":

Gas! Gas! Quick, boys!—An ecstasy of fumbling,
Fitting the clumsy helmets just in time,
But someone still was yelling out and stumbling
And flound'ring like a man in fire or lime . . .
Dim through the misty panes and thick green light,
Under a green sea, I saw him drowning.[53]

Intense Allied research began on defenses against gas attack and, for pre-emptive strikes, warfare gases that could be employed against the Central powers. The Germans had the head start, especially with such a brilliant industrial chemist as Haber marshaling the resources of the Kaiser Wilhelm Institute. But the Allies, particularly the British, had resources and expertise of their own.

The leading scientific figure on the British side of the gas warfare effort was Haber's polar opposite, John Scott Haldane. With the demeanor of a reader at Oxford, which he had been for many years in fact, Haldane certainly contrasted in style with the Prussian Haber, who had been a professor at a *technische Hochschule,* the Karlsruhe Technical University, during the same years Haldane had been at Oxford.

More important than the superficialities of stylistic dissimilarities, however, were critical differences in training and scientific discipline between the two men. Eight years Haber's senior, J. S. Haldane was not a chemist but rather a physician by training. In practice, he was arguably the greatest physiologist of the first half of the twentieth century, with a record of elegant and innovative experimental studies that provided fundamental insights into key aspects of respiration and metabolism.

The outbreak of the war found Haldane the director of an independent research laboratory studying the physiology of miners' diseases. Expertise in miners' health may seem remote from any knowledge needed to start up a crash program in chemical warfare defense. Yet Haldane was, in fact, very well placed to do so precisely thanks to this work, because miners have the longest history of breathing toxic gases of any occupation.

The very term *gas,* originally derived from the word *chaos,* was introduced in the early seventeenth century to describe miners' exposure to "gas metallicum" (metal vapors) and "gas sylvestre" (carbon dioxide gas). The gases, or "damps," in the mines were several and all too familiar to the colliers working the coal seams of England. Carbon dioxide, or *choke damp,* was also known as *suffocating damp* and *black damp.* Choke damp could extinguish a life as easily as it could put out a flame. *Fire damp* or *fulminating damp,* which was methane, killed by violent explosion or by postconflagration suffocation through buildup of *after damp,* or carbon monoxide.

J. S. Haldane was part of a long lineage of British scientists who felt it their duty to address the practical dangers of the collieries. Not only had Humphry Davy contributed his safety lamp, but Davy's most famous student, Michael Faraday, together with the renowned geologist Charles Lyell, had also headed a governmental investigation of one of the major nineteenth-century mine explosions.[54] One of their recommendations was that the miners be better educated about the scientific basis of the dangers to which they were exposed.

J. S. Haldane was following in this tradition when he embarked on a series of mining studies from the 1880s onward. He delineated the mechanisms by which mine gases exert their adverse effects, and he focused on the best means of preventing these effects. Rather than staying in the laboratory, he ventured frequently into the field.

J. S. Haldane would even take his young son on his research visits to the mines. To teach the younger Haldane (who grew up to be the biologist J. B. S. Haldane) how methane gas is lighter than air and accumulates near the ceilings of mine galleries, he had young J. B. S. stand up in precisely such a gas pocket. He then asked him to begin reciting Mark Antony's oration from *Julius Caesar.* Shortly after "Friends, Romans, countrymen," as his father had anticipated, the boy fainted, regaining consciousness only once prostrate on the more oxygen-rich floor.

Haldane senior's physiological studies of mining conditions broke important new ground in understanding the blood's mechanisms of carrying oxygen and the role of carbon dioxide in driving respiration. Haldane also carried out critical investigations of the toxic mechanisms behind the potentially lethal effects of increased barometric pressure. The high barometric pressure problem, due to nitrogen gas that dissolves in the blood under these conditions and later is released as toxic bubbles, was critical for underwater divers and for bridge and tunnel construction workers. Among underwater divers, the condition is known as *the bends. Caisson disease,* the name for the same condition when it occurs in bridge and tunnel construction workers, has actually claimed far more lives. Haldane's decompression tables to prevent the bends, developed in 1907, provided the first scientifically based guide for worker protection from this hazard.[55]

Because of his applied work in these fields, Haldane understood the mechanics of breathing and the requirements and limitations in face-mask protection of various designs. He was also acutely aware of the life-saving role of supplemental oxygen therapy in the face of respiratory compromise. Although he had never experimented directly with chlorine, a scientist with a better set of skills to attack the problem of gas warfare could hardly have been invented.

From the beginning, Haldane's Chemical Warfare Medical Committee and the military superstructure within which it operated appear to have suffered from a serious disconnection. Haldane's group condoned the widest possible dissemination of accurate knowledge about the effects of war gas poisoning and its treatment. The military higher-ups, in contrast, wished to limit such strategic information to as select a group as possible. For example, a thirty-two-page pamphlet, *Memorandum on Gas Poisoning in Warfare,* presents quite detailed and accurate information on chlorine and its effects. It also notes on its cover page, "This Memorandum has been drawn up by a Committee of Consultant Physicians and Physiologists for the information of Medical Officers. IT IS TO BE TREATED AS CONFIDENTIAL AND *SHOULD ON NO ACCOUNT BE TAKEN INTO THE TRENCHES*" (caps and emphasis in original).[56]

In contrast to this restricted pamphlet, the widely circulated pocket-sized *Soldier's Gas Notes* informs and reassures its reader with the kind of misinformed guidance that Haldane would not have tolerated. "GAS IS A DANGER only to the unprotected, undisciplined and badly trained soldier."[57]

Structured as a simple, enumerated catechism—"6. How do you recognize the following: chlorine (bleaching powder)?"—it has twenty-two questions and answers on the correct methods for decontaminating vehicles following a gas attack but only twelve on health effects and first aid. In addition to recommending that the soldier refrain from smoking or taking alcohol following his gassing, *Soldier's Gas Notes* suggests sips of hot sweet tea as a reasonable palliative in the event of poisoning.

DEVELOPING EVER MORE TOXIC GASES

Despite the limitations the military imposed on disseminating appropriate information that it feared might unduly alarm the troops, Haldane and his team were quite effective in rapidly developing respiratory protection against chlorine gas. By May 1915, gas masks had replaced the urine-soaked handkerchiefs of April. Meanwhile, progress was afoot on both sides of the war in introducing other gas agents. These other agents are linked to chlorine gas not only because of their shared history but also because they involve many of the same long-term health risks that all such toxins carry.

By December 1915, Haber's group on the German side had made phosgene gas operational.[58] This deadly agent differs from chlorine in that it is less immediately irritating to the eyes, nose, and throat but ultimately more damaging to the lungs. By the armistice of 1918, both sides possessed a panoply of gas masks and other protective gear, matched bilaterally with an armamentarium of toxins designed to penetrate any defense. Bromine gas, closely related to chlorine, had been briefly employed but was found unwieldy; chloropicrin, another irritant, was found to be marginally effective. The use of hydrogen cyanide was entertained, but it was believed to be too difficult to control.

Fairly late in the war, sulfur mustard was introduced. Also called Yperite (because the Germans first used it in Ypres, Belgium), its devastating effects were even more horrifying that other agents'. A dispersed liquid rather than a true gas, mustard blisters the skin and blinds by burning the cornea, in addition to eating into the airways when inhaled. It even has the strange effect of attacking the bone marrow, although those severely exposed rarely survived long enough to manifest this toxic effect.

In an important sense, with the success of the mustard agent Fritz Haber had won the chemical warfare battle, even if Germany lost the war. Nonetheless, Haber did pay a personal price for his contributions. His wife, Dr. Clara Immerwahr, herself a talented chemist, was so distraught at her husband's war gas work that she took her own life in 1915. Despite any personal loss, Haber's professional trajectory soared. He received the Nobel Prize in 1919 for his prewar work on the synthesis of ammonia, and he remained head of the prestigious Kaiser Wilhelm Institute, continuing to pursue an interest in toxic gases. In 1924, drawing on his past work, Haber dispassionately compared war gas agents:

> A simple and practical measure for toxicity can be obtained that suffices for all practical purposes. For each war gas, the amount (c) present in one cubic meter of air is expressed in milligrams and multiplied by the time (t) in minutes necessary for the experimental animal inhaling this air to obtain a lethal effect. The smaller this product (c × t) is, the greater the toxicity of the war gas.[59]

The formula Haber suggested, which later came to be called *Haber's law*, is now universally accepted by toxicologists and underlies most of the strategies of chemical risk assessment currently employed by public health agencies worldwide, including the Environmental Protection Agency and the World Health Organization. Hydrogen cyanide gas, for instance, which is widely available and easy to produce, yields one of the smallest cross products among war gas agents when Haber's law is applied to it, making it, by Haber's criterion, one of the most toxic. These qualities made cyanide an attractive fumigant for pest control, but, by the same token, such profound toxicity meant that cyanide was hard to use in actual practice when this fumigation was attempted commercially in the 1920s and 1930s. This was the same limitation that earlier had prevented cyanide's field application in World War I as a poison gas.

In the years after the war, Haber was consulted on the matter of cyanide by representatives of Degesch (short for the Deutsche Gesellschaft für Schädlingsbekämpfung), or the German Society for Pest Control. With Haber's input, they were able to refine a formulation for a powdered precursor agent that was easy to transport and capable of releasing cyanide gas on site. The product was licensed under the trade name Zyklon.

As war once more loomed over Europe in the late 1930s, the widespread expectation was that chemical warfare agents would be used again on the battlefield, despite international agreements to the contrary. Intense chemical warfare research was carried out by both the Allied and Axis powers.

Neither Haldane nor Haber lived to see World War II. Haldane died in his home in Oxford in 1936. Haber died as a refugee in Basel, Switzerland, in 1934. He had refused to follow orders to dismiss all Jewish scientists from the Kaiser Wilhelm Institute. Rather than do so, he resigned as director in October 1933. Referring formally to himself in the third person, Haber concluded in his letter of resignation, "I do not think that you can expect from a 65 year old man that he changes the ways that served him so well during a 39 year long career. . . . I assume you will therefore understand that the pride with which he served his German homeland requires that he ask for his retirement."[60]

Fritz Haber's future at the institute was in all likelihood dim, even had he wished to stay. Although he had never practiced the religion of his Jewish forefathers and had even gone so far as to formally convert to Christianity in 1903, he would have been unlikely to have proven himself sufficiently Aryan in the long run to have remained in Berlin. Not long before he died, Haber met with Chaim Weizmann and was considering immigration to Palestine.[61]

The industrial chemistry and technology of manufacturing and handling chlorine gas, developed for bleaching in the nineteenth century, had far-reaching effects in the first half of the twentieth century. The work with chlorine was the proving ground for battlefield chemical warfare in World War I, and it ultimately inspired the research and development that facilitated mass civilian extermination in World War II. But the technology of bleaching itself did not remain static. With innovations came additional health concerns. In the years following World War II, the bleaching industry entered into a new period of development. In the wood pulp paper industry, chlorine dioxide, rather than chlorine, assumed an ascendant position as the bleaching gas of choice.

Chlorine dioxide was not a newly discovered agent, but it had not been widely used previously. It was synthesized initially by Humphry Davy in the early nineteenth century, shortly after his first isolation and naming of chlorine.[62] Chlorine dioxide had no commercial application for more than a hundred years, in large measure because of its instability and extreme potency, even relative to its parent agent, chlorine gas. By 1950, following its new use, chlorine dioxide gassings became more commonplace, similar to chlorine but even more dangerous.[63]

Meanwhile, water chlorination using traditional chlorine gas was widely introduced in this period as a key element of public health protection. This practice evolved, taking the form of an industrial-scale process using large amounts of compressed chlorine gas at central water treatment facilities. The same system was also introduced at much smaller sites, even down to the level of neighborhood swimming pools. By the late 1940s, chlorine gas had also become a major industrial feedstock in plastics and other chemical manufacturing. Railroad tank cars laden with compressed gas crisscrossed most industrialized countries.

The expanding list of potential exposure scenarios is reflected in the medical reports of chlorine gas poisoning that began to appear in the years during and following World War II. In 1944, for example, a gas cylinder leak in New York injured 418 persons, 208 of whom required hospitalization.[64] A truck carrying the cylinder had just crossed over into Brooklyn from Manhattan when its driver became aware of a problem. Unfortunately, he pulled over just next to the ventilation grating for a subway station.

On 31 January 1961, the first exposure from a large train derailment to be well documented in the medical literature occurred in La Barre, Louisiana, just east of the town of Morganza.[65] Over one hundred people were injured, many of whom required hospital treatment. An eleven-month-old child died. On 26 February 1978, at two o'clock in the morning, another chlorine-laden train derailed just north of Youngstown, Florida. This time, the release was even more disastrous. The train tracks paralleled a roadway. Drivers unwittingly drove into a chlorine gas cloud that was so thick it was reported to stall the car engines. Three automobiles drove off into ditches; other drivers abandoned their cars on the road. Eight of the motorists died. By 9 A.M., seven hours after the initial release, the chlorine gas cloud was three miles wide and nearly two miles high.[66]

Industrial releases and freight train derailments proved not to be the only sources of public danger from chlorine. In 1981, a municipal water treatment facility in Zaragoza, Spain, released compressed chlorine gas, injuring 164, of whom 76 were children.[67] In 1982, the *Southern Medical Journal* published details of a group of four victims exposed in a chlorination mishap in a public swimming pool.[68] In 1983, the journal *Archives of Environmental Health* published findings among twenty-eight victims exposed when chlorine gas leaking from an outside tank was sucked up into the ventilation system of a school dormitory in Lebanon.[69]

These large- and medium-scale exposures to chlorine are more dramatic and better publicized than routine gas releases in industrial paper mills or even households, which generally affect one or two persons at a time. The net effect is the same, however. Worldwide, thousands of people are exposed each year, one way or another.

CHLORINE EXPOSURE AS A CAUSE OF ASTHMA

In 1985, medical researchers reported a new syndrome. Its etiology had important implications for exposure to chlorine, which is essentially an attack by a war gas agent, whether it occurs through massive environmental release, workplace gassing, or personal use of consumer products. On the basis of initially just ten patients, researchers described a novel asthmalike condition. Its sufferers experienced ongoing shortness of breath, wheezing, or coughing and required treatment with the same kinds of medicines used in other forms of asthma. Unlike common asthma beginning in childhood or even allergic asthma that can come on slowly in adulthood, this illness begins abruptly, following a brief but intense exposure to any of a variety of different chemicals. All of the chemicals have in common the physical property of being irritant vapors or gases. The researchers named the syndrome *reactive airway dysfunction syndrome,* giving it the acronym RADS.[70]

The proposed syndrome of RADS engendered immediate controversy among medical specialists. Was this really a new, distinct syndrome or merely a variant of asthma? As other investigators reviewed their own patient files, they began to find other case histories similar to those in the original RADS series. Although the exposures had been to a heterogeneous group of materials, many of the patients shared a common exposure: chlorine.

The case of a twenty-five-year-old man who came into a Philadelphia emergency room in the midst of an asthma attack is typical of RADS. It was not his first such emergency visit. Over four years he had experienced frequent hospitalizations for poorly controlled asthma despite a potent medication regimen. As a child he had briefly suffered from mild asthma but by age five no longer had any symptoms. Then, at age twenty-one, he was overcome by chlorine gas while working in a sewage treatment plant. His symptoms at the time were much like those of a World War I gassing victim: coughing up blood, trying to catch his breath, wheezing. The wheezing never left.[71]

The medical researchers interested in RADS had the opportunity to exploit a "natural experiment." They were aware that workers in pulp paper mills and other chlorine-handling industries are intermittently gassed with either chlorine or chlorine dioxide. Health researchers suspected that these workers would be an ideal group in which to study whether repeated gas exposures or even a single large irritant exposure can lead to asthma. Medical teams working in British Columbia, Quebec, and New Hampshire went on to show exactly that. The workers they studied, evaluated by sophisticated tests of lung function, exhibited all of the characteristic findings of asthma. This included narrowing of the bronchial airways, particularly in response to triggering stimuli, combined in some of the cases with the asthma symptoms of breathlessness, coughing, or chest tightness.[72] Despite this new evidence, the debate over RADS continues. Industrial insurers in particular remain reluctant to embrace a new syndrome that recognizes the possibility of persistent aftereffects from a brief, even if overwhelming, exposure.

An ongoing natural experiment of another sort has been taking place in Turkey. In eastern Anatolia, housewives intentionally mix concentrated hypochlorite bleach and hydrochloric acid in a misguided belief that the irritant gas given off provides better cleaning power. This practice has become so common that a single hospital emergency department in the region treated sixty-six cases of chlorine inhalation over a three-year period. A number of those treated went on to develop RADS.[73]

The irony is that RADS is not new. The largest population of persons exposed to high levels of chlorine and other irritant toxins—the gassed veterans of World War I—already established the condition. Within months of the April 1915 chlorine "cloud gas" attacks, medical journal reports began to document the initial effects of exposure. By July of that year, the *British Medical Journal* had already published "Observations on 685 Cases of Poisoning by Noxious Gases Used by the Enemy."[74] Even this early report described a "bronchitic stage" of symptoms in the days following survival from the acute gassing, although it did not further elaborate on this point. The first report of *ongoing* lung damage appeared in the same journal a month later, in its 14 August issue. Major Walter Broadbent, M.D., described an intriguing case of a soldier in whom the effects of the acute gassing had resolved but who, despite this, continued to manifest severe respiratory symptoms. He also described a second case, which he compared to silicosis, the chronic lung scarring that results from mining dusts:

> When the man began to get out of bed, he was intensely short of breath. He was kept in hospital some time, being sent out in a bath-chair every day, but he could never walk more than about two miles an hour without getting out of breath. I have at present another man in hospital with the same dyspnoea [shortness of breath] and no abnormal physical signs, who was treated in France for gas poisoning. The condition is very similar to that of a case of South African miners' phthisis [silicosis], which I saw some years ago. . . . The outlook for these men must be very bad.[75]

With the American entry into World War I in 1917, U.S. physicians also had the opportunity to treat firsthand the victims of the entire spectra of war gas toxins. More important, the U.S. Army, with unusual foresight, required systematic follow-up of all hospitalized gassing cases by a medical examining board. Immediately following the war, a review of two thousand such cases evaluated at Camp Grant, Illinois, reported that approximately half the group had findings consistent with either bronchitis or emphysema. In the other half of the group, gross physical examination found nothing abnormal. Yet the military medical evaluators were befuddled precisely because these soldiers, despite normal stethoscope sounds, nonetheless complained of ongoing lung symptoms. The report commented on this paradox. "And in the face of these apparently normal physical findings, there is oftentimes a complaint of cough, shortness of breath on exertion, all of which presents a disconcerting problem. With the complaint of respiratory distress and without definite physical findings, and no apparent pathology, we have no guide toward a logical prognosis." Despite the staggering burden of ongoing disease that this report documented, its evaluators nonetheless concluded, "We, too, feel that there is no apparent reason why these subjects should not regain normal respiratory function and rid themselves of their gradually disappearing symptoms."[76]

Laboratory tests also seemed to support this overly optimistic view, revealing little chronic pathologic change in test animals that managed to survive an acute gassing. These studies, underwritten with U.S. government funding, were performed by a large war gas research operation that had been established at Yale University. The Yale researchers studied chlorine gas, mustard gas, and the other major warfare agents. By 1920, the Yale University Press had already published ("with the consent of the Surgeon General, U.S. Army, and the Director, Chemical Warfare Service," as it notes on its title page) M. C. Winternitz's impressive tome, *Collected Studies on the Pathology of War Gas Poisoning*, complete with forty-one elaborately colored plates.[77]

This was not, however, the last word on the subject. By 1933, both the U.S. Army Chemical Warfare Service and the U.S. Veterans Administration had been established. Jointly, they carried out a follow-up study among the 3,000 U.S. veterans who had been disabled by gas by the end of the war (of the 70,742 total documented U.S. gassings).[78] Their landmark study, just like the 1919 Camp Grant survey before them, found ongoing lung disease with both chronic bronchitis and asthma. The asthma cases that they documented, a fairly common residual compliant, would today be recognized by medical specialists as a classic presentation of RADS.

MODERN EXPERIENCE WITH WAR GASES

Of all the World War I warfare agents, including chlorine, sulfur mustard came to be most feared, and for good reason. Although not used in World War II, this scourge has not been eradicated. In the 1980s, Iraq used mustard, against both Iran and its own Kurdish citizens. Recent medical studies from Iran have been able to show that this irritant, too, just like chlorine, can cause RADS asthma and chronic bronchitis as well.[79]

Mustard has many of the attributes most valued in a warfare agent: a low constant using Haber's law (although it is not technically gas but rather a fine liquid aerosol), a rapid debilitating effect, and the capacity to overpower protective devices. Still, throughout the twentieth century, governments hoped for even more lethal chemical weapons. Government chemical warfare programs around the world, both before and then escalating after World War II, continued to search for ever-deadlier toxins.

A simple chemical substitution in the basic structure of sulfur mustard led to a new group of agents, nitrogen mustards. Like the original toxin, nitrogen mustard is also a blistering agent, through either inhalation or skin contact. It also has an even more potent capacity than its parent compound to attack blood-forming cells. When the data from the U.S. nitrogen mustard experiments conducted during World War II were finally declassified in the 1950s, this information allowed nitrogen mustard to be developed into one of the first effective chemotherapy agents for lymphoma.[80]

All of the mustard toxins were found to share a common mechanism: they attack DNA, binding to this critical molecule and thus interfering with its function. Although this accounts for nitrogen mustard's potency in killing dividing cells, such as the cells of a tumor, it also gives nitrogen mustard the ability to cause genetic mutations. Thus the potential benefits of nitrogen mustard were also found to be linked to a new risk: second cancers appearing in long-term cancer survivors.

At about the same time that this side effect began to be appreciated in treated cancer patients, similar illnesses among former munitions workers also came to light. These employees had labored in the war industries that were making and stockpiling mustard gas during World War II. Twenty years after the war's end, they too were manifesting alarming rates of cancer. Nitrogen mustard may never have been used as a weapon in battle, but low levels of the poison absorbed by munitions workers on the job were finally claiming their first war gas victims.

Nitrogen mustard is not the only by-product of chemical warfare research. The entire organophosphate pesticide industry is also the result of this war effort. Sarin, the prototype organophosphate chemical weapon, is one of the most potent agents of this class. It was the agent used in the famous Japanese subway terrorist attacks in the mid-1990s. Sarin and other toxins of this group are versatile. They need not be inhaled to do their damage. A drop on the skin is enough to kill; once absorbed, it then blocks breathing by paralyzing the muscles of respiration. But sarin is also lethal through its damage to the brain. Given their remarkably low Haber constants, sarin and closely related poisons will remain major chemical terrorist threats for the foreseeable future.[81]

None of the other major World War I chemical warfare agents is likely to have future military applications, but each still exists commercially. Phosgene is an important chemical intermediate in key industrial sectors, especially in pesticide manufacturing. More important, phosgene is easy to make on the spot, by accident. This can occur when certain chlorine-containing hydrocarbon solvents are broken down by intense light or heat. The most striking cases have occurred when an electric arc welder works on a piece of metal that has just been cleaned or "degreased" with such a solvent. Because phosgene gas induces little to no immediate irritation, the unfortunate welder can continue with the work, unaware that he or she is creating a deadly atmosphere. Only hours later may symptoms first become manifest. The clinical picture of this kind of episode is identical to the kind experienced by a World War I gassing victim and can be just as deadly.[82]

Chloropicrin, an irritant and another World War I chemical agent, is now widely used in combination with another agent in household termite fumigation. Chloropicrin's purpose is not to treat the infestation so much as to warn away anyone prematurely entering the treatment premises. Pure chloropicrin is also the soil fumigant of choice for some crops such as strawberries, and its application has caused illness by drifting into nearby communities.[83] Bromine, which was used as a war gas but was never a major factor on the front lines, has made a comeback, of sorts, in home water decontamination. Although *hot tub disinfector's lung* has not yet been named as such, a number of case reports have documented irritant lung damage following mishaps with bromine when it is used in this manner. Some of these cases have the classic symptoms of RADS.[84]

THE FUTURE FOR CHLORINE

Unlike the other former war gases that have come out of retirement to find new roles in serving demands in novel commercial markets, chlorine seems to be more and more on the defensive. This is most true in its industry of highest use, pulp paper manufacture. The problem that has finally come to limit chlorine-based bleaching is not the gassing of the employees who work in the mills but, rather, the recognition that chlorine bleaching produces a wide variety of persistent toxic wastewater contaminants that can reach deep aquifers and degrade the environment.

Scandinavia, which has always been a leader in the chlorine bleaching industry, has played a key role in reducing its use in wood pulp paper processing. The chlorination of drinking water is also problem ridden because of chemical by-products created in this process, including suspected cancer-causing agents that remain in water as it runs through the pipeline. Although not yet dominant in the market, ozone gas has become an increasingly popular industrial substitute for chlorine and chlorine dioxide, both as a bleach and as a water disinfectant. Ozone at ground level presents a different set of problems from those encountered when it is found low in the atmosphere (photochemical smog; *too much* ozone is bad) or when it occurs high in the atmosphere (naturally present as an important filter of radiation; *too little* ozone is bad).

At intense ground-level concentrations, ozone causes severe lung damage after it is inhaled. It acts much like phosgene, with a delayed onset followed by profound distress. Ozone was introduced in the Swedish wood pulp paper industry in 1992. The first reports of ozone-related lung injury among workers employed in this new paper process are just beginning to appear. Not surprisingly, the acute effects of high-level ozone toxicity seem to be similar to those of chlorine inhalation, and, not surprisingly, RADS-type asthma is a chronic aftereffect.[85]

If industrial users are having second thoughts about chlorine, it is largely in response to the controls of national and international regulatory agencies. These bodies have a critical role in controlling the occupational and environmental hazards of chlorine from industrial uses. Tank transportation of toxic gas is an ongoing hazard. This was dramatically underscored by a January 2005 conflagration resulting from the derailment of a chlorine-laden freight train that was switched onto a spur dead-ending at a textile mill in Graniteville, South Carolina.[86] Nine persons died, and 529 others sought medical care. A number of those killed were workers on the night shift at the factory who could not successfully escape the cloud of green gas that enveloped them when the train derailed. Major releases of chlorine gas during railroad transit have also occurred in Texas (2004; two killed, forty-one others injured) and Missouri (2002; sixty-seven injured).[87]

Controlling the quiet epidemic of household gassings presents a different challenge. In the home, chlorine bleach products are more popular than ever. Aerosol sprays make it possible to generate a fine mist of hypochlorite bleach without ever having to produce chlorine gas through combination reactions. New household rust removers containing hydrofluoric acid allow the unintentional home chemist to manufacture highly irritant fluorine gas along with chlorine. Acetic, oxalic, phosphoric, and muriatic acids for cleaning tiles, tubs, and surfaces provide a veritable smorgasbord of agents that can facilitate custodial misadventure. The myriad home-product exposures attributable to hypochlorite bleach used alone or to accidents involving the mixture of chlorine and an acid constitute a public health problem that begs for broad-based prevention. Should chlorine gas be too mundane for the hapless house cleaner, the combination of bleach with products containing ammonia can create chloramine compounds, another group of toxic irritants. Moreover, recent research indicates that chloramine exposure is endemic in heavily chlorinated swimming pools. Nitrogen-containing human body sweat and urine, which commonly contaminate pools when children are swimming, also combine with the chlorine to make chloramines. Chloramine exposure at swimming pools is associated with increased risk of childhood asthma.[88] On top of all of this, a recent trend has emerged in deliberately mixing hypochlorite with other agents to make homemade "chemical bombs." These seem to be used prominently in school pranks gone sour: in one October 2001 event at a high school in Rhode Island, twenty-three persons (five teachers and eighteen students) required hospital treatment for breathing symptoms.[89]

Better product labeling is important to protect against some of these problems, yet this alone is not likely to be sufficient. Several years ago we carried out a simple study testing an educational pamphlet among 120 lower-income household-product consumers. One in ten had actually experienced an exposure to a bleach-mixing irritant. Despite that, more than one-third did not believe such practices were dangerous. Even after going through the educational pamphlet, nearly one-quarter still did not rate the practice as dangerous.[90] Rather than affixing warning labels, we may need to restrict the components of cleaning products in certain instances or modify or outright prohibit specific delivery devices, especially delivery systems that form very small droplets of bleach suspended in the air. It is also important for us to recognize that consumer consumption of chlorine is driven by mass marketing. The advertising industry is not sacrosanct; alcohol and tobacco restrictions provide ample precedent for actions that can be taken in deference to the higher priority of public protection over unfettered commercial access.

We are all heirs to more than two millennia of a collective need to bleach everything in sight as white as driven snow. Once the airwaves carried a singsongy commercial for a laundry detergent in which an irritating voice repeatedly recited, "Ring around the collar, ring around the collar."[91] The commercial's darker echoes of "Ring around the rosy," originally a rhyme of the plague years, may have been unintended, but nonetheless it should give us all pause. The discovery of chlorine was a technical breakthrough that had immense effects on those who produced and used bleaches and related products in the workplace. Chlorine led the way as the twentieth century's first mass poison and as an environmental threat through massive releases and through subtler contamination effects. And, as much as anything else, chlorine has provided ongoing generations with its most powerful weapon in a two-hundred-year chemical war against stains. It is a weapon we have yet to bring fully under adequate control.

FIVE

Going Crazy at Work
Cycles of Carbon Disulfide Poisoning

CASE NOTES FOR THREE VICTIMS

From the case history of a twenty-seven-year-old man, previously healthy, committed to the Hudson River State Hospital for the Insane, April 1887: "I have no hesitation to diagnose his case as acute mania. . . . At times will not answer questions put to him, at others, raves incoherently . . . at other times in constant dread that some one will kill him. . . . He will undress himself entirely naked, lie for a moment in that state upon the floor, and then will get up and dress himself again."[1]

The published report refers to him only by his initials: C. S. The strange illness afflicting C. S. became even worse, rapidly progressing to a complete loss of mental faculties. His treating physician, Dr. Frederick Peterson, diagnosed acute mania progressing to dementia, or, in modern clinical terms, psychosis. Dr. Peterson expected that C. S. would remain in this sorry state for the remainder of his days, like so many fellow unfortunates that populated institutions like the Hudson River State Hospital. Then a very strange thing happened. Against all odds, slowly but unequivocally, Dr. Peterson's patient began to improve. Mr. S. was discharged, completely cured, a year and five months after commitment for insanity. It was as if a life sentence had been commuted through some unknown and beneficent agency.

The underlying cause of this mysterious, acute dementia and its unanticipated recovery was obscure. At least, this was so at first. Dr. Peterson's curiosity was aroused soon after the commitment of C. S., when a strikingly similar case, W. J. K., arrived only twelve days later. W. J. K. also had been a fit man in his prime, a factory laborer, and now he was raving and pitiful. Dr. Peterson recorded Mr. K.'s delusions in chilling detail. "A sense of oppression in his chest, which has led him, in spite of his reason, to imagine his lungs were gone; and so peculiar sensation in his mouth that in spite of himself he sometimes thinks his tongue is gone. . . . On several occasions the ideas with regard to his tongue and lungs being gone have so overmastered him that he has nearly gone into maniacal excitement" (325).

The greatest coincidence, however, was not the two patients' similar medical presentation but rather that they were personally known to each other. Despite the huge population from which the inmates of the Hudson River State Hospital were drawn, these patients had been workmates in a particular factory.

W. J. K. was not as far gone as C. S. Despite the severity of his delusions, he began to wax coherent in only a matter of weeks. There was good reason for this, as it turned out. Although he had worked at the same factory as the first patient, he'd been employed there for only two months. In fact, he had left the job because he was already troubled and getting worse. Since this was some weeks before he was committed to the asylum, he appeared to have avoided the full severity of what otherwise would have been further progressive injury.

When lucid enough to tell his tale, it was the patient himself who called his doctor's attention to the likely cause of the illness. W. J. K. was not alone in his trouble, he reported. Five or six other men working in the same factory department had also all gone insane. As if to prove the point, in August 1887, a third case from the factory was also committed. In staccato medical phrasing, Dr. Peterson captures him as "M. B., male, age thirty-one, married, a Hebrew, born in Austria" (326). Two days prior to his transfer to the asylum, M. B. had been found "in a condition of great mental excitement, disturbing the neighborhood by loud noises and violent praying."

As it turned out, C. S., W. J. K., and M. B. shared more than just a workbench. They were linked by exposure to what was then a relatively new, but already commercially important, synthetic chemical.[2] By 1887, that chemical had already reshaped one manufacturing industry on two continents. A generation later, it would give birth to an entirely new industry worldwide, helping to create the first interlocking set of modern, truly multinational enterprises. It is a chemical that is still widely used today, with novel applications and new sources of exposure being added to those already in place. We do not know even the first name of C. S. or W. J. K. or M. B. They may have been Carl, Wilhelm, and Moses. But the toxin that drove them insane certainly does have an identity, even if few other than working chemists may have ever heard of it. It is called *carbon disulfide*.

Dr. Frederick Peterson was a prominent physician working in a major medical center. As chief of clinic of the "Nervous Department" of the College of Physicians and Surgeons in New York, he was well positioned to publish his report of three cases of carbon disulfide poisoning in the *Boston Medical and Surgical Journal* (later renamed the *New England Journal of Medicine*). Nonetheless, despite his authority and his position, he found it incumbent to conclude his paper with the following critique:

> I have delayed in publishing these cases for some years, thinking that I might hear of other similar ones, or that I might acquire more information from the owners of the factory or from doctors in attendance upon their employees, but it is astonishing what a large amount of ignorance and secretiveness develops among the authorities connected with any factory, when questions arise as to the unhealthful conditions under which the operatives pursue their vocation.[3]

CHEMICAL PEDIGREE

Carbon disulfide can trace its lineage back almost a century before the case report from the Hudson River State Hospital; more than one hundred years after Dr. Peterson's observations, carbon disulfide still poses a risk. The story of carbon disulfide is like a slow-motion recording of a collision, run over and over again. It is a familiar disaster scenario: a massive sailing vessel, made possible by the latest in welding methods, fitted steel, and piston efficiency, ignores an iceberg; a huge dirigible, sustained aloft by new ways to mass-produce lighter-than-air gases, gives insufficient concern to its flammability. The apt vehicle for carbon disulfide in this metaphor is a long-haul truck, laden with the cheap consumer goods that this chemical has made possible over the years: colored balloons, knockoff designer party dresses, crisp candy wrappers, and faux satin sheets. In the carbon disulfide disaster, there are no front-page dispatches, no emotional radio commentaries. No program is interrupted. It is the same humanity, but the deaths taking place one by one are easy to ignore.

Little in the fundamentals of carbon disulfide suggests that it would sit at the intersection of so many different industrial applications or pose the threat that it does. Carbon disulfide is a deceptively simple and elegantly symmetric little molecule. It is composed of a single carbon and two sulfur atoms, CS_2 in standard chemical notation. Because it is carbon based, carbon disulfide falls within a very large category of substances, all of which are considered *organic* compounds.

A number of years ago, on hearing that I was working one semester in the research laboratory of an organic chemist, the mother of a friend affirmed my wise vocational choice with the pronouncement, "Lots of good things to eat!" For chemists, needless to say, *organic* means something different from what it means for Whole Foods. Not all organic molecules, even very simple ones, occur spontaneously in nature and, whether natural or not, each carries its own risks.

A single carbon atom linked to four of hydrogen, for example, forms methane, which is a common, naturally occurring gas that seeps out of coal seams. Methane is not very toxic in and of itself, but kills when it smothers out all oxygen or when it ignites in a coal mine explosion. One carbon linked to four atoms of chlorine instead of four atoms of hydrogen constitutes carbon tetrachloride. Carbon tetrachloride never existed on earth until it was first artificially synthesized in the laboratory. It is a highly toxic organic chemical, profoundly damaging to the liver, among other body organs. Unlike methane it is nonflammable, which made carbon tetrachloride attractive early on as a filler for fire extinguishers. Among its many other commercial applications, it was also one of the first dry cleaning agents.

Carbon disulfide falls somewhere in between methane and carbon tetrachloride. It does indeed occur in nature but only in trace amounts and, even then, under rather unusual environmental conditions. Carbon disulfide can sometimes be found, for instance, near the mouth of an active volcano. Oceanic carbon disulfide can be detected as well, possibly as a metabolic by-product of certain planktons. Because of its tenuous natural pedigree, carbon disulfide was unknown until it was first synthesized in a laboratory late in the eighteenth century, one of the many offspring left by the founding generation of modern chemists.

The parentage of carbon disulfide is directly attributed to a relatively obscure German chemist named Lampadius. He reported his findings in a brief scientific letter published in 1796.[4] At a time when chemical terminology was only just becoming standardized, Lampadius described an odd substance he had synthesized that seemed to contain sulfur but had other qualities as well. It was a liquid, he noted, a noticeably volatile liquid. Lampadius reported most faithfully what he had done but described most confusingly what he had found. It wasn't really his fault. Up until his discovery, every other organic molecule that had been either synthesized or found in nature (and pulled apart to discover what it was made of) showed carbon linked to hydrogen, oxygen, or nitrogen, solely or in combination. Other elements, including sulfur, might also be present, but at least one of the big three, it seemed, was invariably present as a part of carbon-based substances.

Chemists were always on the lookout for novel compounds, and Herr Lampadius's weird sulfur hybrid did not go unnoticed. At first the compound proved difficult to reproduce experimentally, invoking a certain amount of skepticism about whether it existed at all. When the substance finally was re-created, debate ensued about what its true structure might really be. Two groups of opposing French chemists each claimed to have solved this minor chemical mystery, and both were wrong, mistakenly inserting various combinations of oxygen, hydrogen, or nitrogen into a structure that actually contained none of them.[5] An absence of any apparent use for sulfur-alcohol did not seem to reduce its scientific cachet.

The French controversy caught the attention of the one investigator most likely to set the record straight, the British scientist Humphry Davy. He first experimented only briefly with carbon disulfide. Although Davy published his initial results, the work was equivocal and preliminary: sulfur was indeed present, but it was not clear whether either oxygen or hydrogen was in the molecule.[6] There certainly was no nitrogen. When he was unable to give the question the attention he felt it deserved, Davy enlisted a protégé, Alexander Marcet, in solving the structural riddle of the unusual new chemical that did not seem to be following the rules.

Marcet's assignment fortuitously coincided with an extended working visit to England of the great Swedish chemist Jons Jacob Berzelius.[7] It was the summer of 1812. Working intensively over a period of only weeks, Marcet and Berzelius precisely and conclusively worked out the identities and ratios of the elemental constituents of carbon disulfide.[8] They dismissed the descriptor *sulfur-alcohol,* which many were using, and coined the name *sulphuret of carbon* to make clear that sulfur and carbon were the molecule's only elemental constituents. *Sulphuret of carbon,* through the evolving nomenclature of early chemistry, was replaced by the term *bisulphide of carbon* until early in the twentieth century, when *carbon disulfide* was finally settled on. Even though the terms may have changed, the chemical composition of carbon disulfide was never seriously questioned after the work of Marcet and Berzelius.

A NEW CHEMICAL SOLVENT

Marcet and Berzelius's work did more than just nail down the chemical structure of carbon disulfide. The potent solvent properties of carbon disulfide also became clearly evident for the first time through their experiments. Solvents are important experimentally and commercially. The most obvious, abundant, and simplest solvent in the world is water. Indeed, in natural systems, from single-celled organisms to human beings, water is *the* solvent.

For the new experimental chemists of the early nineteenth century and for those who sought to find practical applications for their discoveries, however, water proved to be a rather poor solvent. Most of the novel compounds being extracted, modified, or synthesized de novo mixed poorly with water at best, and often they did not go into an aqueous solution at all. The old-fashioned alcohols, grain and wood, provided a useful second-string roster of alternative solvents, but they often failed, too.

At the time, relatively few other chemical solvents were known or could be commonly used. Ether (a simple carbon-oxygen-hydrogen compound) was at the top of the short list of solvents, and it was the benchmark with which all other new candidates were compared. Carbon disulfide was every bit as potent as ether, and then some. To this day, carbon disulfide is still one of the solvents of choice in experimental chemistry; it was certainly there under the workbench fume hood during my one-semester stint as an organic chemistry student.

Ether had not yet been introduced as an anesthetic by 1812, but those who worked with it were well aware of its marked propensity to vaporize. Along with its solvent properties, this, too, was a characteristic that carbon disulfide seemed to share with ether. Although this attribute would later prove to be pivotal in the toxicity of carbon disulfide, for Marcet and Berzelius it earned only fleeting mention. A small footnote in their paper published in the *Philosophical Transactions of the Royal Society London* observed, "The volatility of this liquid is very remarkable; it exceeds considerably that of ether."[9]

Even as late as 1849, the major text of the day on applied industrial chemistry, a two-volume French work of more than six hundred pages, by

Anselme Payen, mentions carbon disulfide only in a single footnote alluding to the chemical curiosity.[10]

Footnote status could have aptly summed up carbon disulfide altogether, given how little attention it received. Scattered observations were made from time to time. Carbon disulfide became easier to make as synthetic chemistry grew more sophisticated during those decades. Also, the ability of this odd, volatile solvent to dissolve even sulfur and phosphorous was first noted during this period, although initially this was just another experimental oddity attributable to the orphan compound.

VULCANIZATION

One simple commercial application turned out to be the Daddy Warbucks that changed everything for carbon disulfide. The chemical came to have a pivotal role in a new, relatively limited industry that was poised to become gargantuan. Had the nebbish hero of *The Graduate* been coming home to Manchester, England, circa 1845, in lieu of Los Angeles circa 1965, the obnoxious family connection would have collared him with the single word of advice, "Rubber!"

The financial stakes in the new rubber industry were huge. A technological breakthrough had finally been found that could actually make rubber good for something. Left as is, natural *India rubber,* as it was then called, was a next to useless material. In hot weather, it decomposed to a gooey mess. In cold weather, it cracked, shattering into pieces. The technological solution changed rubber into a resilient wonder material of remarkable flexibility and adaptivity. Thus one writer of the time could describe, in a slightly self-mocking tone, her feelings about what we now call rubber bands:

> How people can bring themselves to use India-rubber rings, which are a sort of deification of string, as lightly as they do, I cannot imagine. To me an India-rubber ring is a precious treasure. I have one that is not new; one that I picked up off the floor, nearly six years ago. I really tried to use it; but my heart failed me, and I could not commit the extravagance.[11]

In 1845 there was one and only one technological route for successfully treating rubber on a commercial scale. Vulcanization proved to be a straightforward process in the end, but the search for a way to do what vulcanization did had been something of a mythic quest among inventors throughout much of the first half of the nineteenth century. Competition on both sides of the Atlantic was especially intense, and the fight over the claim of success became particularly bitter. In the end, similar processes were patented separately and nearly simultaneously (depending on your position in the matter) in the United States by Goodyear and in the United Kingdom by Charles Macintosh and Company.[12] The process that each company claimed and ferociously protected came to be called *hot cure* vulcanization. Mixing natural rubber with sulfur, then exposing the combination to controlled heat, could bring about the near miraculous transformation to a stable, pliable form of rubber.

The technology of hot vulcanization could not have become commercially viable in isolation. Hot vulcanizing succeeded industrially because it was linked to mechanical innovation that made possible the heavy equipment needed for mixing and rolling rubber feedstock. Within the cavernous rubber factories of the day, giant mixers operated like grandiose versions of modern countertop food processors. These fed into massive calendar presses operating on a principle of mammoth interlocking rolling pins, squeezing out sheets of rubber that then went on to oven curing. This hell's kitchen of hot vulcanization was a nineteenth-century paradigm of capital-intense, large-scale factory manufacturing. It was an arena in which Goodyear and Macintosh and Company could easily dominate.

Yet beneath the feet of these hot-vulcanization behemoths, a little cold-blooded creature was scurrying. On 25 March 1846, Alexander Parkes filed a British patent for an entirely new process for treating India rubber that could be carried out at room temperature, yet rendered a product that was both malleable and stable for a variety of applications. The patent was quickly approved.

Parkes was a chemist and an inventor.[13] His true métier was another new technology, electroplating. It was this work that initially drew him to revisit the long-ignored solvent properties of carbon disulfide. In 1843, he patented a process for electroplating particularly delicate objects, accomplished by dipping them in a solution of phosphorous dissolved in carbon disulfide. This was followed by an immersion in silver nitrate and then by electrolytic deposition of metal. Parkes's creations of metal-coated ferns and flowers greatly appealed to the Victorian aesthetic. His highest accolade was to present a silvered spider's web to Prince Albert for his inspiration and amusement.

Parkes's invention of the new vulcanizing process was directly related to his electroplating experience with carbon disulfide. The technique was simple in the extreme. The goods to be treated required only dipping into a solution of carbon disulfide in which sulfur had been dissolved. The powerful solvent carried the sulfur into the rubber, where it acted, without heat, to vulcanize the material. The goods to be dipped had to be small items, generally, but this meant that they could be shaped with simple tools. No mixers, no calendar rolling presses, no ovens, and almost no overhead.

Charles Macintosh and Company rightly saw this upstart process as a real threat to its market domination. Thomas Hancock was Macintosh's chief scientist, its chief operating officer, and something of a corporate Rumpel-stiltskin, obsessed with a process he controlled that could spin India rubber into marketplace gold. It was Hancock who had claimed preeminence in the discovery of hot vulcanization, and it was he who had led the patent charge in battle with Goodyear. Within the year, Hancock acquired the patent for the new Parkes method. But even as the new owner of the process, he would not deign to call it cold vulcanization, as the method was becoming more widely known. Hancock would insist on referring to it only as a rubber "converting" method, to differentiate it from the true religion of hot vulcanization.

It was a semantic distinction that time has not honored. The acquisition of the patent for the Parkes method also proved to be a tactical maneuver that was not wholly successful. The Parkes technology was simply too low to hold on to. Just about anyone could do it, and just about everyone who wanted to, did. By its very design, cold vulcanization was best suited to small-scale workshops producing items such as baby nipples, balloons, rubber toys, and other small consumer items. Moreover, it soon became apparent that carbon disulfide could have other off-patent rubber applications as well. For example, carbon disulfide allowed rubber sheets to be made malleable for splicing together, either for simple repairs or in more complicated fabricating. Carbon disulfide could also be applied in rubber-based fabric waterproofing, another new manufacturing process that was just coming on line at this time.

TROUBLE IN FRANCE

It was exactly this kind of rubber vulcanization micromanufacturing that could find a particularly receptive niche in and around Paris, well beyond the troubling particulars of British patent law. The technology of the process dictated its small-scale nature, allowing cold vulcanization and other carbon disulfide treatments of rubber to be carried out in poorly maintained workplaces that were often little more than sheds and sometimes even less. At the same time, it was the physical properties of carbon disulfide that guaranteed heavy exposure to all those who worked with it, saturating the air through its volatility and penetrating the skin through its solubility.

Hints of trouble began to emerge as soon as the new industry established itself. In 1851, the title page of the second edition of Payen's French textbook noted its augmentation with chapters covering a number of new chemicals and their applications, including carbon disulfide in the rubber industry.[14] Payen warned that the use of carbon disulfide in the "cold vulcanization" of rubber can be both inconvenient and even dangerous to workers on account of its vapors and cautioned further that the work is best done in an open space with good ventilation. Payen was not specific about the dangers involved, except to emphasize the risk of fire given the solvent's inflammability.

Two years later, the first medical notice of carbon disulfide was recorded on the part of the great French physician Duchenne de Boulogne (after whom Duchenne's muscular dystrophy would later be named). His presentation, to the Medical-Surgical Society of Paris, was on the general subject of progressive muscle atrophy in the context of other neurological and psychiatric illnesses.[15] Almost in passing, while listing several other disease entities, Duchenne mentioned that carbon disulfide exposure in vulcanization can cause an illness whose symptoms resemble that of the general paresis of the insane.

Then on 15 January 1856, a thirty-seven-year-old Parisian physician, Auguste Delpech, read a brief scientific note before an afternoon meeting of the French Academy of Medicine.[16] It was the first paper fully focusing on a syndrome that, with better description, clearly was not simply a variant of a recognized disease. It appeared to be a syndrome entirely new to medical science. Protean in its manifestations, this novel illness was restricted to employees in the relatively young industry of rubber working. Moreover, Delpech was convinced there could be no other explanation for the cause of the outbreak, save one. The source of this illness, the agent to which all of these workers were subjected, was carbon disulfide.

The constellation of symptoms was indeed unusual and frightening. Carbon disulfide induces headaches, muscle weakness, and bodily numbness, Delpech reported. At night, the victim experiences disturbed dreams, agitated sleep, or frank insomnia. On the day that follows, he is racked by torpor, a state of inertia, or somnolence. None of this is as striking as the cognitive deficits from carbon disulfide: compromised memory, confusion, and even maniacal behavior.

In May of the same year, Delpech again publicized the dangers of carbon disulfide, writing in a widely circulated medical newspaper. This time he focused on a single case, a twenty-seven-year-old unfortunate named Victor Delacroix. His specific job had been using carbon disulfide to patch and repair rubber objects. Previously in perfect health, within three months of first exposure, young Delacroix began to experience a variety of complaints, predominantly neurological and very much toxic in nature. In fact, Delpech emphasized that some of the findings resembled the manifestations of lead poisoning. Delpech found Delacroix, ten years his junior, a preternaturally aged and broken man, noting in particular that his patient's "sexual desire and erections were abolished." After being sent out to the countryside to convalesce far from the workshops of Paris, he did improve somewhat. Nonetheless, Delpech specifically highlighted that Delacroix's impotence did not remit.[17]

Delpech was ideally suited to take on the case of carbon disulfide. He had already been made professor of medicine at the University of Paris, having completed a dissertation on paralysis.[18] He was of an age and in a place where the biological model of medicine first became preeminent. Moreover, toxicological science was providing many of the key building blocks for that model. Indeed, Claude Bernard was preparing his seminal text *Leçons sur les effets des substances toxiques et médicamenteuses* for publication just as Delpech was beginning his work on carbon disulfide. In the same spirit, Delpech himself carried out animal toxicology experiments with carbon disulfide, quickly killing two pigeons but managing to keep a rabbit alive long enough to manifest paralysis.[19]

Delpech's studies of carbon disulfide poisoning, matching narrative descriptions of human illness with an experimental model of the disease reproduced in the laboratory, fit particularly well with the scientific concerns and worldview of his medical contemporaries. Although his initial reports on carbon disulfide were well received, Delpech seems to have been pretty much going it alone as he took on the plight of the French rubber workers. Following his Academy of Medicine presentation, he published an expanded, seventy-nine-page summary of all his work up to that time.[20]

Only one other independent report of carbon disulfide poisoning was published during this early period. In it, a clinician named Beaugrand tells of a sixteen-year-old named Bois.[21] Beaugrand confirmed much of the symptom complex described by Delpech, including a passing remark on the adolescent boy's ongoing sexual impotence.

By 1863, Delpech was able to turn out a 116-page scientific paper in which he detailed twenty-four clinical case histories of carbon disulfide toxicity.[22] For this project, Delpech focused on a single subset of cold-vulcanization workshops, the "inflated rubber industry." The nature of this particular trade involved mechanical distension of rubber up to a desired thinness and elongation. This was followed by treatment with carbon disulfide into which sulfur chloride had been dissolved and then by open-air drying. This last step usually took place in the same crowded room as all other work activities.

The inflated rubber industry involved two principal products. One, colored balloons, Delpech identified matter-of-factly. The second he would not name explicitly. Rather, he provided a euphemism for it in italics: *preservatif.* This, he added, should "indicate sufficiently its usage, that and its especial destiny for export."[23] The decade of the 1850s was precisely the period when the term *French letter* to mean condom first appeared in the English slang lexicon.

The twenty-four cases Delpech described serve both as a more complete rendition of what he had already sketched out in his initial reports and as a framework to which he could add important variations to an established theme. It is here that Delpech first documented two cases of exposure-related insanity. Ominously, he also alluded to the suicide of a rubber worker, a case that was outside the series he had examined personally. The woman had become progressively abnormal from ongoing exposure, in the end deliberately self-asphyxiating using carbon disulfide vapor.

TROUBLE IN ENGLAND

Although Delpech's initial 1856 report seemed to have had little impact, his 1863 paper was more widely appreciated. On 26 September 1863, the *London Times* even carried a small item entitled "Unhealthy Trades," following in the same column under an irate letter on vandalism that had damaged the old yew tree in Darley Dale churchyard. Under the byline of a correspondent named Galignani, the brief article alluded to Delpech's recent report. Galignani noted that carbon disulfide could "even lead to lunacy, and at all events will cause obtuseness and imbecility. . . . It is one of the most dangerous substances known in chemystry *[sic]*, but unfortunately also one of the most useful."[24]

The timing of the *Times* notice, even brief and buried on page twelve with a tree vandalism item, posed a potential risk for Macintosh. Only in April 1863, he had hosted a representative of the Commissioners Appointed to Inquire into the Employment of Children and Young Persons in Trades and Manufactures Not Already Regulated by Law. The factory tour had gone well. Carbon disulfide was never mentioned, although the commission visitor had to be reassured at one point. "That pungent smell and taste which you notice is caused by naphtha, used in dissolving rubber for spreading on to cloth."[25]

Three days after the *Times* article, it seemed that further damage control was warranted. Mr. Herbert Birley, one of the partners at Macintosh, quickly transmitted a letter to the commission, reassuring them, "Our use of bi-sulph. carbon extends over a period of 16 years, and, so far as we are aware, without injuriously affecting the health of those engaged in it."[26] The problem lies with the French, Birley goes on to imply, because the workers there tend to work and live in the same poorly ventilated buildings. The commission did not pursue that matter further. The sweet smell of success wafting over Macintosh, whether from naphtha or carbon disulfide, was not dissipated.

CARBON DISULFIDE HYSTERIA

The wide notice of Delpech's 1863 paper was well deserved; it remains to this day a classic descriptive account of carbon disulfide poisoning. Delpech took pains to demarcate between two separate phases of carbon disulfide poisoning, assigning mental disturbance to an initial period of intoxication and relegating to a later stage many of the associated distal nervous system effects, such as weakness and numbness of the arms and legs. Within the initial phase of illness, Delpech prominently features multiple examples of inappropriate male sexual arousal, taking note, for example, of Case X, a twenty-year-old troubled with genital overexcitation. The second phase of carbon disulfide poisoning invariably follows the first. Its principal sexual manifestation is marked by the impotence Delpech had already reported in his first descriptions of the disease seven years earlier.

These sexual manifestations were not limited to males. Delpech was also able to include a number of females in his new series. Among them was Madame D., Case XIX, in whom carbon disulfide induced "aphrodisiacal excitation" and, as a clear indication of feminine susceptibility to this type of toxic effect, abnormal menstrual bleeding.[27] Any psychosexual if not prurient tinge to these early descriptions of carbon disulfide intoxication is not necessarily out of the mainstream for Delpech's times. This was a period when neurology was clearly establishing itself as a distinct discipline; psychiatry, as such, did not exist yet.

Consistent with a general biological model of disease, in which toxin-based examples were considered particularly valuable for their mechanistic insights, poisons to the nervous system (neurotoxins) were especially noteworthy to the clinicians of Delpech's day. This was all the more true in the study of mental derangement, a mechanistically impenetrable group of neurological conditions, ranging from melancholy to madness. For this reason, early texts on the subject of insanity took special note of the two toxins already well known to affect the mind, mercury and lead. For example, Esquirol's classic 1845 text on insanity pointed out, "The vapor of lead, produces in Scotland a species of insanity, in which the maniacs lacerate themselves at every opportunity and which the Scotch peasants call, mill-reeck."[28]

In the generation that followed Delpech, the neurological landscape began to shift, even if the earthquake of modern psychiatry had not yet struck.[29] The field of neurotoxicology sat right on the fault line. The mental manifestations of toxicological insults were still of interest to the scientists of this period, but they were invoked only insofar as they might serve to reinforce grander theoretical constructs. Furthermore, in the field of proto-psychiatry as the 1880s came to a close, there was really only one critical doctrine, and its proponent was the great neurologist Jean-Martin Charcot.

Hysteria is the diagnosis with which Charcot is most closely identified. He initially promoted the existence of this condition, and it was his many medical acolytes who sustained *hysteria* as an accepted label through a diagnostic epidemic persisting more than a generation beyond Charcot. Hysteria, as defined by Charcot and his followers, was a peculiar affliction. It was characterized by a variety of different physical complaints seemingly of a neurological nature. In particular, paralytic symptoms were typical in the hysteric patient. Moreover, the onset of the condition was often abrupt, even apoplectic.

When a treating neurologist delved deeper into a case history, he could uncover other associated dysfunctions. These were frequently of a sexual nature. The physical examination in cases of hysteria, however (and this was key to the diagnosis), would reveal inconsistencies with any known constellation of injury to key neurological-anatomical pathways insofar as they had been mapped out by medical science.

Charcot and all others who worked in his shadow also repeatedly made one other observation: hysteria was almost always, albeit not universally, a female disease. Thus it is easy to see why carbon disulfide, with its aura as a neurological and psychosexual toxin, might have held a particular allure for Charcot and his circle.

Hysteria was already a well-established diagnostic label by the time Charcot personally weighed in on the subject of carbon disulfide. He featured it as the first case of the day in his Tuesday lesson of 6 November 1888. He was then near the end of his long and illustrious career, but Tuesdays with Jean-Martin Charcot were not feel-good sessions teaching the deeper meaning of life. Think, rather, of Gene Wilder's impish and off-handedly sadistic lecturer in the movie *Young Frankenstein.* These were classic teaching rounds, with the patient/subject presented in the flesh to illustrate the relevant points. Charcot began his presentation that day:

> You have without doubt, gentleman, more or less heard talk of the carbon disulfide industry. This industry includes the preparation of carbon disulfide itself, as well as subordinate industries, among which one must cite the example of the fabrication of vulcanized rubber. Hygienists and clinicians are concerned with these industries because of certain accidents, principally neurological, to which its workers are subject. . . . The patient you have before your eyes offers a perfect example of this genre.[30]

Charcot's presentation, preserved as dutifully transcribed for later publication, must have taken more than an hour, even if gone through as a nonstop didactic exercise. And this does not count the *demonstration,* that is, Charcot's public examination of the patient before him, illustrating to the assembled clinicians the physical abnormalities to be shown.

In his background comments as he gives his lecture, Professor Charcot is generous in acknowledging the contributions of the then late Dr. Delpech, whose first report of carbon disulfide intoxication had been issued more than thirty years before. Charcot is also gracious in his comments to his junior colleague, Dr. Pierre Marie (later of the triply eponymous *Charcot-Marie-Tooth disease,* a rare but debilitating degenerative neurological condition), acknowledging him as the person who had recruited the case in question.

As Charcot nears the actual demonstration, the patient is first introduced by name, appearing in the transcribed text as "*P . . . on,* always a sober man, never partaking to excess, of alcohol or otherwise, with a simple and tranquil manner" (44). The patient is referred to neither as *Mr.* nor by an overly familiar first name. As later readers of the transcription, we are allowed to fill in the blank between *P* and *on* as if playing a kind of voyeuristic game of hangman. For example, it could be *Mr. Pigeon,* should we so wish. The patient on the stage is never directly spoken to at all. In the transcription, he is always alluded to in the third person, even though in the actual demonstration itself he must have been given at least simple instructions, for example, told when he should stand, sit, put forward an arm or leg, and so forth.

The circumstances of the exposure are noteworthy. The patient had worked on and off in the rubber trade for seventeen years. It was only in the last few months, however, that he had taken on the particularly nasty job of cleaning out vulcanization vats. These must have been heavily contaminated with carbon disulfide. On 24 September 1888, a mere six weeks before the examination, the exposure had been so heavy that he was actually knocked out on the job. Charcot takes pains to emphasize that, prior to losing consciousness, the patient first experienced a sensation of burning in his scrotum. He remained comatose for approximately half an hour, only after which could he be aroused, although he remained a bit dazed. He had to be carried home and was bed-bound for the two days that followed the accident. Only after he could get out of bed did the leg weakness develop, accompanied by a patchwork of decreased sensation, facial twitching, and partial vision loss. The "poor devil," Charcot recounts, also experienced recurring nightmares involving fantastic and terrible animals, among other images.

To Charcot all of this could mean only one thing: they had before them an unfortunate victim with all of the classic manifestations of hysteria. The odd physical complaints, he tells us, were the key to the puzzle, with their bizarre mix of disruption to seemingly unrelated neurological structures. The psychic distress was just the icing on the cake. This presentation, in fact, was all the more diagnostic because male hysterics (granted, the exceptional minority) often exhibited just the sort of despondency manifested by *P . . . on.* In contradistinction, female hysterics, who were predominantly from the petite bourgeoisie, usually displayed an inappropriately detached, indifferent attitude to their debilitating condition. No doubt, Charcot surmises, the gender and working-class origins of these male cases, often associated with a traumatic accident, drove such a mental attitude. To a modern reader of the case report, we would add to the list of gender, class, and trauma the obvious fact (unacknowledged by Charcot) that the hysterical-depressed working stiff is out of a job.

In our own time, we can be easily repulsed by the label *hysteria* and all of its apparent social significations. In particular, the modern critique of hysteria is predominantly and justifiably feminist. Attempts to understand the diagnostic fad of hysteria—if not excuse it—view this construct and its widespread acceptance as an epistemological necessity within the development of psychoanalytic thought. After all, Freud early in his career studied with Charcot and was greatly influenced by him. (The winter he spent with Charcot occurred two years before the lesson on carbon disulfide was taught, but Freud surely read the case presentation in print later.) This line of reasoning argues that Charcot needed to ask the scientific questions that he did, even if the diagnostic construct of hysteria was applied, or perhaps misapplied, in a manner that reflected the social norms of the day.

The unstated ethos informing such a "contextual" understanding of hysteria is that of scientific neutrality, approaching the question without anachronistic disdain or indignation but rather with an attitude of detached indifference (ironically, the very state of mind that fits in with Charcot's standard psychological profile of the female hysteric). It is precisely in the neutral light of scientific review, however, that Charcot's clinical misinterpretation of carbon disulfide intoxication becomes most clearly illuminated, highlighting profound flaws in the fundamental presumptions of hysteria.

Needless to say, diagnosing hysteria to explain away symptoms following an occupational injury is a kind of victim blaming that would quickly fill Charcot's dance card at the Workers Compensation Defense Attorneys' Ball. That is not the key point here. Rather, it is that Charcot was fundamentally and dogmatically wrong about the biology of carbon disulfide as a poison. Instead of considering the evidence at hand, Charcot's observations bent reality to make it conform to the preset demands of the diagnosis he needed to make. Each and every one of the patient's principal problems is explicable by the toxic effects of carbon disulfide on the nervous system already documented a generation previously by Delpech. Moreover, in the specific case of *P . . . on,* the blatant nature of the overexposure he experienced (to the point of an acute coma) underscores the direct toxic link between cause and effect.

We know Charcot from a photographic image taken in the full power of his career: distinguished, professorial, and certain in his demeanor. In the *carte d'visite* he inscribed to the young Dr. Freud in 1886, he is even standing Napoleon-like, with his right hand sliding into his double-breasted coat.[31] In the same period, the images of many of his patients were documented in a massive documentary project on mental illness carried out by a leading photographer of the day. Captured in the same albumin emulsions, Charcot and his erstwhile clients seem more alike today than different from one another.

Although *hysteria* was diagnostically eclipsed by the terminology of modern psychiatry not many years after Charcot's death, its legacy lived on in the industrial medical term *Charcot's carbon disulfide–hysteria* (especially in the German medical literature) well into the twentieth century.[32]

Charcot's influence continued to be felt in other ways, too. Carbon disulfide poisoning held an ongoing fascination for the French neurologists who followed him. The veritable name-that-syndrome who's who that wrote on carbon disulfide included Gilles de la Tourette (Tourette's syndrome) and Guillain (Guillain-Barré syndrome).[33] Marie, Charcot's bulldog for hysteria, wrote a widely cited paper about carbon disulfide, further expanding the case presented in Charcot's lesson. "Genital problems are, however, frequent in carbon disulfide hysteria, and can consist of genital excitation or, conversely, impotence."[34]

Despite France's powerhouse of heavy-hitting neurologists, its medical domination in the study of carbon disulfide began to weaken. In Britain, medical writers marked out with precision the ways in which carbon disulfide damages the nerves of sensation, especially the faculty of vision (whose impairment Charcot had seen as a clear mark of hysteric symptoms, not as a toxic injury).[35]

It was also an Englishman who first attempted to warn the masses about the dangers of carbon disulfide. Benjamin Ward Richardson was a physician, writer, advocate of both temperance and tricycle riding for health, and something of an all-around eccentric and public health polymath. In 1879, he wrote a small tract on the subject of occupational health, intended for the working man and published under the aegis of the Society for Promoting Christian Knowledge. In it Richardson wrote, "Toy balloon makers . . . are subject to much danger from the inhalation of the vapours of bisulphide of carbon. . . . The workers become depressed in spirits, they lose appetite, they are emaciated, and some of them are actually rendered imbecile and insane."[36]

Despite these dangers, Richardson (also an early animal rights advocate) was a great promoter of the use of carbon disulfide for the painless euthanasia of unwanted pets.[37] Carbon disulfide was recognized as an anesthetic agent and was even used briefly in clinical practice. An 1859 pharmacopoeia cautioned, "This fluid is extremely volatile, and hence has been suggested as an anesthetic agent. But thus far, experiments with it have not shown any superiority over other and safer liquids."[38]

Carbon disulfide was used for still other therapeutic purposes, as the same pharmacopoeia advises. For rheumatism, for example, one could combine carbon disulfide with ethanol and ingest four to six drops, every two hours. Either hypertrophy of the stomach or contraction of the esophagus calls for a sweeter mix: cow's milk, six fluid ounces; sugar, two drachms; and carbon disulfide, one scruple.

POOR CONDITIONS IN THE RUBBER TRADE

As the nineteenth century drew to a close, the working conditions for those in the cold vulcanization trade continued to be appalling, not only in France, but elsewhere as well. It was the British rubber industry that gave the English language its first use of the word *gassed* in its true modern sense, when an 1889 article in the *Liverpool Daily Post* noted that "gassed was the term used in the india-rubber business, and it meant dazed."[39]

Even in his very first report on the subject, Delpech recommended that carbon disulfide vulcanization be completely forbidden in small rooms. For larger factories, he proposed that direct contact with the toxin should be reduced if it could not be eliminated. In his later paper (1863), he promoted the use of a protective device invented by one of the workers he treated, a kind of glove box apparatus such as that ultimately used a hundred years later for handling radioactive materials.

In 1902, the level of ongoing carbon disulfide poisoning was captured in the writing of a leading British physician of the day, Dr. Thomas Oliver (later Sir Thomas). His description of the working conditions of the day makes clear that laissez-faire policy, assigning all health protections to the ultimate prerogative of the employer, could ultimately lead only to a dead end. It was a terminus demarcated by metal window bars, intended to protect poisoned workers by keeping inside those who might otherwise be at risk of killing themselves by jumping out:

Girls have told me that on leaving the factory at night they have simply staggered home, they have even fallen as if drunk, or at the end of a day's work they have had a splitting headache, and on reaching home have sat down, tired out, and fallen asleep before touching their evening meal. This sleep is heavy and non-refreshing. In the morning they drag themselves to the factory feeling ill and headachy, and, like people who are accustomed to the intemperate use of alcohol, they only get relief and recover their nervous equilibrium by renewed inhalation of the vapour of the bisulphide of carbon. Sad as this state of things is, it is nothing to the extremely violent maniacal condition into which some of the workers, both male and female, are known to have been thrown. Some of them have become the victims of acute insanity, and in their frenzy have precipitated themselves from the top rooms of the factory to the ground. In consequence of bisulphide of carbon being extremely explosive, vulcanisation by means of it has generally to be carried on in rooms, one side of which is perfectly open. This open front is usually protected by iron bars.[40]

In France, dating as far back as the Napoleonic period, some rudimentary mechanisms existed to address noxious workplace conditions. In the traditional French fashion, such exposures were classed into three levels according to the perceived degree of hazard. This was intended to guide local police actions but only insofar as neighborhood contamination was concerned. For example, a tallow maker, falling within the noisome but not hazardous class, should be situated outside a residential neighborhood. The French classification of hazardous trades, which was drawn up before any industrial use of carbon disulfide, was not regularly updated and revised, but controls could be applied to any hazard on the basis of these general principles.

Britain, in contrast to France, did not have a system that allowed a generic approach to hazards. It took on issues one at a time when it did so at all.[41] Finally, contemporaneously with Dr. Oliver's description of the poor conditions rampant at the time, British authorities took on vulcanization. In 1897, Arthur Whitelegge, her majesty's chief inspector of factories, promulgated a set of rules, numbered one through fourteen, that put into place detailed regulations over carbon disulfide's use in the industry.[42] These rules banned children and young people altogether from work with the toxin. They required automatic machining for certain tasks, specific ventilation and enclosure controls, and monthly medical examinations for all workers. By 1902, even the German Bundesrat (Federal Council) had promulgated a new rule specifically limiting daily carbon disulfide exposure to a maximum of four hours for each rubber worker. Although this rule was not nearly as detailed or as proscriptive as the British rules, it marked another turning point in regulatory control.

Even as belated controls were being introduced, the rubber industry was fundamentally reengineering the vulcanization process, bypassing the need for carbon disulfide. A number of new sulfur-containing chemicals, known as rubber accelerators, were first introduced in this period. Many are still used today. Ironically, carbon disulfide serves as a key starting material in the synthesis of many of them, thus guaranteeing some ongoing role for the toxin. Nonetheless, by 1910 carbon disulfide had all but disappeared from vulcanization mixing rooms.

Other applications of the solvent did remain in scattered industries, such as the industrial extraction of certain fats and oils. The nature of such processes, however, did not seem to lead to frequent heavy exposure for either workers or secondary users. Thus, in the early years of the twentieth century, medical experts shared a sense that the scourge of carbon disulfide had passed, viewing this as a public health victory that was incorrectly credited to improved regulatory controls, when actually the reduced use of carbon disulfide in vulcanization was due to new technologies, not governmental action.

ARTIFICIAL SILK

Any real victory over carbon disulfide use, however, was illusory. As vulcanization dependent on carbon disulfide was phasing out, a new and far larger source of contamination was coming forward. This time, the technological innovation propelling the use of carbon disulfide was introduced in the textile industry.

Rubber making had been an entirely new industry, mechanically and chemically engineered with little in the way of antecedent methods on which it could be based. The textile industry was quite different. Even at the time the rubber industry was born, textiles were already the grand old dame of mechanization. The "factory system" was, at its core, predicated on textile manufacturing. This industry, in reality a group of industries, was every bit as much technology driven as microelectronics is today. A confluence of innovations in the eighteenth century drove textile manufacturing with new technologies that were powerful and transformative.

Yet despite its innovations, the textile trade could not break out of a confining box, bounded by the same four basic starting materials: cotton, wool, silk, and flax. Despite all of the changes in textile manufacturing, these fundamentals seemed to be immutable—the same textiles had been woven and traded since antiquity. Roman inscriptions document occupations such as maker of woolen cloth *(lanarius)*, linen dealer *(negotiator lintiarus)*, and silk worker *(sericarius)*. The ancient civilizations of the Nile and Indus rivers first cultivated cotton; the silk routes from the East had been well trodden for millennia.

The Book of Leviticus takes an unequivocal stand against fooling with Mother Nature when it comes to textile innovation, proscribing the mixing of wool and linen threads in the same garment. The edict hardly seems necessary; attempts at something new never amounted to much. Ramie, a linenlike Asian fiber, is sometimes purported to have made it as far as Egypt for use as an outer wrapping for mummies, but this claim appears to be more fancy than fact.[43] Consumer demand for another fiber, sackcloth, has always been narrow too, even in the ancient world. The opening of the New World to the Old produced a major deflection on the culinary charts (with potatoes, maize, and tomatoes, for example) but yielded only the minor blip of alpaca wool among raw materials for textiles.

Locked out of fundamental change, what the textile industry did pursue aggressively was innovation in ersatz, using the limited materials that were available. In practice, this meant producing a cheap cotton version of more expensive commodities. Velvet, in its richest form a silk product, is nice, but cotton modified to look like velvet is *almost* as nice. Substitutes were first introduced in 1769, initially as *velveret,* then later as *velveteen,* a name that has stuck. Not too long after, a cotton-based substitute for satin silk, *satinette,* was created. Still a bit later, a cotton imitation of linen was run up the flagpole. Very few, however, saluted *linenette.*[44]

Finally, late in the nineteenth century, industrialized cotton-weaving technology was able to produce an imitation of wool flannel. Flannel has its origins in the British Isles (the word most likely English, although Welsh is a possibility); the world's first known written recording of it is as a Privy Purse expense for Elizabeth of York in 1503. Flannel stayed pretty much untouched until the late 1880s, when *flannelette* was introduced. The fabric is so familiar now as cotton flannel that most consumers might not even think of wool as the original raw material used for it. No less than Sir

Thomas Oliver himself addressed the hazards of this new product, writing in 1908:

> Flannelette . . . is nothing else than cotton cloth, one surface of which has been picked by sharp points and caused to be fluffy like flannel, but in which there is no wool at all. As I have mentioned flannelette, I need only add that it is an extremely inflammable substance and as it is cheap and frequently forms the underwear and nightdresses of children, it has been, and still is, every year, unfortunately, the cause of death of large numbers of children by their garments catching fire.[45]

Over several thousand years of human civilization, no one had invented an entirely new textile: the best we could come up with was *velveret, linenette,* and *flannelette.* It is against this backdrop that the manufacture of novel synthetic fibers for spinning and for weaving cloth must be understood. Could the manufacture of synthetic fibers be accomplished, it would be a technological accomplishment of tremendous significance.

RAYON

Because of its value, silk was the most desirable target for a textile substitute, just as it had been for the cotton knockoffs. When a breakthrough in synthetics did come, the change was immediate. Consistent with the rapidly accelerating pace of chemical engineering accomplishments of the later nineteenth century, several successful methods for synthesizing silk were perfected in quick succession. In France, a research assistant working with Louis Pasteur patented one of these methods in 1884 and began industrial-scale manufacturing in 1889. Only three years later, a competing process was patented in England. This latter process was to become the dominant mode of production worldwide. Called the viscose method, it allowed conversion of the abundant and cheap starting material, cellulose pulp from ground-up wood, into a finished textile product rivaling silk. Viscose synthesis is a chemical-intensive process with several different steps, but its most salient feature is that it is entirely dependent on carbon disulfide as its key constituent.[46]

The production of artificial silk, led by the viscose process, was the chemical industry's premier mass-market success in the twentieth century. In the first decades of the century, artificial silk manufacturing worldwide expanded exponentially, growing more than a hundredfold. Although the fabric was a success with consumers, the term *artificial silk* seemed less than ideal. Such a thoroughly modern product required a sleeker appellation. It was shortened to *art silk,* implying a subtle, avant-garde elegance, and was further varied as the German *Kunstseide.*

At one point *glos* was proposed as an alternative, but this name, which sounds so clearly made up, did not take hold. By 1924, with the United States a leader of the pack in worldwide production, the National Retail Dry Goods Association of America took charge, recommending a completely new name for the product. From now on, it was to be called *rayon.*[47]

The first cases of disease from rayon manufacturing were reported even before the new name was invented. Medical science had been alerted by the French to the poisonings caused by carbon disulfide in the rubber industry. This time it was American physicians who sounded the alarm. In a paper read before the College of Physicians in May 1904, the doctors took pains to describe the novel industrial process in which their patients worked, in particular the churning rooms, where exposures seem to be the worst:

> In the process cellulose is treated with caustic soda, making alkali-cellulose, and then with bisulphide of carbon. In the second part of the process the alkali-cellulose and the bisulphide are contained in tight casks and the mix is tumbled. When this is finished the bisulphide is blown out of the casks and into the external air with air. The product, sulphocarbonate of cellulose, is now dumped into vats and again mixed with caustic soda. It is here and when the casks are cleaned that the workmen are subjected to the strongest fumes. Nearly all of them are affected more or less, but only two of them have come under observation.[48]

This was the first U.S. manufacturing facility for artificial silk of the viscose process and one of the earliest anywhere in the world. It was located in Lansdowne, a suburb of Philadelphia six miles from the city center, which had only just incorporated in 1893. It was a real estate– and industrial development–friendly borough. One of the new friends it found was the General Artificial Silk Works, also newly incorporated. We learn the following about the first patient the specialists at the University of Pennsylvania treated:

> His work kept him in the bisulphide room all day. When he would first go into the fumes he would feel exhilarated, became loquacious, and passed for a jolly fellow. When he cleaned the casks he would be almost overcome.

. . . After he had been at the work for about a month he began to have headache. . . . He was depressed, taciturn, and irritable when he would go home; his memory was poor, and his appetite failed, for he tasted and smelt the carbon bisulphide almost constantly. . . . These symptoms continually became worse. . . . He was so debilitated that he had great difficulty in getting up stairs. His sexual power was lost. (193)

The second patient, who came in not long after the initial case had presented, seemed a little better off, although he complained of excitement alternating with weakness and irritability. When the doctors heard from him again a few weeks later, he told them that after an episode of passing out at home he had quit his job. The first case underwent a treatment regimen that included administration of phosphorous, iron, strychnine, and quinine. He returned to work after ten weeks, no thanks to the treatment and despite the following recognition by his physicians: "If the patient is not removed from influence of the bisulphide, cachexia [wasting away] may set in and cause death" (196). Near the end of their report on the two cases, the treating physicians also recalled the words of one of Delpech's own patients, fifty years earlier: "He who works in carbon bisulphide is no more a man" (196).

Not long after this initial scientific notice, a second publication further documented the hazards of carbon disulfide in artificial silk manufacture by reporting additional Lansdowne cases.[49] Thereafter, a remarkable silence on the subject fell over the medical profession. The hush in U.S. medical journals was joined by the British, French, German, and Italian journals, all of which were also completely mute on the topic of artificial silk.

Meanwhile, the manufacturing sector was active. The Lansdowne mill closed, but its U.S. patent was acquired by the British viscose magnate Courtauld. It initiated American Viscose Company operations in Marcus Hook, Pennsylvania, late in 1910. In 1920, patent rights changed hands again, now taken over by DuPont. DuPont, in addition to being aligned with Courtauld, had interconnected artificial silk arrangements with other European manufacturers. The motivation for these arrangements was straightforward—between 1922 and 1925, DuPont's net profit margin on what had only just officially become "rayon" averaged 32 percent.

When the medical publications' nearly twenty-five-year de facto moratorium on examining the effects of carbon disulfide in rayon manufacturing was finally broken in 1928, the change occurred almost in passing. The British *Lancet* carried a small item quoting the home secretary in its Parliamentary Intelligence section. In response to a query on the health conditions in Britain's artificial silk factories, Sir William Joynson-Hicks rose up before the members and stated firmly and without any equivocation whatsoever,

> I have received reports by the Medical and other Inspectors of Factories who have been visiting these works. It appears from these reports that the conditions generally are satisfactory, but cases of conjunctivitis have occurred at one or two works, and there have also been some cases of dermatitis. Suitable precautions have been taken in each case and the hon. Member may be assured that the conditions will continue to receive the special attention of the Medical Staff.[50]

Put diplomatically, Joynson-Hicks's reassurances were inconsistent with the actual facts of the matter. Specifically, the honorable M.P.'s assertions were contradicted by his own chief governmental inspector, Thomas Legge. Until 1926, Legge had been the senior inspector of factories and was worried about a new pattern of carbon disulfide poisoning he was seeing. Between 1925 and 1931, Legge noted sixteen reported cases of carbon disulfide poisoning in Great Britain.[51] Of these, eleven had been among workers processing artificial silk in churning rooms. The earliest case was officially reported in 1925, fully three years prior to the home secretary's false assurances that minor eye and skin problems were the only documented hazards of the trade.

YET ANOTHER NEW SOURCE OF EXPOSURE

Legge also noted two additional cases of poisoning occurring in another emerging manufacturing process dependent on carbon disulfide—the production of transparent packaging paper. This consumer product was developed commercially by a Swiss chemist in 1908. Later its patent rights were assigned to a new French industrial concern created in 1917 solely for the purposes of manufacturing the product in question. That corporation was named La Cellophane société anonyme.

In the years that followed World War I, the rapid expansion in cellophane on both sides of the Atlantic paralleled that of the rayon textile industry. Total sales for the wrapping product were far smaller than for rayon, but cellophane had other market advantages, in particular the opportunity for tight control over who might be allowed to manufacture and sell the product. In the U.S. rayon industry, DuPont found that other makers were beginning to crowd in on the action, despite the interlocking international affiliations designed to prevent this from happening.[52] By 1930, thirty rayon producers existed in the United States, with an average industrywide profit of a mere 5 percent, albeit on a huge-dollar business. DuPont was not about to make the same mistake with cellophane by allowing a number of competitors, no matter how small, to siphon off part of the profits. It did not want simply to dominate the market; it wanted to *be* the market.

According to court records,

> On December 26, 1923, an agreement was executed between du Pont Cellophane Company and La Cellophane by which La Cellophane . . . granted du Pont Cellophane Company the exclusive right to make and sell in North and Central America under La Cellophane's secret processes for cellophane manufacture. Du Pont Cellophane Company granted to La Cellophane exclusive rights for the rest of the world under any cellophane patents or processes du Pont company might develop.[53]

It was quite a Boxing Day present. Over the next decades the dollar value of the product increased approximately fiftyfold. When a second competitor finally entered the U.S. market in 1930, DuPont quickly entered into a cross-licensing agreement rather than risk a patent squabble that might have nullified both claims, thus further opening up the trade. Even during the Depression years, DuPont's average profit margin on cellophane was approximately 30 percent.

IN THE AGE OF FASCISM

As the 1930s progressed, new scientific medical papers finally began to appear confirming the hazards of viscose rayon. This scientific record is notable in and of itself but is remarkable also as a barometer of the political climate of the times. One of the most thorough investigations of carbon disulfide toxicity in this period was carried out in factories of Pennsylvania, where the industry remained geographically concentrated ever since it had first been established.

Dr. Alice Hamilton of the Harvard Medical School, the leading occupational physician in the United States at the time, had been calling for such a systematic investigation for years. In her memoirs, she notes how she would regularly hear of possible referrals of carbon disulfide cases, only to be stymied in her pursuit of more information by factory managers.[54] Her experiences underscore an effort orchestrated by an industry eager to keep a lid on a brewing problem.

Finally, state authorities in Pennsylvania, at Dr. Hamilton's insistent urging, agreed to a medical survey of the rayon industry. At this time a federal presence in workplace hazard evaluation was virtually nil. All standards for occupational protection were promulgated on a state-by-state basis, if at all. One of Dr. Hamilton's chief collaborators in the Pennsylvania investigation was Dr. F. H. Lewy, a former chief of the Institute for Neurological Diseases in Berlin, now living in exile.[55] Dr. Hamilton took great pride in the Pennsylvania study, particularly in the irony of being able to present some of the results (prominently acknowledging Dr. Lewy as her coauthor) at the 8th International Congress for Industrial Surgery and Occupational Disease. This was the last such international occupational health meeting before World War II, held under Nazi aegis in Frankfurt am Main in 1938.

In Europe, carbon disulfide manufacturing was every bit as big as in the United States. Belgium and France were both major producers of rayon. In Belgium, for example, a special train car was set aside to transport women workers exposed to carbon disulfide, so that they would not be brought into contact with other commuters, presumably on account of the carbon disulfide workers' licentious behavior.[56]

Some of the richest occupational medical literature on carbon disulfide exposure during the 1920s, 1930s, and 1940s emerged from Italy. The political-economic state apparatus in the Fascist regime was an important contributor to large-scale overexposure, despite firm medical evidence of the hazards of carbon disulfide. Much of the data on carbon disulfide's adverse effects was painstakingly collected by an occupational medicine system supported by the authorities. The regime, whose rhetoric highlighted workers' centrality to the state, apparently saw no contradiction in collecting such occupational health data at the same time that exposure conditions were deteriorating under its oversight.[57]

In 1925, when the Fascist regime had been in power only a few years, the chief of the Italian Medical Labor Inspectorate oversaw a detailed inspection of the viscose rayon industry. His report was blistering. When exhaust systems were operative at all, the report noted, they were usually misdirected so as not to draw away the carbon disulfide effectively. Moreover, the exhaust systems often discharged the toxin that was collected into neighboring workrooms.

The viscose industry in Italy continued to grow rapidly throughout the 1920s, becoming second in production only to the United States. Despite the Depression, production continued to increase, albeit not as steeply. Employment in the industry fell sharply, although productivity (production per employee retained) nearly tripled in the same period.

In 1930, an Italian research investigator first reported the link between carbon disulfide exposure and a new chronic neurological illness resembling Parkinson's disease.[58] By 1934, a follow-up to the 1925 study by a new chief medical inspector reported that the work speedup was leading to a new wave of carbon disulfide poisoning.[59]

Another source of documentation on working conditions in the Italian viscose rayon factories during the Fascist period came from the secret police. Concerned about possible underground organizing in the mills, the state secret police infiltrated the viscose factories with planted operative-informants. To the frustration of the authorities, the main focus of their operatives' reports was not the identity of clandestine communists but rather denunciation of the working conditions that the labor spies were enduring for the sake of the Fascist Party and the state.

It was during this time that a new engineering discipline, "industrial hygiene," was first able to provide quantifiable chemical measurement of workplace contaminants on a regular basis. Using the techniques of this discipline in 1940 in Turin and again in 1943 in Milan, an Italian investigative team documented the degree of carbon disulfide overexposure that was taking place in rayon factories in those two cities. Air concentrations of the toxin were routinely ten to twenty times greater than the levels accepted at the time. The research team, however, was unable to publish the findings until 1946, after the liberation.[60]

Similar issues also came to the fore in Nazi Germany. One of its priority uses for rayon textile was for lining officers' dress uniforms. The economic and strategic importance of rayon in Germany, however, went far beyond textiles. Its greater importance lay in a new technological offshoot of the rayon textile industry that the German chemical industry had initially developed in the 1920s and in which Germany had dominated during the years that followed: the production of *rayon staple*.

The new manufacturing process took standard viscose filament and cut it into regular short lengths. The cut fibers, typically just emerging from the viscose precipitation bath and soaking with residual carbon disulfide, were then carried away by a conveyor belt to be baled, almost like cotton. Rayon staple can serve many uses, especially as batting or cloth insulation and as the raw material for other nonwoven textile applications. Unfortunately, the additional processes of cutting and conveying the fibers drenched in carbon disulfide provide a powerful vector for exposure, even greater than that experienced in traditional filament spinning in rayon manufacturing for woven textiles.

Koln-Rottweiler AG was a leader in making rayon staple, which the Germans specified as *Zellwolle* (literally, "cellulose-wool," sometimes translated as "artificial wool") to differentiate this product from standard rayon *(Kunstseide)*. In 1920, in its Premnitz plant, Koln-Rottweiler began producing cellulose-wool at a rate of two metric tons a day. In 1926 Koln-Rottweiler merged with IG Farben. By 1938, fifty thousand metric tons of staple had been produced.[61]

The increased hazards from such rayon production were acknowledged at the highest level as a necessary expedient for the ramped-up production of armaments and related matériel. On 7 February 1939, in the speech "Industrial Hygiene and the Four-Year Plan," Professor Dr. Hans Reiter, president of the Reich Health Office, included rayon staple production as a specific example of a key production method.[62] Such methods were needed, he emphasized, to produce substitutes for the raw materials that were denied the Fatherland because of its limited domestic natural resources. Reiter was a prominent National Socialist official and the author of a major Nazi text on racial purity but is remembered today largely through the chlamydia-caused sexually transmitted disease named after him, Reiter's syndrome.

By 1940, the first report of carbon disulfide poisoning specifically due to rayon staple manufacturing in Germany appeared.[63] It described a forty-year-old man who began working in the industry in April 1936 and one year later was so intoxicated that he was hospitalized with a diagnosis of schizophrenia. In 1944, the International Labour Office published the special supplement *Industrial Health in Wartime,* not only singling out carbon disulfide for inclusion among a small group of selected hazards, but also highlighting *artificial wool* and citing the German experience.[64]

Perhaps the darkest chapter in the history of carbon disulfide involved a cellulose wool (rayon staple) plant established by the Germans in occupied Lodz, Poland. Widzewska Manufaktura operated from February 1941 until January 1945. The work schedule was later described in the following terms: "Employees worked eight hours a day, seven days a week with one day a month off, providing the employee worked during three consecutive Sundays for eleven hours. No voluntary labor turnover was permitted."[65]

On 7 July 1943 and again on 14 October 1943 a German chemist working at the plant precisely quantified the degree of overexposure to carbon disulfide that was taking place. He filed the results in a confidential report with his superiors. Measured levels were 326 and 451 parts per million, approximately ten times higher than German-recommended levels at the time, at least for Aryan workers. After one in four among six hundred workers had already been diagnosed with carbon disulfide poisoning, the authorities directed that any more forced laborers to become ill should be sent directly to a psychiatric facility. This order was carried out. Most, if not all, were later put to death because of their mental defect.

POST–WORLD WAR II

In the first years after the end of World War II, much stayed the same in the rayon industry, albeit with minor adjustments. IG Farben was broken up, but the former Koln-Rottweiler, under state control in the German Democratic Republic, simply became the Friedrich Engels Chemical-Fiber Works. The U.S. rayon industry also remained strong. A major rayon facility producing filament for textiles opened in 1948, and an adjoining rayon staple plant went into operation in 1956.

As time progressed, however, major changes occurred in where and how carbon disulfide was used and, consequently, who suffered the greatest exposure. Some of these shifts reflected larger trends in synthetic chemicals. Rayon was not the only kid on the block. Nylon, commercially introduced in the 1940s, was the harbinger of a slew of new synthetic textiles, many of which are based on petroleum by-products. These feedstocks, although obtained from a nonrenewable resource, have been priced inexpensively, even relative to cotton, the cheapest natural textile, and to cellulose pulp, the feedstock for rayon.

Thus, in the postwar era, cotton and rayon both began to face serious competition from polyester and its petrochemical synthetic brethren. Underscoring the weakness in the rayon industry, the one U.S. rayon filament plant that was only just opened in 1948 had already ceased production entirely by 1974.

Despite a loss in total market share, however, the rayon industry still had room for growth, particularly in Asia. Rayon manufacturing had already expanded greatly in Japan before World War II. In the 1960s the

Japanese began to export their industry (including secondhand equipment) to Korea, which experienced its own epidemic of carbon disulfide poisoning in the years that followed. So many cases occurred with such long-lasting effects that the Koreans opened a special hospital dedicated solely to treating carbon disulfide poisoning, documenting over eight hundred poisonings through 1999.[66] China also joined in the rayon manufacturing boom in a big way.[67] It received some of its initial production machinery as hand-me-downs from the Koreans, thus perpetuating a chain of toxic industrial recycling. While these new Asian producers were entering the market, the rayon-manufacturing industrial centers established before the war, particularly Italy, still remained players.

Using these working populations as a field laboratory, researchers began to carry out ever more sophisticated epidemiological studies, examining the health of the modern labor force exposed to carbon disulfide. Although levels of intoxication had been lowered to the extent that the rayon churn rooms were no longer incubators of frank raving insanity, the new wave of epidemiological studies began to uncover other, subtler health threats. The association between carbon disulfide and Parkinsonism, first reported by the Italians before World War II, was confirmed and expanded with additional findings of even more complex manifestations of other nervous system damage.[68] Even these findings were not as disturbing as those of another pattern of disease that began to emerge with the systematic study of death records. It became apparent in a number of epidemiological studies that chronic low-level carbon disulfide exposure could lead to hardening of the arteries, cerebral vascular disease, and stroke.[69]

Cellophane was having an even harder time than rayon. In 1947, the federal government filed a complaint against DuPont for violating the Sherman Anti-Trust Act through its cellophane deals. The legal battle was tied up in the courts for years, going all the way to the U.S. Supreme Court.[70] In a 1956 split decision (with Warren, Black, and Douglas dissenting), the Court sided with DuPont. Much of the case centered on whether wax paper, aluminum foil, and cellophane all constituted the same market. The lower court trial judge went so far as to visit the 1952 Annual Packaging Show at Atlantic City in order to research this issue personally. DuPont won its case, but Saran Wrap and other noncellophane plastics, such as polypropylene, were about to make the issue irrelevant.

Despite a declining market, cellophane is still king when it comes to certain wrapped goods (such a candies, cigars, and gift baskets) for which that special see-through crumple is, by now, traditional. In the 1950s, cellophane even got a much needed market boost when Arnold N. Nawrocki, working for the Clearfield Cheese Company in Curwensville, Pennsylvania, invented the first apparatus for wrapping individual slices of processed cheese in cellophane.[71]

Other specialty applications have also remained for cellophane. In 1985 the U.S. National Institute for Occupational Safety and Health was called in to investigate an alarming cluster of heart disease cases among a relatively young group of workers in a sausage factory outside Chicago, Illinois. It turned out that since 1957, carbon disulfide had been used in the plant. Owned by a company called Teepak Inc., the factory produced Wienie-Pak packaging for skinless hot dogs.[72]

NIOSH inspectors reviewed multiple air samples that had been taken in the plant for carbon disulfide: one in twenty was over the legal limit, and the average concentration was five times higher than NIOSH's recommended safety level. Moreover, this may be a conservative estimate, because no air samples were taken before 1980, when exposures were probably even higher per the typical historical trend. As limited as the estimate of exposure was, NIOSH had an even harder time pinning down the extent of heart disease that had occurred, since its inspectors were not provided access to health records for most of the former employees. In the end, all that NIOSH could or would say about carbon disulfide exposure and the heart disease deaths at Teepak was that "among younger workers (50 years old or younger) there appears to be an association."[73] The observed rate of heart-related deaths that led to this modest conclusion was about twelve times higher than the predicted rate for workers not exposed to carbon disulfide.

Even when relegated to cheese slices and wienies, cellophane has given DuPont a healthy return on its investment. Better yet, in textiles DuPont held the patent on many of rayon's synthetic competitors. In 1951 the du Pont family's Delaware residence, Winterthur, opened its doors to the public, a premier museum of American decorative arts. The Courtauld fortune, built almost entirely on rayon, had earlier established a museum in London in the 1930s, completed with a final bequest on Samuel Courtauld's death in 1947.

OTHER SOURCES OF EXPOSURE

Also in the postwar period, rubber vulcanization gained renewed relevance as a source of carbon disulfide toxicity, albeit indirectly. Carbon disulfide had long since been phased out of vulcanization, although the rubber industry continued to consume the toxin as a precursor for its specialty accelerator chemicals. Then, in the 1950s, a new discovery was made regarding one of these substances: disulfiram. This chemical has the unusual property of interfering with alcohol's breakdown in the body. The effects of this metabolic disruption are dramatic and can even be life threatening, manifesting in severe nausea, vomiting, and, in extreme cases, shock and cardiovascular collapse.

Precisely these effects were seized on as the pharmacological justification for licensing disulfiram as the drug Antabuse. It is still prescribed as a cornerstone of "aversive therapy" for alcoholics.[74] Problems have been noted with long-term Antabuse use, however. One of its side effects can be damage to sensory nerves, which should not be surprising. Although Antabuse acts by blocking the breakdown of alcohol, the drug itself is metabolized in the body, just as most medications are. A major by-product of the metabolization of Antabuse, it turns out, is carbon disulfide.[75] The unfortunate experience of both rubber and rayon workers has shown us that carbon disulfide is a potent toxin precisely to sensory nerves.

Although the rubber, rayon, and cellophane industries have traditionally dominated the use of carbon disulfide, the toxin also has a long history of use in agriculture. Because of its volatility, which accounts for so much of its danger in manufacturing, carbon disulfide has most often been employed agriculturally as a fumigant. In the 1880s, during the famous phyloxyra epidemic that devastated the wine industry, carbon disulfide was promoted at one point as a potential miracle cure for the fungal disease. Carbon disulfide's main use over the years was as a grain fumigant, an application linked with substantial exposure, which was not discontinued by the U.S. Environmental Protection Agency until 1985.[76]

This phase-out of a marginal use of carbon disulfide has been dwarfed by a huge new application. A novel fumigant called *metam sodium* (also known as *metham* or *carbam* in some countries outside the United States) was just coming on the market in the late 1980s. Carbon disulfide is its main starting ingredient. Metam sodium is intended not for the limited market of grain storage but as a soil treatment to be used against a variety of agricultural pests in a number of different crops.

Virtually no one had ever heard of metam sodium until a train accident one night in 1991. Coming around a sharp turn next to the Sacramento River and near the small town of Dunsmuir, California, a tank car carrying thousands of gallons of the pesticide derailed. Nearly forty miles of river turned into a kill zone for most aquatic life.[77] This might not have been surprising, given metam sodium's potency as a pesticide. The effect that could not be explained at first was the intense respiratory irritation experienced by those exposed near the river. It began with the train crew and emergency cleanup crews, then spread out in concentric circles of distress, enveloping the local residents of Dunsmuir.

Initially, State of California health officials had only fragmentary information on the relatively new chemical. Only as days passed and a pattern of disease emerged, indicating an outbreak of newly induced asthma among those most heavily exposed, did more data emerge. It turned out that metam sodium breaks down quickly in the environment, producing a number of other chemicals. One of the most important is a potent irritant chemical called methyl isothiocyanate, very closely related in structure to the lethal toxin released in Bhopal, India, in 1984. Another spontaneous breakdown by-product of metam sodium is the chemical precursor from which it is made, carbon disulfide. Every time metam sodium is applied agriculturally, methyl isothiocyanate and carbon disulfide are released into the air. More than fifty million pounds of metam sodium are used per year in the United States, and the market is growing.

Given the limited number of sites of rayon and cellophane production left in the United States, even if we factor in the growing use of the pesticide metam sodium, carbon disulfide should be no more than an obscure and fleeting general air pollutant. Unfortunately, the reality is otherwise. Every year the U.S. Environmental Protection Agency makes available as a public-use database something it calls the *Toxics Release Inventory*. Its most recent data do indicate a reduction in carbon disulfide air emissions. By 2002 they were below a third of what they had been ten years earlier. Part of the reduction may be accountable, indirectly, to the phasing out of freon. For a relatively brief period spanning the 1970s and 1980s, carbon disulfide was a major raw material for the manufacture of such propellants.[78]

This "success" in reduction of carbon disulfide pollution relates to the current amount reportedly released into the air annually: only thirty million pounds or so. This amount, however, is only about 10 percent of the 350 million pounds of carbon disulfide produced per year in the United States and is about three times the amount annually exported. In fact, carbon disulfide has consistently been among the top EPA-listed toxic-release air contaminants year after year. Moreover, these data are based on industry-supplied numbers, not on actual measurements. Those contributing these data include the biggest producers of carbon disulfide in the United States, such as Akzo Nobel (formerly Akzo Chemicals) in Axis, Alabama, PPG in Natrium, West Virginia, and Total Petrochemicals in Houston, Texas (formerly Atofina, which was formerly Elf Autochem). But the EPA database also includes over a hundred other sites reporting carbon disulfide releases. And this listing *excludes* secondary breakdown, such as that which occurs following metam sodium use.

The health effects that might be attributed to any toxin, even if it is potent, are very difficult to pin down with any certainty once it is diffused at relatively low levels throughout the environment. Cause and effect are nearly impossible to establish when a disease is common, potentially attributable to multiple factors, and no different in form whether caused by a suspect toxin or occurring through another mechanism. This is the case with stroke, for example, as well as heart attack and Parkinson's disease, all of which are common health problems that have been linked to carbon disulfide.

Moreover, despite carbon disulfide's many years of study, possible new dangers from it continue to emerge. In September 2000, the *American Journal of Kidney Diseases* reported the case of a man who first came to medical attention at age forty-five, suffering from diffuse vascular disease, kidney disease, and neurological complaints. Over the ensuing ten years he worsened, requiring dialysis and developing severe dementia prior to death. He had worked for fifteen years in the spinning department of an unnamed U.S. viscose rayon plant. Exposure levels in the plant were documented to be as high as two hundred to five hundred parts per million (around the same level as that reported for the plant in Lodz in 1943). In order to obtain this exposure information from the plant owners, his treating physicians had to invoke the Freedom of Information Act.[79]

THE RECURRING CYCLE

The history of carbon disulfide has been a story with a recurring theme: An episode of concern emerges as the dangers of carbon disulfide are recognized. Then, over time, fears are allayed by a false sense of security that the exposure either has been brought under strict control or that it has even been eliminated altogether. Later, new concerns are brought to the forefront as another epidemic of disease emerges.

Much of the up and down nature of carbon disulfide exposure and its accompanying disease outbreaks has been dictated by changing patterns of use, driven by cycles of technological innovation. Just as important, these fluctuations in carbon disulfide exposure have been paralleled by alternating failure and success in translating public health warnings into concrete actions leading to effective controls.

In the mid-nineteenth century, Delpech not only discovered the problem but immediately made practical recommendations for reducing carbon disulfide exposure in the vulcanization workshops. Although his advice was not heeded at the time, later in that century some of the earliest detailed work rules geared to health protection were promulgated specifically for the rubber trade, even if later supplanted by innovation that made carbon disulfide vulcanization largely obsolete.

The rayon industry, in contrast to the rubber trade, emerged at a time when at least a rudimentary apparatus was in place for worker health protection in industrialized countries. Once again, medical reports very quickly identified the hazard. The blunted response to these findings, absent any effective controls for at least several decades, demonstrates the power that economic-political forces can successfully exert in retarding public health interventions in the industrial sector.

Even at the close of the twentieth century, as the recent case report documents so clearly, OSHA seemed incapable of effectively enforcing the standards that have already been promulgated. This only begs the question of why the current OSHA standard for maximum carbon disulfide exposure, set at twenty parts per million of the toxin in air, has stayed in place unchanged as long as it has. This legal level has remained static, despite the ongoing recommendation from NIOSH (under the aegis of the Centers for Disease Control), dating back to 1977, that carbon disulfide exposures be kept to no more than one part per million, a standard twentyfold more stringent.

Beyond recommending this new standard more than twenty-five years ago, NIOSH itself has been far from proactive when it comes to carbon disulfide. In 1979, it carried out a study among workers in a rayon staple plant, finding that almost every job it examined involved exposures above its own recommended limit. In some areas, average samples were above even the OSHA standard, and key peak values were ten times again higher than that standard. In 1981, however, when NIOSH investigators authored their first scientific publication to come out of that investigation, it equivocally concluded that "further study may be needed to define the relationships between effect and exposure with sufficient certainty for regulatory use."[80]

More than ten years later, NIOSH finally published a detailed scientific analysis of the principal cardiovascular endpoints it had evaluated back in the 1979 field study.[81] The analysis contained important findings of both increased blood pressure and higher blood lipids correlating with higher carbon disulfide exposure, a relationship that might help to explain carbon disulfide's epidemiological link to heart disease.

Since its 1985 visit to the sausage factory outside Chicago, NIOSH has not completed a single evaluation of a rayon factory or any other facility of primary carbon disulfide use through its Health Hazard Evaluation program. It came close to doing so once. In March 1996, NIOSH received a request for technical assistance from the Department of Public Health of the State of Alabama, which was looking into claims of adverse health effects made by the employees of a rayon plant in Axis, Alabama. The plant was owned by Courtaulds Fibers, Incorporated; the workers were represented by the Union of Needletrades, Industrial, and Textile Employees (UNITE). A few days after receiving the state's request for assistance, NIOSH received a confidential Health Hazard Evaluation request from an employee of the plant, also seeking NIOSH action. Under normal circumstances, either request alone would have been sufficient to instigate a NIOSH investigation. Two NIOSH representatives, a physician and an industrial hygienist, did make a brief visit to the plant in April of that year. But on the basis of their initial assessment, they suggested a more detailed survey with questionnaires and air sampling in follow-up, a routine NIOSH approach to such studies.

When NIOSH submitted an outline of a proposed study to Courtaulds officials in June 1997, more than a year had elapsed since the plant visit. Courtaulds responded with an eight-page cover letter and twenty-seven pages of supplemental comments from five hired consultants. NIOSH temporized: the physician originally on the project was no longer with the agency; once a new a team was assigned, follow-up would be undertaken. In December 1997, NIOSH wrote a lengthy letter to the Alabama Department of Health (copied to Courtaulds and to UNITE) explaining why it would not, after all, be studying the plant. One of the chief reasons NIOSH cited was that the employees at the facility knew too much about carbon disulfide, which might impact the validity of any questionnaire survey.[82]

NIOSH has continued to be on the defensive when it comes to carbon disulfide. Its belated cardiovascular report was roundly criticized in a 1996 industry-sponsored data reanalysis.[83] This "fresh look" at the data attributed an observed carbon disulfide dose response to being the result of an exposure-race interaction that misled NIOSH, thus distorting its findings. Orchestrated by the Carbon Disulfide Panel of Chemical Manufacturers Association, the companies supporting the reanalysis included, among others, Teepak, Inc. (the corporate giant, if you recall, of the Wienie-Pak), Akzo Nobel Chemicals, Inc., and Courtaulds Fibers, Inc. Two years later, in 1998, Akzo Nobel acquired Courtaulds, launching a newly named entity at the Axis, Alabama, site: Accordis Cellulosic Fibers, Incorporated. This entity was later divested by Akzo Nobel to CVC Capital Partners. But by whatever name, the operation releases about ten million pounds of carbon disulfide into the atmosphere each year.

Perhaps, above all else, the story of carbon disulfide should alert us to a continuing regulatory disconnect between the experience gained in the workplace, even if belatedly and at a terrible human cost, and the more subtle threats to human health borne by exposures through air, water, foodstuffs, and medications.

What potential margin of benefit would support continued approval of a medication such as Antabuse that, once ingested, generates carbon disulfide in the body and appears to be associated, even at "therapeutic doses," with some of the classic findings of carbon disulfide toxicity? Why are so few restrictions placed on the transportation and application of a fumigant (metam sodium) that routinely releases carbon disulfide into the air? How is it that carbon disulfide, as a leading toxic air pollutant, does not rank higher as a priority for abatement? How can public education on chemical hazards be so poor that one can still purchase on the Internet a how-to kit for a classroom exercise called "the barking dog" experiment, in which phosphorous is dissolved in carbon disulfide that evaporates into the room so that the phosphorous ignites with a "woof"?[84]

It seems that the only group paying attention to carbon disulfide is the writing staff of *General Hospital*. In 1991, they introduced a story line in which an evil cartel sought to control global business through the use of carbon disulfide it was manufacturing in a converted cannery right in the TV soap opera hometown of Port Charles.[85] The cartel was eventually thwarted in its evil plans, and the carbon disulfide threat receded.

In the final analysis we must still come back to the unabated threat of carbon disulfide in real workplaces. International tariff agreements proscribe trade in prison-made goods but take no heed of the conditions under which rayon textiles continue to be made in many parts of the world. It is true that this is not an outright prison labor issue. But for more than 150 years, the control strategies for carbon disulfide have all resembled, in one form or another, the bars an English factory owner installed in his workplace so that his workers, demented from carbon disulfide exposure, would not jump out.

SIX

Job Fever

Inhaling Dust and Fumes

EXPERIMENTAL WELDING

A few years ago, my colleagues and I embarked on a series of research experiments that had a fairly simple design, verging on simplistic. The participants in the study, referred to as experimental human subjects in the formal design, had a straightforward task to carry out. They came into the laboratory and performed electric arc welding on steel plates. The period of welding varied from fifteen minutes to one hour. There was nothing special or sophisticated in the welding itself. It was basic "stick" welding, which means that the welding rod used is a stiff electrode consumed in the heat of the process. Such welding is routine for thousands of people every day. Not only is it a standard work task carried out by skilled workers in factories and building sites, but it is also performed in barns by farmers and in home garages by ad hoc repairmen and hobby tinkerers. Most people who do stick welding have had little if any formal training beforehand. Weekend welders can simply rent the needed equipment, assuming they have a 220-volt outlet. In fact, that is how we approached the experimental protocol.[1]

One complication that we did face was in telling the volunteers what to weld, since we weren't trying to make or fix anything. The main goal was to create as much welding fume as possible. The welders were instructed to go over the metal piece to produce a lot of bead, which is the line of molten metal marking where the rod mixes with the base steel. For the experiments, we had access to an enclosed, climate-controlled chamber usually used for studies of air pollution exposure. In this way the welding fume could be vented to the outside, although not too efficiently. The air in the chamber was intended to be smoky enough to mimic most makeshift, semienclosed welding situations.

The welding operation had one other specific aspect that was key to the study: it employed galvanized steel, which is standard metal that has been covered in a very thin layer of zinc, an excellent corrosive preventive. Galvanized metal has a silvery sheen. The coating is most familiar on metal used where corrosion is most likely, such as in fencing, garbage receptacles, and the like.

When galvanized steel is welded, a particularly intense blue-white fume is produced as the layer of zinc covering is vaporized. In the air, the pure zinc metal fume exists momentarily and then is immediately converted into zinc oxide by joining with the oxygen present in the atmosphere. When zinc oxide is inhaled, as any welder who has ever worked on galvanized steel can tell you, it has a very predictable effect. At first, it does nothing, although some welders associate zinc oxide fume with a slight metallic taste. The welder finishes the day routinely, although the foreman may recommend a glass of milk with lunch to the novice.

That evening, however, the welder begins to feel a bit achy and unwell, just as if he or she is "coming down with something," which is indeed the case. A chill comes on, followed by a fever, which breaks with a sweat in the night. Although headache and a bit of nausea may also accompany the worst phase, breathing complaints other than a slight cough are unusual. By the morning, all of the symptoms begin to resolve as quickly as they came on.

METAL FUME FEVER

The preceding scenario describes a self-limited bout of illness that, for all the world, seems to be a "twenty-four-hour bug." It goes by a number of different names among welders, including galvo, galvanized fever, welding fever, and, finally, the particularly noteworthy name, Monday morning fever. A more general medical term for the syndrome is *metal fume fever*.[2]

Scientific understanding of how and why zinc oxide inhalation produces a flulike illness remains incomplete. The explanation is of potential importance, not only because of the way in which the condition starts, but also because of the consistent manner in which it seems to stop itself in its tracks. Other inhaled materials can also cause systemic bodily reactions; unfortunately, few of them are self-limited, even following a single exposure. For example, heavy inhalation of the metal cadmium, which can occur through sheet metal work, also causes fever and, along with it, severe damage to the lungs, which can be fatal. Low-level, repeated cadmium inhalation can cause slow destruction of the lung, leading to emphysema. In contrast, zinc oxide, whether inhaled on a one-time or a repeated basis, does not cause lasting damage. The lessons to be learned from the fever and flu symptoms caused by zinc oxide, if they could be applied to other syndromes, might be used beneficially to cut short life-threatening disease processes.

Fume fever is also relevant to a less severe but far more common problem. Galvanized metal may not produce a better mousetrap, but it could theoretically help to cure the common cold. Metal fume fever is not the basis for the widespread use of zinc supplements as an over-the-counter remedy for the flu, but there is a connection.[3] Zinc oxide, applied as an ointment, paste, or poultice, is a centuries-old topical remedy for inflammation of various sorts.

The key signs of inflammation form a quartet of redness, warmth, swelling, and tenderness. Recognizing these cardinal signs of disease has been a central catechism of medical teaching for at least as long as zinc oxide has been in the pharmacopoeia. Inflammation can be localized or can spread to multiple parts of the body. It can be caused by infection (such as a viral flu) or injury (a scald or burn, for example), or it can occur without any trigger (as in various forms of arthritis or other autoimmune diseases).

The introduction of the microscope into the systematic study of pathology in the eighteenth century led to the discovery that the hallmark of inflammation is an influx of the body's own white cells into the affected tissue. Early in the understanding and acceptance of the role of microbes in infection in the mid-nineteenth century, at least one trigger of inflammation came into even better focus.

Various experimenters established not only that viable bacteria can induce inflammation but also that, even when frank infection does not take hold, dead bacterial cells and even parts of cells can induce inflammation as well. The prototype substance derived from infectious organisms was eventually purified from the cell walls of certain bacteria. It was named *en-*

dotoxin to capture its potency as a stimulating factor in the native inflammatory response to infection.

As we began our welding experiments, we had fully in mind the known effects of purified endotoxin and how these might relate to metal fume fever. Just like fume fever, exposure to endotoxin causes fever, chills, and malaise. Their courses of action over time are similar, too. Although endotoxin, when injected, causes a fairly immediate onset of symptoms, its inhalation (like that of zinc oxide galvanized welding fume) is followed by a delay of some hours before its effects are manifest. We also knew, from cases in which a white blood cell increase had been measured, that metal fume fever runs its course accompanied by the same inflammatory response. Not only does the body's total white blood count briskly elevate, but also white blood cells increase in concentration in the lung, just where the zinc oxide fume has deposited. The same had been shown to be true of inhaled endotoxin.

Endotoxin is a more potent stimulant of inflammation than zinc oxide inhalation is. Nonetheless, in low doses endotoxin fever is self-limited, like zinc oxide. In fact, as my coresearchers and I reviewed the available data on the two substances, the similar dose response appeared to be another link between endotoxin and zinc oxide.[4] A key first step in dissecting any toxic mechanism requires teasing out its dose response. In the simplest relationship, increasing exposure with each test predictably induces a greater response. This straight-line step-up, however, is far from universal.

Some substances manifest a complex dose response. For example, once allergic sensitization occurs, minute exposure to an otherwise nontoxic material can induce a life-threatening response: *anaphylaxis*. Endotoxin and zinc oxide fume share an unusual dose response that is, in a sense, the reverse or mirror image of anaphylaxis caused by sensitization. Repeat exposure to endotoxin and zinc oxide fume manifests a pattern of blunted effect; this dose response is termed *tachyphylaxis*.

Welders recognize this phenomenon, because one of their common names for the problem, *Monday morning fever,* is based on a tachyphylaxis pattern of response. Monday morning fever occurs in circumstances in which the inhalation of zinc oxide is a daily matter (as might occur in shipyard welding). An episode of fume fever is most likely to occur on the evening of the first day back to work after an exposure hiatus, often as short as a weekend break.

Workers in another industry also suffer from an endemic occupational disease that goes by the identical name, Monday morning fever. In this industry there is no zinc oxide, but there is abundant endotoxin. Just as with metal fume fever, this form of Monday morning fever is a self-limited, flu-like illness coming on in the evening hours after work, most commonly on the first day back after a weekend or holiday or when newly joining the trade. In this other line of work, Monday morning fever is also known by an alternative name: *mill fever.*

The cotton- and linen-weaving industry, in which mill fever occurs, is far larger and older than the welding trade. Episodic fever in textile mills has a long history. But from the beginning, its recognition as something distinct and work related has been ridden with problems. The symptoms of mill fever do not distinguish it from a spontaneous outbreak of contagious disease. An outbreak of infectious illness can be a frequent event in any large employed population, but, although facilitated by on-the-job contact, it is unrelated to exposures specifically generated on the job.

In 1784, an alarming outbreak of fever occurred in the mills of Radcliffe, near Manchester, in the emerging industrialized textile center of England. A committee of medical experts was convened, headed by Dr. Thomas Percival, a leading physician of his time. The committee's report noted:

> We have fully satisfied ourselves, either from actual observation, or authentic testimony, that a low, putrid FEVER, of a contagious nature, has prevailed many months in the cotton mills, and among the poor, in the township of Radcliffe. . . . We are decided in our opinion, that the disorder has been supported, diffused, and aggravated, by the ready communication of contagion to numbers crowded together; by the accession to its virulence from putrid effluvia; and by the injury done to young persons through confinement and too-long-continued labour; to which several evils the cotton mills have given occasion.[5]

The committee voiced determined optimism that "these evils . . . are not without remedy," going on to make a number of specific recommendations for better ventilation, more frequent cleaning of the physical plant, shorter work hours, and improved personal hygiene among the workers. The report also included a very specific suggestion that rancid machinery oil be changed, given its likelihood as a "copious source of putrid effluvia."

In retrospect it is clear that the major fever outbreak at Radcliffe was predominantly due to an infectious cause, most likely typhus. Neither the severity of the outbreak nor the spread of illness beyond the workforce (to the unemployed poor) is consistent with mill fever of the Monday morning variety. But mill fever probably also occurred sporadically in Radcliffe. Perhaps for this reason the committee singled out contaminated machining oil for remediation. Such oils are prone to bacterial growth that generates endotoxin, an ideal trigger for outbreaks of mill fever.

The medical report on the 1784 outbreak can be seen today as an opening shot across the bow in what ultimately was to become a two-hundred-year engagement of forces in the health protection of textile workers. The timing of this initial skirmish is far from coincidental. By the 1780s, textile industrialization had consolidated the benefits of a first generation of technological breakthroughs. These technological innovations had interrelated effects, not only on the means of production, but also on the health of employees. Moreover, as of 1784 none of this change involved steam power, still a decade away in any widespread application to the textile industry.

COTTON CARDING

The holy trinity of the Industrial Revolution in cotton manufacturing was composed of the flying shuttle, the spinning jenny, and the water frame spinner.[6] The flying shuttle, which was the first of the three introduced, proved to be a key innovation that increased the efficiency of cloth weaving. Despite its importance, the flying shuttle did not fundamentally alter the mechanism of the loom, and, more saliently, it served only to aggravate the shortcomings that already existed in cotton thread spinning. In the mid-eighteenth century, even after the introduction of the flying shuttle, spinning was still a slow, labor-intensive, cottage-based production process. The jenny and the water frame, attacking the same problem with very different mechanical solutions, changed cotton spinning fundamentally. Individual spinning wheels linked to single spindles were replaced by massive, multi-spindled mechanical devices. The huge physical space required for such devices, as much as the capital investment and the economies of scale involved, dictated the emergence of the expansive factory shed and the eclipse of the weaver's cottage.

The novel, high-volume spinning technologies begat new demands for the raw materials needed to feed into the manufacturing flow. Spinning was not the first step in mill processing, even taking into account that the cotton had already been raised, harvested, ginned, baled, and shipped. Preparing cotton for spinning first requires its cleaning to rid it of gross debris, a process called scutching. Then the cotton fibers have to undergo an initial crude alignment to facilitate their spinning and twisting into yarn and thread. This latter step is known as *carding*, a term that originated from the shape of the very first hand-held equipment used to accomplish this task. Hand-operated carding, however, could not possibly meet the needs of the new spinning machines; the new technology of mechanical carding quickly emerged in the mid-1770s.

The mechanization of cotton carding has been relegated to marginal standing in the canon of the Industrial Revolution, an apocryphal status compared with the earlier patriarchal roles of the loom and the spinner and the later, nearly messianic appearance of the steam engine. From the standpoint of textile workers' health, however, carding mechanization has dominated all of the other technological changes in the cotton industry, leaving a grim legacy of disease and disability. The process of mechanical carding generates great quantities of cotton dust—fine, penetrating fiber fragments that float in the air and settle on every surface, including the membranes of the airways. The dust is taken in with every breath. Mill fever is one potential complication of inhaling cotton dust.

Mill fever has two exposure prerequisites: first, relatively high levels of fiber dust and, second, conditions in which bacteria or fungal mildew contaminate the material handled. Since textile manufacturing is not a sterile process, some degree of bacterial or fungal residue is always present. Mill fever breaks out when the levels of dust and contamination are both high enough, conditions made possible by carding.

BYSSINOSIS

A bad case of mill fever may be briefly debilitating, yet in and of itself it does not seem to be a harbinger of any residual illness. But the same workers who are at risk of contracting mill fever are also at risk of a more chronic and insidious disease that also comes from inhaling cotton dust. This disease is linked to other natural fibers as well, especially flax used in linen making. It is a lung condition characterized by a chronic cough, wheezing, and shortness of breath, and it is progressive and debilitating. Among cotton and other textile workers in the trade, the disease is commonly known today as brown lung. In more formal medical terminology, it is referred to as *byssinosis.*[7]

Mill fever and byssinosis are not the same condition, but they are interrelated. A growing number of research studies over recent years have supported the scientific view that endotoxin and other biologically active substances derived from the cell walls of bacteria and fungi play a pivotal role in both mill fever and byssinosis. Long-term exposure to contaminated dust at levels too low to cause mill fever acutely may nonetheless be capable of inducing byssinosis. Such factors of exposure level and duration may account for the differences between the two conditions. It is also possible that while endotoxin alone can induce mill fever, other natural constituents in cotton, flax, and certain other fibers cause byssinosis with endotoxin simply being a cofactor or a marker of contamination.

Whatever the precise mechanisms of disease induction, byssinosis and mill fever, beyond question, are both real health risks of cotton and other natural-fiber manufacturing. Yet despite the obvious connection, the textile industry has resisted recognition of a direct link between exposure and disease for as long as mechanical carding devices have been turning.

For more than 150 years, the principal battle line in the struggle for textile workers' protection has been demarcated by the fight over byssinosis. The most extreme line of argument advanced by the industry has been that no such condition exists at all, even going so far as to claim that cotton dust inhalation might actually be beneficial to health. When this position finally could be held no longer, an alternative strategy was adopted. Scientific support was marshaled in an attempt to box up byssinosis within an exposed salient that would make the diagnosis vulnerable to a line of attack different from a crude denial of its existence. Byssinosis was labeled as an allergic or "hypersensitivity" disease. If byssinosis could be isolated as a phenomenon occurring only among susceptible workers, it follows that contraction of the disease would be poorly predictable, sporadic, and even idiosyncratic. In occupational and environmental disease, *idiosyncratic* has always been all too easily translated as *unpreventable.* Thus, the specter of regulation for dust exposure and the risk of inspection to enforce such regulation could be effectively overthrown.

If byssinosis has been central to textile workers' health and safety, mill fever has been a far more marginal issue. Mill fever periodically appeared in the scientific literature, fell into obscurity, and then reappeared as if a newly discovered medical curiosity. Yet despite the greater importance of byssinosis, its scientific course can be described in terms very similar to that of mill fever, albeit not quite as extreme in its ins and outs.

The meandering paths of the two conditions, byssinosis and mill fever, almost seem to parallel each other as they trek down through years of shared neglect. Moreover, to a remarkable degree their story also illuminates the history of zinc-caused metal fume fever. Each is closely linked to new technologies introduced closely to one another in time and space, with many of the same medical researchers pursuing the root causes of the conditions. Perhaps most important, each case has involved a recurring reluctance to accept that a problem even exists, lest its recognition lead to mandated controls.

In the early years of the Industrial Revolution, Great Britain did not hold a monopoly over textile manufacturing, even though it dominated the industry. Within the first twenty years of the nineteenth century, both continental European and North American industrial manufacturing centers for textiles sprang up on the model of the British factory system. It was in France, not England, that the adverse effects of inhaled cotton dust were first noted scientifically.

In 1822, a French physician named Philibert Patissier published *Traité des maladies des artisans,* based in part on a translation of Ramazzini's classic Latin treatise on occupational diseases. Ramazzini's text, predating the Industrial Revolution, was by then more than a century old. Patissier updated it with numerous original observations of his own and citations from other medical writers of the time.

Ramazzini's text had already described chronic cough among hand carders of flax, hemp, and silk in 1700. Patissier supplemented this with other citations, including autopsy findings among flax workers reported by the great anatomist Morgagni in the early eighteenth century. But it was in regard to cotton that Patissier added key new information based on the experience of French factory workers. Of cotton spinners, he wrote, "These workers continually inspire air charged with a very fine cotton debris that excites the bronchi, provokes cough, and induces chronic irritation in the lungs. Those affected are obliged to change profession to prevent phthisis [consumption]."[8]

Patissier's text was well received and widely circulated. It could not have escaped notice by English medical readers of the day, but nonetheless his observations on cotton dust went without comment for almost ten years, a period of near exponential growth in the textile industry. Finally, in 1831, an English writer named William Rathbone Greg published a forty-page tract, *An Enquiry into the State of the Manufacturing Population and the Causes and Cures of the Evils Therein Existing.* Greg was particularly well positioned to comment on this subject. Although not a physician, he was a Manchester cotton mill owner, as were his brother and his father. In his *Enquiry,* Greg cites Patissier's observations on cotton dust, expanding on them to warn, "The small particles of cotton and dust with which the air of most rooms of factories is impregnated, not unfrequently lay the foundation of distressing and fatal diseases. When inhaled, they are a source of great pulmonary irritation; which if it continues long, induces a species of chronic bronchitis, which, not rarely, degenerates into tubercular consumption."[9]

Greg was well acquainted with another contemporary leading figure of Manchester, the physician Dr. James Phillips Kay (much later Sir J. P. Kay-Shuttleworth). Indeed, Greg cited Kay's work on the health effects of cotton dust alongside Patissier's, and for good reason.

Kay had recently cofounded a new Manchester-based scientific publication, the *North of England Medical and Surgical Journal,* contributing his own article concerning *spinner's phthisis.* In this article, Kay was insightful in emphasizing cotton carding as the manufacturing process responsible for the greatest exposure. "The carding of cotton employs a great number of workmen and their younger assistants, and in some coarse mills, the atmosphere is so loaded with foreign particles as to prove a source of pulmonary irritation to a visiter [sic], who spends even a few minutes in the rooms."[10]

In describing spinner's phthisis is the same review, Kay explicitly captures the nature and progression of a lung disease he found particular to cotton workers. To this day, Kay's personal observations hold up as a classic description of the early to middle stages of a new disease that only later came to be called byssinosis:

> The disease induced has appeared to me to differ from ordinary chronic bronchitis. In the commencement of the complaint, the patient suffers a distressing pulmonary irritation from the dust and the filaments which he inhales. Entrance into the atmosphere of the mill immediately occasions a short dry cough, which harasses him considerably in the day, but ceases immediately after he leaves the mill, and inspires an atmosphere free from foreign molecules. These symptoms gradually become more severe; the cough is at length very frequent during the day, and continues even after its em-

ployments have ceased, disturbing the sleep, and exhausting the strength of the patient; but it is accompanied with little or no expectoration. (360)

Kay also called attention to the feasibility of engineering controls for cotton dust, although this was relegated to a footnote documenting that "several gentlemen, impressed with the necessity of adopting some system, have invented methods of ventilation and of covering the machines, which have considerably diminished the evil" (359 fn.).

Active ventilation was a particularly relevant issue at this time because of another technological innovation that was coming into play in the textile industry: centralized steam heating systems. These systems were especially important in the cotton mills, because controlled heat and humidity were necessary to prevent cotton fibers from breaking under the strain of spinning. To save on fuel expenses, mill operators often cut back on ventilation that was supplemented with outdoor air, even though engineering solutions were available to address this problem.

OTHER TEXTILES

In 1831, the same year as Greg's *Enquiry into the State of the Manufacturing Population* and Kay's observations, the first original general English-language text wholly devoted to the subject of occupational disease was published: *The Effects of the Principal Arts, Trades, and Professions, and of the Civic States and Habits of Living on Health and Longevity*. Its author, Charles Turner Thackrah, had completed his medical studies in London but had taken up practice in his hometown of Leeds. Like Manchester, Leeds was also a northern textile-manufacturing city, but a center of the wool rather than the cotton industry.

Thackrah's book was an immediate success. He quickly prepared an expanded second edition, which appeared in 1832. Thackrah based most of his descriptions on firsthand observation, limiting his citations as much as possible to data derived from direct personal informants rather than from published texts. For this reason Thackrah has little to say about the cotton mills, except to report a single visit that he made to Manchester, where he was impressed by the size and relative cleanliness of the lone factory he saw with his own eyes. Thackrah has a great deal more to say about other textile work, especially in the woolen and linen trades that were closer to home. For example, he described a particular branch of the wool textile trade in which old woolen rags were reprocessed into yarn for reweaving:

Persons commencing or returning to the employ, are so generally attacked with head-ache, sickness, dryness of the fauces [back of the mouth], and difficulty of breathing, that the complaint is known in the district by the name of the "shoddy fever." This disorder subsides in six or eight hours; but cough and expectoration of dirty mucus, chiefly in the morning, generally remain, and indeed are almost universal, in a greater or lesser degree, among those who long and steadily attend to the machines.[11]

In this description, Thackrah was the first to clearly document a form of mill fever. This manufacturing process was called *shoddy grinding,* and it used machines aptly named *devils* to tear up old woolen cloth. Shoddy grinding generated considerable amounts of fiber dust, much of it from rags that were likely heavily contaminated with endotoxin.

Thackrah was also meticulous in detailing a number of specific occupations in the textile trade in which a high proportion of lung disease could be attributed to fiber dusts, especially linen weaving. To make linen, a key process in preparing the flax fibers for spinning was called *heckling.* Being the dustiest operation in the trade, hecklers were the textile workers to whom Thackrah turned his greatest attention, detailing case findings in a series of such workers. Thackrah was eager to apply a relatively new tool to his investigation—the stethoscope. Because the factory was too noisy to use the device adequately, he had the workers sent to his home for examination. One was W. S.

A heckler, aged 33, entered the flax manufacture . . . at the age of 13, became a heckler by hand at 16 or 17. . . . Of late he has been employed in the heckling by machinery, which he conceives to produce more dust than the process by hand. . . . For the last seven years has suffered a difficulty of breathing. It commenced like a common catarrh [chest cold], and affected him chiefly in the evening and night. . . . Of late he has become thinner, and stoops in his gait. (75 fn.)

W. S. was meant to be a representative from the healthier of two groups of workers Thackrah examined. The second group was selected on the basis of longer-term employment, and all were diseased. For these, in addition to applying the stethoscope, Thackrah also used a device called a *pulmometer* to quantify the amount of air exhaled in a single breath on forced expiration. In what is one of the earliest, if not the very first, medical reports measuring lung function in a group of industrial workers, Thackrah records, "I may also remark, in reference to the capacity of the lungs, that no fully formed man, in good health, throws out less than 200 cubic inches at a forced expiration. Large men expire 230–280. One only of the flaxmen in the preceding statement [i.e., among the long employed] surpassed the minimum standard, no other reached it, and the last person examined could throw out but 80" (75 fn.).

The early 1830s marked a time of active agitation for factory reform in the major industrial centers in Britain. The reformers, among whom were a number of progressive physicians like-minded with Thackrah, emphasized the pressing need to address poor working conditions. Understandably, the focus was on the long hours of mill employment, especially insofar as these might be detrimental to the health of children. Overcrowding and confined air, with the risk of contagion, were also cited as potential hazards, echoing the concerns voiced by Dr. Percival's committee at the time of the Radcliffe fever outbreak fifty years earlier.

The reformers turned to the law to solve these social ills, and the Ten Hour Bill was meant to be the legislative centerpiece of the reform effort. The bill proposed restricting the hours of mill employment to ten per day, meal times excluded, for all those under eighteen years of age, while banning altogether from mill work those under age nine. The principal advocate in Parliament for the Ten Hour Bill was M.P. Michael Sadler. In Sadler's 1832 parliamentary speech introducing the second reading of the bill, he cited from Thackrah's text, which he held in his hand.[12]

Thackrah, for his part, actively supported the legislation. Along with other leading physicians, including Hodgkin of the eponymously named lymphoma, Thackrah testified at parliamentary hearings in its behalf. The hearings were organized by Sadler to provide a "scientific" underpinning for the proposal and thus blunt political attacks on the controversial social legislation.

The importance of the medical arguments in favor of the Ten Hour Bill is underscored by the prominence this line of argument was given by populist supporters of the proposed law. One of the best known of these was Richard Oastler, also known as the Factory King because of his leadership in agitating for factory labor reform. In the fall of 1832, Oastler began to write for a new halfpenny newspaper for workers, not much more than a weekly leaflet, named the *British Labourer's Protector, and Factory Child's*

Friend. A number of its issues were taken up with direct quotes from Thackrah's and other medical testimony.[13]

A surviving transcript of a public meeting held in Leeds in 1832, in the run-up to the parliamentary vote, captures Thackrah's oration in what must have been a great moment of optimistic belief in the power of popular-based change. Speaking to the crowd, he put forward a formal resolution in support of the Ten Hour Bill:

> Gentlemen, I beg leave to move "That it is the opinion of this meeting that an act of Parliament to limit the labour of children employed in factories to ten hours a day for five days in the week, and to eight hours on Sunday, would be founded in justice, humanity, and policy; would be well calculated to produce the beneficial results desired, as ten hours a day is as long a period for children to labour as is consistent with the preservation of health, the allowance of necessary relaxation and rest, and the well-being of society at large." [Cheers are noted in the transcript.] Gentlemen, the resolution adverts to the policy of the measure. Of this I am no judge. Whether ten or eleven hours or any other number may suit trade, or how such limits may affect wages, I know not.[14]

Thackrah then goes on to offer his own personal observations on the issue as a physician:

> I came forward merely as a medical man and a friend of humanity; and as such I consider that ten hours a day for children to be kept at labour in a confined atmosphere and forced to attend on machinery, is enough, and more than enough. [Cheers.] I would protest against children labouring at all, if the necessity for it could be obviated. . . . The present system is in my opinion destructive alike to the health and comfort of the present, and the hopes of future generations. [Loud applause.] But does the health of children suffer—are diseases immediately produced? . . . The vital principal in children is much stronger than in adults. It longer resists the baneful effects of circumstances and the various agents of disease. Hence children in flax and shoddy mills bear the dust much better than adults. But the vital itself suffers: the strength of the constitution is gradually exhausted. . . . The proposed measure of limiting the hours of labour is therefore recommended alike by patriotism, justice, and humanity. [Cheers.] Allow me once more to say, for fear of being misunderstood, that I think ten hours is enough, and too much. [Loud cheering.]

Thackrah's optimism was misplaced and the cheering short-lived. Sadler's existing seat was pulled out from under him as part of a parliamentary reform. He stood and lost in a new district. The mill owners quickly seized the initiative, calling for further hearings on the Ten Hour Bill. This time, the investigation was orchestrated through a special commission whose meetings were not open to the public and whose witness list was dominated by mill owners and operatives. It was little surprise that the commission recommended strongly against the Ten Hour Bill.

The substitute legislation that was put into law, the Factories Regulation Act of 1833, gutted the core of the original Ten Hour Bill's protection: for children aged thirteen and above, no time limit whatsoever was set, and for those nine through twelve, a nine-hour day was set (to be phased in over several years). Mill employment for those under nine years of age was prohibited, exempting silk mills. The Factories Regulation Act did carry with it one important innovation: the creation of the new position of factory inspector appointed by the Crown, totaling four inspectors for the entire United Kingdom.

The supporters of the Ten Hour Bill were in disarray or worse. Michael Sadler's health failed after his election loss. He retired from public life and died shortly thereafter, in July 1835. The *British Labourer's Protector* had already ceased publication in April 1833. Its chief writer, Richard Oastler, continued to agitate for reform, but by the end of that decade he was in jail on a politically orchestrated charge of bad debt.[15]

The enthusiasm of the physicians who had advocated so forcefully for better factory conditions also seemed to dampen. The *North of England Medical and Surgical Journal,* in the statement of purpose introducing its premiere issue, had committed itself to publishing "investigations illustrative of the influence of local circumstances, particularly of the employments and the diversified moral and physical habits of society on health and disease."[16]

In 1831, the journal shut down after publishing only one volume. Its cofounder, Dr. James Phillips Kay, went on to publish a highly influential book, *The Moral and Physical Condition of the Working Classes Employed in the Cotton Manufacture in Manchester.* In his new book, Kay strongly stated his *opposition* to the Ten Hour Bill. He argued that not only would this legislation depress wages, but also factory children would gain no benefit from getting out of work after only ten hours because "if this measure *were unaccompanied by a general system of education,* the time thus bestowed, would be wasted or misused" (italics in original).[17]

In later years, Dr. Kay largely abandoned his interest in physical health, including the study of lung disease, focusing almost exclusively on moral well-being, especially insofar as this might be fostered through public education. The *North of England Medical and Surgical Journal* had been in print just long enough to review Thackrah's text on occupational disease on its initial publication in 1831, highlighting his original observations on the illnesses of flax workers as particularly noteworthy.

Dr. Charles Turner Thackrah died on 23 May 1833, one day past his thirty-eighth birthday.[18] He did not live to see the defeat of the Ten Hour movement or its aftermath. The loss of Thackrah was major. No British figure comparable to him in professional stature in the field appeared for at least a generation. Thackrah's absence can be felt keenly in the medical literature on the subject of occupational disease of the next decade. The little that was published in the period immediately following his death is best epitomized by the work of Daniel Noble, a Manchester-based physician. Noble's eighty-one-page *Facts and Observations Relative to the Influence of Manufactures Upon Health and Life,* published in 1843, was little more than a polemic, actually purporting the health *benefits* of working in the cotton mills.[19] Spinner's phthisis is singled out by Noble for particular scorn. He dismisses this disease as little more than a fiction of agitators for social reform and their few and misguided medical allies.

PUBLIC HEALTH WITHOUT OCCUPATIONAL HEALTH

In contradistinction to the retrenchment in occupational safety and health protection, the movement for general public health and sanitation seemed to take off at the very same time. In 1842, Edwin Chadwick released his landmark *Report . . . on an Inquiry into the Sanitary Condition of the Labouring Population of Great Britain.* In over 450 pages, including appendices, the report lays out, in voluminous detail, national needs for better housing, increased nutrition, and general sanitary improvements. Chadwick's report set the British public health agenda for the remainder of the nineteenth century.

If Chadwick proclaims the benefits of decent housing and sanitary living conditions in a stentorian voice, it is reduced to a mere whisper when it comes to the workplace. Industrial health and safety is almost entirely missing from the pages of his report. The few entries that are devoted to the "prevention of noxious fumes and dust" in the workplace are primarily concerned with lead-exposed workers in France. Most of the attention to textile workers is given to their housing, with a particularly noteworthy subsection entitled "Instance of a superior moral and sanitary condition enjoyed by workers in a cotton factory." Here we learn of one mill where all the workers, "more especially the females are not only in the possession of good health but many of them (quite as large a proportion as we have seen in any of the extensive well-regulated similar establishments in country districts) are blooming."[20]

Chadwick is explicit in the view that the living conditions of the workers (combined with the poor moral influences to which they are exposed), rather than working conditions behind the factory door, account for almost any illness that might be associated with occupation. After all, he already could claim some specific expertise in this subject. Ten years before, Edwin Chadwick had been one of the three commissioners who oversaw the report killing the Ten Hour Bill.[21]

One only has to turn to the popular literature of the time to be reminded that the contemporary reality was far from English mill girls in bloom. In Elizabeth Gaskell's novel *North and South,* first published in 1854 but set in a period about ten years earlier, a consumptive named Bessy is befriended by the novel's heroine, Margaret. Both are nineteen years old. Making a sick call on the wasting girl, Margaret tries to distract her from her troubles by asking her about what her life was like before she became ill:

> "Don't let us talk of what fancies come into your head when you are feverish. I would rather hear something about what you used to do when you were well."
>
> "I think I was well when mother died, but I have never been rightly strong sin' somewhere about that time. I began to work in a carding-room soon after, and the fluff got into my lungs and poisoned me."
>
> "Fluff?" said Margaret, inquiringly.

Gaskell has Bessy explain to Margaret and to the reader exactly what fluff is:

> "Fluff," repeated Bessy. "Little bits, as fly off fro' the cotton, when they're carding it, and fill the air till it looks all fine white dust. They say it winds round the lungs, and tightens them up. Anyhow, there's many a one as works in a carding-room, that falls into a waste, coughing and spitting blood, because they're just poisoned by the fluff."
>
> "But can't it be helped?" asked Margaret.
>
> "I dunno. Some folk have a great wheel at one end o' their carding rooms to make a draught, and carry off th' dust; but that wheel costs a deal of

money—five or six hundred pound, maybe, and brings in no profit: so it's but a few of th' masters will put 'em up."[22]

In France and Belgium, there seemed to be more willingness to consider the potential risks of cotton manufacturing. In 1839, the leading demographer of the time, Louis-René Villermé, was commissioned to report to the French Académie des sciences morales et politiques on the "physical and moral state" of workers employed in the silk, cotton, and wool factories of Lyon, a major textile manufacturing center. Villermé reconfirmed and expanded upon Patissier's earlier observations regarding the French textile industry. Villermé was not afraid to use the term *cotton phthisis* to describe a lung condition among cotton mill workers in which "cough is the first symptom of a slow acting and formidable disease of the chest."[23]

He emphasized that this cotton phthisis is pathologically distinct from tuberculosis. Villermé, like Kay before him, also called attention to potential engineering controls that could, by lowering dust levels, reduce the risk of disease among the mill workers. In 1845, Belgian investigators in the textile center of Ghent followed in Villermé's footsteps, pointing out that respiratory symptoms among mill workers tended to be most intense early in the week on return to factory. This temporal pattern is important because it marks a key intersection in the temporal patterns of disease for the first stages of byssinosis and Monday morning or mill fever.[24]

Finally in the early 1860s, after British medical researchers maintained a complete silence on the subject for nearly twenty years, Dr. Edward Headlam Greenhow began a systematic investigation of the health hazards of the textile trades. Greenhow was working under the aegis of John Simon, who orchestrated a series of public health reports for the Privy Council, a governmental body in which Simon served in a role somewhat analogous to that of the U.S. surgeon general.

Greenhow was commissioned to carry out a number of field investigations, collecting data on respiratory diseases among a spectrum of manufacturing towns in England. On the basis of Greenhow's findings there, Simon reported to the government:

In cotton-factories, the carding-rooms are by far the most injurious. They employ many operatives—sometimes even a third of the whole establishment. All employed in these rooms inhale a dusty atmosphere, with much cotton-fiber diffused in it. . . . The influence of the ordinary carding-room atmosphere on persons regularly employed in it is such, that, apparently, few carding-room operatives reach fifty years of age without having acquired an amount of chronic bronchitis which at no distant time disables them. Yet evidently the evil is in great part controllable. . . . [It] is lessened in proportion as the room is lofty and ventilated, in proportion as the carding-engines are closely covered, and in proportion as means are used to modify the more dust-producing processes.[25]

Greenhow's data, summarized in Simon's Privy Council reports and appended to them in their entirety, contributed to a renewed interest in the actual employment conditions of workers, not simply in their housing and social habits.

One result of this new interest was a series of British legislative initiatives that strengthened and extended the limited controls of earlier factory acts (including the 1833 Factories Regulation Act, which had gutted the ten-hour limit, the interim Factory Act of 1844, and the final successful passage of such work-hour limits in the Ten Hour Act of 1847). No legislative reform, however, mandated technical controls to reduce cotton or other mill dusts.

Greenhow's work would have fallen into complete obscurity except for one particularly avid reader of British governmental reports who spent most days sequestered in the Readers' Room of the British Museum. That reader was Karl Marx. Yet even Marx, when citing Greenhow in *Das Kapital*, uses the text to document the role of the factory system in generating the surplus value of labor, not to illustrate the health hazards of dusty trades per se.[26]

In 1877, Dr. Adrien Proust (father of Marcel) published a major French textbook on public health and hygiene, including a substantial section devoted to occupational diseases.[27] In this book, Proust addresses lung disease among cotton textile workers, which he describes in stages starting with chronic cough and progressing over time through inflammation to a terminal phase, which, at autopsy, reveals lungs that are "shriveled."

A few years earlier, German pathologists had first introduced the term *pneumoconiosis* to subsume lung diseases caused by inorganic dusts. *Silicosis* and *asbestosis* are later variants of this original terminology. Proust eruditely noted that a German medical authority on occupational disease, in suggesting that the lung disease among textile workers might best be called *lyssinosis*, mistakenly substituted an *l* for what should have been a *b*, for *byssos* (Greek for "fine fiber"). Proust's correction to *byssinosis* went on to become the accepted medical term.

It is ironic, but fitting, that the first appearance of the term *byssinosis* in an English-language text, in a scientific article on pneumoconiosis published in 1881, was little more than a dismissive aside.[28] The author of the article was a medical student named Thomas Harris, who was clearly reflecting the standard teaching of his day. He rejects *byssinosis* as a term with little specific meaning, since any lung disease that might be associated with cotton inhalation, he claimed, did not differ from "ordinary" phthisis (that is, tuberculosis). The critical inference in this line of reasoning is that the absence of any disease peculiar or particular to exposure in cotton work indicates little is warranted in the way of specific controls.

The presumption that byssinosis did not exist at all or that, if it did, it was only tuberculosis called by another name conveniently ignored the preponderance of clinical and pathological data that had already accumulated on both sides of the Channel. Yet despite the weight of the evidence to the contrary, this was the ill-founded view that continued to dominate British thinking on the subject of cotton workers' health.

The students of Harris's class aged into practitioners and teachers a few years later, in the 1880s and 1890s and on into the early years of the twentieth century. It was not much of a leap from saying that work could not cause a disease like phthisis to arguing that consumptive types might be identified and culled from the workforce, a eugenically inspired prevention strategy that was to become popular in industrial public health.

JOB FEVER REDISCOVERED

Near the end of the nineteenth century, seventy years after Patissier first documented the lung disease of cotton spinners, Dr. John Arlidge, a leading British expert on industrial disease, wrote pointedly, "It is singular that in this country, where cotton-spinning is carried out on a scale surpassing that found in any other, there is a complete dearth of information respecting the morbid anatomy of the disorders due to the work."[29]

In the same textbook on occupational disease, Arlidge covered many of the textile trades that Thackrah had highlighted so many years before in his own textbook. Arlidge revisited the subject of wool shoddy making, personally inspecting the trade and finding important improvements since the fever-causing workshops of Thackrah's day. "My own examination of shoddy-making and its machinery furnished no evidence of the prevalence of this disorder at the present time, and I trust that 'shoddy fever' has become, like not a few other industrial diseases, a thing of the past."[30]

Arlidge acknowledges that although he presumed shoddy fever had gone extinct, "this anticipation may be too hopeful," because a recent governmental monograph on a closely related manufacturing process described a condition called *flock fever*. Flock, like shoddy, was also made by pulverizing old woolen cloth, in this case cloth of such poor quality it was unfit even for shoddy. Flock fever seemed to be remarkably akin to the febrile illness Thackrah had described fifty years earlier. Arlidge notes:

> The symptoms described are those of a severe catarrh of the bronchial passages, viz., shivering, difficulty breathing, cough, soreness of the chest, and expectoration of mucus charged with dust. In about a week's time, if the man continues at work, a tolerance of the dust is established, and the symptoms subside, and do not recur so long as he keeps at the same work; but on leaving it off, the tolerance for dust is soon lost, and on returning after an absence for a week or two, the workman suffers again as at first.[31]

Like Thackrah, Arlidge was also concerned with the question of flax exposure in linen manufacturing. He notes that chronic cough was endemic among veterans of the trade. The young mill workers, called doffers, suffered a different malady:

> This disturbance is known as "mill fever." It attacks them within the first few days of employment, and is looked upon by the workpeople as a "seasoning" which has to be passed through. It is ushered in by chills, nausea, and vomiting, quickly followed by headache, thirst, and heat of the skin; and is, in short, a true febrile disorder. After from two to eight days it spontaneously disappears without medical intervention, leaving the patients weak and languid.[32]

Immediately following this description, Arlidge goes on to make an important broader connection. "A similar temporary derangement, little regarded, befalls the young hands on first entering other textile factories; but not, we believe, of equal severity with that observed in the flax-mills" (376).

In highlighting shoddy and flock fever (due to wool work) and mill fever (predominantly due to flax work but also seen in other textile mills—that is, cotton), Arlidge was the first to consider the inhalation of contaminated organic fiber dust as a generic common denominator of fever at work. Nonetheless, the connection to cotton dust is downplayed, and Arlidge seems not to have come to the realization that byssinosis and mill fever might be somehow interrelated.

Eventually, yet another generation after Arlidge, attention began to turn again to the British cotton industry. First in 1910 and then again in 1911 and 1912, sporadic outbreaks of a troubling "new" illness began to occur in a number of different English textile mills. The symptoms were similar in all cases, with an onset at work of chest tightness followed by cough, progressing by nighttime to an asthmalike attack of breathing difficulty accompanied by aches, fever, and chills. All of the mills in which the outbreaks occurred shared certain technical features of cotton weaving: the thread had been coated, or *sized,* with starch and then maintained under conditions particularly conducive to mildew overgrowth prior to weaving.

Edgar Collis, a British physician who investigated these outbreaks and did much to bring renewed interest to the question of lung disease among cotton textile workers, voiced understandable frustration in concluding his report. "The occurrence of these cases is, I think, of interest; they exhibit a distinct and definite train of symptoms, always associated with an occupational environment suggestive of the cause. Yet medical men attending them, each seeing only one or two cases, have not considered them unusual, but have passed them by as ordinary cases of bronchitis, asthma, or even incipient phthisis."[33]

Because the mill fever that Collis investigated involved an intermediate stage of processing, after carding and spinning and during the weaving of thread into cloth, the relationship to byssinosis was not clear cut. Nonetheless, by the late 1920s and especially in the 1930s, a series of British governmental reports, initiated by the Industrial Fatigue Research Board and followed up by others, began to assess the health of cotton textile workers systematically across trades.[34] These reports delineated two stages of illness among cotton mill workers: an initial period of mill fever, and a late stage of incapacitating byssinosis. The reports belatedly represented the first official British governmental acceptance of a specific entity of dust-caused disease in the cotton industry.

BELATED MILL FEVER IN THE UNITED STATES

The United States lagged behind Great Britain, following a century-long tradition of claiming that laborers in American textile mills were virtually disease free insofar as dust was concerned. As early as 1833, as part of a lengthy overview entitled "Influence of Occupation on Health," which appeared in twelve published parts over six months in the *Boston Medical and Surgical Journal,* Dr. E. G. Davis observed:

Those employed in cotton mills are exposed to the inhalation of filaments of this substance. This inconvenience exists principally in carding rooms, in which the operatives are constantly exposed to an atmosphere filled with the fine particles of this substance, which from its lightness will remain suspended for a long time. The effect of this, however, is slow in manifesting itself; and in our own establishments, where a single branch of labor is seldom pursued steadily for a great length of time, I am not aware that disease ever occurs which can distinctly be referred to this cause.[35]

Shortly after this, echoing and even amplifying contemporary British views, a prize-winning essay on occupational health, written in 1837 by a New York physician named Benjamin McCready, acknowledged the growing economic importance of the textile industry while minimizing its health risks:

It is only within a few years that the manufacture of woolen and cotton cloth has been introduced to any extent into the United States. . . . Lately the business has rapidly increased, and now there are factories scattered through many of the states of the Union, while in New England a very considerable population depend upon them as a principal means of obtaining a livelihood. . . . The evils of factory labor, so far as I have been able to form an opinion concerning it, depend less upon circumstances not necessarily connected with it, but which in England at least, have been found invariably to accompany its progress. Of these evils, the length of time which the operatives are employed, the confined and ill ventilated apartments in which they reside, their intemperate and inactive habits, and the bad quality of the provision which they consume, are the principal.[36]

Over the next hundred years, despite all of the changes that took place in the U.S. textile industry in the aftermath of the Civil War, little else was written on the health of its cotton workers. The general view held that American shores were free from the disease rumored to be rampant in the European mills.

In the end, it was not a medical journal that defied tradition and broke the story but rather a trade publication called *Textile World* (offices in New York, Boston, Atlanta, and Greenville, NC). In its March 1940 issue, squeezed between the pieces "Knowledge of Dobby Designing Aids Weavers" and "Hints on Cloth Room Layout," a single-page article appeared entitled "Card-Room Fever: Strict Control of Dust Will Eliminate Health Hazard from Low-Grade Cotton."[37]

Its author, a governmental industrial hygienist named M. F. Trice, in North Carolina, reported on an outbreak of illness in mills brought on by the use of compressed air to blow dust off carding machines, especially when *low-grade,* discolored cotton was processed. An investigation was triggered when a symptomatic worker filed a compensation claim. When the treating doctor was called to testify, he not only documented that the worker had an acute inflammatory condition of the throat and lungs manifesting in cough and fever but also added that he had cared for twenty-five to thirty similar cases from the same mill. The worker, however, was denied compensation, since he had neither silicosis nor asbestosis, the only two dust diseases then compensable in the state.

Shortly after the North Carolina outbreak, the U.S. government embarked on an unintended experiment that established beyond any reasonable doubt the link between cotton dust and mill fever. A program sponsored by the U.S. Department of Agriculture, meant to reduce a domestic cotton surplus and to benefit rural farm families economically, initiated a cottage industry of mattress making.

Participating low-income families, working in small communal workshops, received fifty pounds of raw cotton and ten yards of cotton ticking (fabric) per mattress to be produced. Making the mattress itself involved opening the bales, fluffing or crudely carding the cotton, closing the mattress, and beating the finished product. The hitch was the cotton—it was mostly low-grade, dusty, and *stained* cotton from the 1940 crop. The illness it caused included the classic manifestations of mill fever, most notably chills and fever peaking six to nine hours after exposure.

During 1941, at the peak use of this crop of cotton, the mattress program involved 2,832,885 families in forty-six (of forty-eight) states. The total number of cases of mattress-related mill fever is unknown; seven hundred cases were reported in one state alone. The problem was so widespread that the National Institutes of Health assigned a team to investigate the issue.

The NIH made available considerable laboratory resources at its newly opened Bethesda headquarters in order to identify how and why stained cotton causes this illness. The research team carried out physical and chemical analyses of the cotton, cultured the cotton for mold and bacteria, and injected or applied directly to test animals high concentrations of extracts of the cotton and its bacteriological contaminants. These experiments clearly showed that stained cotton was contaminated with bacteria that produced an endotoxin-like substance capable of inducing inflammation and fever.

The achievement of a more realistic exposure scenario, however, required a different approach. The research team constructed a small cotton-carding apparatus attached to an exposure chamber, wherein test animals could inhale cotton dust in a controlled manner. Altogether in these inhalation experiments they studied thirty hamsters, eighteen rabbits, eight guinea pigs, four kittens, five baboons, and four monkeys. Unfortunately, only the baboon experiments provided any indication of the respiratory or systemic responses anticipated.

One experimental option remained. The researchers placed themselves in turn in the same chamber, each undergoing exposure to sterilized cotton, stained cotton, and then normal cotton intentionally contaminated with suspect bacteria. The sterilized cotton induced no symptoms, but the deliberately contaminated and the naturally stained samples each induced the classic symptoms of mill fever.

The symptoms were most severe from the naturally stained cotton. In that experiment, each subject developed fever (ranging from 101.1 to 102.7 degrees) and an elevated white blood cell count of twenty thousand or more (greater than twice the upper limit of normal). Although the names of the subjects are not stated explicitly, clearly they were the three authors of the scientific report as published in the *Journal of the American Medical Association* in August 1942: Paul A. Neal, M.D.; Roy Schneiter, M.S.; and Barbara Caminita, B.S.[38]

MAKING BRASS

The *JAMA* report on mattress makers by Neal and his colleagues is a classic of its kind. It was very much on my mind and those of my co-investigators as we began to bring welders into the laboratory to study metal fume fever. We knew that welding fume in general, and zinc oxide fume specifically, does not contain endotoxin or any other bacterial contaminant, despite all the similarities between metal fume fever and mill fever.

What goes for welding is also true of brass and brass making, the first zinc-using industry in which metal fume fever appeared.[39] Charles Turner Thackrah, the selfsame British physician who had been the first to study flax workers systematically, was also the first to report fever among brass workers, although he gave this far less prominence and did not connect the two occupational diseases in any way. Almost in passing, in describing the health risks of foundry workers for the second edition of his text (1832), Thackrah noted, "The brass-melters of Birmingham state their liability also to an intermittent fever, which they term the brass-ague, and which attacks them from once a month to once a year, and leaves them in a state of great debility."[40]

In another section of the same text, Thackrah comments on a similar syndrome in brass button makers. Although he never stated this explicitly, it is likely that medical colleagues in Birmingham called the brass fever syndrome to his attention. Birmingham was the center of the British brass industry at the time, while Leeds, where Thackrah was based, had more limited production. What *is* clear is that Thackrah could not have learned of the condition from any previous written source on occupational disease, none of which mentions fever among brass workers.

In fact, even the first edition of Thackrah's text (in 1831) did not mention *brass workers' ague* (fever), although it does describe the occupation in Leeds, noting, "The *Founders* suffer from the inhalation of volatalized *[sic]* metal. In the founding of *yellow brass* in particular, the evolution of oxide of zinc is very great. It immediately affects respiration; it less directly affects the digestive organs. The men suffer from difficulty of breathing, cough, pain at the stomach, and sometimes morning vomiting."[41]

Why did metal fume fever first "appear" in 1832? Ignorance does not explain it; zinc fume fever did not go unreported simply because the potential hazards of metals and the metalworking trades were not well appreciated, for they were, even back to ancient times. For example, the Roman writer Pliny the Elder warns of mercury ore (cinnabar) and lead compounds in his *Natural History*, commenting that "as cinnabar and red lead are admitted to be poisons, all the current instructions on the subject of their employment for medicinal purposes are decidedly risky."[42] In contrast, in the next book of the *Natural History*, Pliny discusses the use of zinc carbonate or zinc oxide (cadmia) as a safe remedy to dry moisture, treat head lesions, stop discharges, and cleanse inflamed swellings. Cadmia was of interest to the Romans for its industrial use as well as its medicinal uses, specifically because of its critical role in making brass.

Brass is an alloy made up of two metals: zinc and copper. In the ancient Western world it was more expensive to make and far less widely used than the alloy bronze, which is composed of copper and tin. But brass has a quality that could never be achieved in bronze—a yellow, almost golden sheen, resistant to tarnish. Brass was never going to be mistaken for gold, even by a fool, but it had a certain flash nonetheless. Livia, the wife of Emperor Augustus, owned mines whose copper was considered particularly suitable for alloying into brass; Livian copper was preferred for minting

Roman brass sesterce (sestertius) coins. The Romans went so far as to classify brass by two names. *Aes* referred to standard brass such as might be cast in coin or other small objects, differentiating this from a truly rare and golden-hued alloy known as *aurichalcum*. It is still a matter of debate whether aurichalcum existed at all or was simply a creation of classical hype.[43]

In order to make brass, the ancients mixed copper with zinc carbonate, a naturally occurring zinc-containing mineral named *smithsonite,* also commonly known as calamine. In the ancient world this natural form of calamine was specified as *cadmia fossilis* to distinguish it from *cadmia fornacis.* This latter material, "furnace calamine," was a form of zinc carbonate that accumulated on the walls of smelters. These accretions were deposited as a by-product in the process of refining other metals such as copper and lead. The furnace calamine scraped off the smelter walls could be further refined, in turn, to produce zinc oxide. This purified end product, known as *popholyx,* was prized by ancient physicians and alchemists alike. Over time, metalworkers realized that prefiring calamine to its zinc oxide derivative facilitated brass making.

Successful processes of metalworking, and especially alloying, evolved through empiric observation, yet the ultimate viability of each method is determined by the physical and chemical attributes of the materials involved. The process of "cementing" copper with zinc carbonate or zinc oxide to produce brass alloy is possible because zinc oxide, when slowly heated in a furnace together with copper and a source of carbon such as charcoal, briefly forms metallic zinc.

The life of zinc as a free metal in fume form is brief. As soon as it is generated, the pure metal unites with the copper to create brass, driven by the vapor pressure of the newly forming alloy. Left on its own, the vapor pressure of pure zinc would cause it to quickly boil away. On the surface of the planet Mercury this might be the end of the story: metallic zinc vapor would simply mix into the atmosphere. But on Earth, or in any other atmosphere containing free oxygen, metallic zinc vapor rapidly converts to zinc oxide fume, which is why it was easy for the ancients to produce *popholyx* and, by the same token, why pure metallic zinc was virtually unknown in the ancient world.

Although scattered references in the classical literature allude to the making of brass and the uses of brass are well documented through various artifacts, including ancient coins, no detailed descriptions of brass making by the cementation process appear prior to medieval and Renaissance sources.

There is little reason, however, to believe much changed in the process between Roman times and those later periods. A series of sixteenth-century metallurgic texts by Italian and German authors, partly scientific tracts and partly how-to "Joy of Metal Cooking" guides, go into great detail on brass founding. Each of these texts makes clear that making brass through the cementation of copper and calamine was a lengthy process, requiring many hours of closely controlled foundry firing.

These same texts are also important early written sources on the health dangers of metals already recognized as hazards by the ancients, in particular lead and mercury. Indeed, the very first printed medical text wholly devoted to occupational disease was specifically on the subject of the health hazards of metalwork. Originally written in the German metalworking center of Augsburg in 1473 but not printed until 1524, the translated title of the eight-page pamphlet is "On the Poisonous Evil Vapours." Its author, a physician named Ulrich Ellenbog, warns in an equivalent archaic German,

> Wherefore when ye masters and men work silver with lead, or gild [which would use mercury], ye shall guard yourselves as far as ye may from the vapour and smoke, for it is poisonous to you, and it is my advice that ye do it in the open air with all diligence, and not in a closed room. Also ye shall not bend too much over this vapour but turn away therefrom and bind up the mouth. This vapour of quicksilver, silver, and lead is a cold poison, for it maketh heaviness and tightness of the chest, burdeneth the limbs and ofttimes lameth them as one often seeth in foundries where men do work with large masses and the vital inward members become burdened therefrom.[44]

Although Ellenbog also mentions the hazards of antimony, litharge (lead oxide), verdigris (copper acetate), and even coal smoke, he does not address cadmia fumes or brass working among his various and sundry warnings. This omission, of course, does not preclude the possibility that illness was occurring from such work but went unnoticed. Ellenbog's brief text is little more than a simple homily for metalworkers, with a few words of commonsense prevention followed by curatives, which in some cases may be worse than the disease. He is a big promoter of wormwood wine (a precursor of absinthe) as a therapeutic, for example.

The single most important text on metalworking from this period is *De Re Metallica,* by Georgius Agricola, who was also a German physician. Unlike Ellenbog's brief text, Agricola's was a near-encyclopedic tome on all aspects of metal mining, refining, and founding, informed in part by his personal experience as a mining town physician. *De Re Metallica* was first published in Latin in 1556 and was quickly translated for German and Italian editions. Only much later was it translated into English, with extensive commentary. Published just before World War I, this translation was the work of the future U.S. President Herbert Hoover and his wife, Lou, both of whom were geologists prior to his entry into political life.

Amid his detailed descriptions of mines and mining equipment, Agricola turns his attention squarely to the health of the miners, acknowledging bluntly, "It remains for me to speak of the ailments and accidents of miners, and of the methods by which they can guard against these, for we should always devote more care to maintaining our health, that we may freely perform our bodily functions, than to making profits."[45] Agricola does mention the mining hazards of a mineral he refers to as *cadmia* in Latin but that, in the contemporary German translation, appeared as cobalt, a metal that has no Latin equivalent and was just then becoming known in the mines of central Europe and was often contaminated with arsenic.

In addition to the dangers of certain metals, Agricola describes asphyxiant gases and traumatic injury from falls and mine collapses and even alludes to the occupational hazard of mine-dwelling demons, underscoring how much these early sources can sometimes mix chemistry with alchemy and medicine with metaphysics.

Although we cannot be certain that absolutely no health-related ill effects were observed in association with brass alloying by ancient and medieval methods, clearly brass made by classic cementation does conform to a fixed range of physical parameters. Specifically, because of the underlying metallurgic chemistry of the process, brass made by cementation has an upper limit on the concentration of zinc that can be introduced into the alloy, namely, just over one part zinc per three parts copper. Even that concentration was hard to achieve, but it was desirable.

As early as the Middle Ages, brass smelters understood that a higher ratio of cadmia could yield a more yellow or golden brass, producing highly marketable items that could compete with silver and even with gold. Thus, although there was certainly an incentive to produce brass with a higher zinc content, there was simply no ready way to do it. Ores of very high zinc content do sometimes occur in nature and may account for the rare appearance of objects with a high content of metallic zinc among archaeological finds. Zinc in the form of a pure metal, however, was unknown and could not be produced by the standard metal smelting technologies of Europe, even up through the late Renaissance.

Brass making in Europe finally began to change in the seventeenth and eighteenth centuries. The impetus for change came not from domestic technology but as a benefit of Chinese innovation. At this time, a novel import from China (often traded via India) began to appear in the West.[46] The new import was an exotic metal called *tutenag* by European traders, who also began to refer to it as *spelter*. Because of this trade, spelter became a common term for zinc, although it is now fairly obscure. One of the earliest published notations on tutenag (after the trade was already well established) is attributable to Carl Ekeberg, a merchant ship officer of the Royal Swedish East-India Company, then a great rival of the Dutch and English. This notation also contains an extremely early allusion to the potential adverse health effects of zinc oxide inhalation. In 1756 Ekeberg wrote, "Of tutenago, which the Chinese call Packyn, most is to be found in the province of Whonam, but some is also found in the surrounding country. . . . Its ore is ash-colored, bluish, slightly glittering like iron-ore. . . . The ore melts easily and emits during the smelting and oxidation a thick stinking smoke injurious to the health."[47]

Chinese sources on zinc refining considerably precede the European. In Chinese, metallic zinc was called *wo-ch'ien,* or "Japanese lead":

> Zinc, a term of recent origin, does not appear in the ancient books. It is extracted from smithsonite [zinc carbonate]. . . . Fill each earthen jar with ten catties of smithsonite, then seal tightly with mud, and let it dry slowly so as to prevent cracking when heated. Then pile a number of these jars in alternate layers with coals and charcoal briquettes, with kindling on the bottom layer for starting the fire. When the jars become red-hot, the smithsonite will melt into a mass. When cooled, the jars are broken open and the substance thus obtained is zinc, with a twenty per cent loss in volume. The metal is easily burnt off by fire if not mixed with copper. Because it is similar to lead, yet more fierce in nature, it is called "Japanese lead."[48]

This quotation was taken from the *T'ien-kung K'ai-wu* (The Creations of Nature and Man), a Chinese technological encyclopedia written by Ying-xing Song in 1637, but the first commercial-scale refining took place even earlier, starting sometime around 1500. The precise origins of Chinese zinc refining technology are unclear and may even have originated in the Indian subcontinent.

The importation of spelter from China to Europe from the mid-seventeenth to the mid-eighteenth century rapidly increased, accounting for many tons of trade annually. During this period, brass continued to be made through the old cementation process in its initial formulation. To produce a yellow, more desirable product, though, the practice of increasing the zinc content of the nascent brass with additional metallic zinc as a final step in the founding process also began in this period, becoming more common as metallic zinc became more available.

The marketplace taste for a finer-quality brass, particularly in England, was further stimulated in this period through a related Chinese import. This material was an exotic and highly desirable alloy that came to be known as *paktong*. It was silvery, lustrous, and, most important, did not tarnish. No one in the West knew how to make anything remotely resembling paktong, and even its chemical composition was at first elusive. Eventually, it was determined that one of paktong's key attributes was its high zinc content, constituting one in two parts or more in some samples. Because most of the remaining composition was copper, paktong at first seemed to be an odd brass variant, perhaps even the mythical aurichalcum of the ancient world.

It was only later analysis that finally identified a significant nickel content in paktong. Nickel was another metal being newly discovered in Europe in the eighteenth century. It would take nearly another hundred years until "German silver" and related zinc-copper-nickel alloys essentially reproduced the mix that the Chinese had invented in paktong.

In the eighteenth century, relatively small amounts of paktong alloy were imported into England and recast into extremely expensive, highly prized consumer goods. Most of these were small objects, especially candlesticks, but for the ultrawealthy even larger items were possible, such as andirons or other fireplace accessories. To this day, paktong objects are especially coveted by collectors of antique British brass and silver.

THE NEW BRASS

At the same time that the potential value of alloys with a high zinc content was gaining wider recognition, Europeans began to recognize that metallic zinc could be found closer to home than China. Paralleling the long-held practice of scavenging zinc oxide as a smelter by-product was the discovery of very small deposits of another metallic substance in the cracks of the furnace wall at times after firing certain lead ores. Advances in metallurgy identified this substance as metallic zinc, which replaced the name *counterfeit,* originally applied to the furnace metal because of its suspect, base nature.

In 1738 an English manufacturer took out a patent for the commercial-scale, industrial distillation of metallic zinc. Zinc would no longer be a limited and expensive import item. The availability of cheap metallic zinc transformed the process through which foundries made brass. Brass did not require cementation, a time-consuming process in which workers cautiously heated copper and calamine together over the course of several days, a process that also limited the zinc content of the alloy and thus its market appeal. Brass could now be produced simply by rapidly melting copper and adding metallic zinc to it in short order. The new technique was fast, provided for high-volume production, and allowed brass to be easily made at a concentration of 35 percent or more metallic zinc.

The new admixing process had only one, small complication: the production of copious zinc oxide fume. The old slow cementation process could occur without the overproduction of zinc fume because of the wide gap between the temperature at which zinc melts (419 degrees Centigrade) and the one at which it boils (930 degrees). Copper, however, melts at 1,083 degrees, a temperature far higher than zinc's melting point and, indeed, one at which zinc readily boils. When zinc is mixed into a pot of molten copper, much of the zinc rapidly boils off. The metallic vapor instantaneously combines with atmospheric oxygen and converts to zinc oxide fume. Because zinc had become so cheap, losing much of it through boiling away in this manner presented little obstacle to the new manufacturing technique. Sufficient zinc, combined with rapid manual stirring, ensured achievement of the desired end product.

For almost a century after the arrival of cheap zinc, the cementation and zinc-copper admixing processes of brass making coexisted. As late as 1790, both foundry processes were treated as standard practice, for example in Richardson's *Chemical Principles of the Metallic Arts, with an Account of the Principal Diseases Incident to Different Artificers,* although this book acknowledged that, either way, some extra zinc must be added to produce "better" brass. "Brass is either made by fusing copper and zinc together; or by fusing copper and the ore of zinc or lapis calaminaris. . . . To obtain better brass either the metals must be used, or the common brass must be cemented with calamine and charcoal dust and sometimes manufacturers add to it, old brass, by which the new is said to be meliorated."[49]

With cotton weaving, the technological changes of industrial process-ing, first and foremost the introduction of large-scale mechanical carding, were the prerequisites of acute mill fever and chronic byssinosis. Metal-working, no less than textile weaving, was also an ancient art. And like mill fever, fume fever emerged because of a key technological change, intro-duced, as it turns out, at about the same time as the change in textile weav-ing. If we return to Thackrah's original description of fever attacking brass foundry workers, the meaning now becomes clearer. In emphasizing that in "*yellow brass* in particular, the evolution of oxide of zinc is very great," Thackrah is implicating the emerging technology of making brass from metallic zinc added to copper. Metal fume fever had never been reported before, not because it had gone unobserved, but because exposure to con-centrated zinc oxide was previously uncommon or altogether unknown.

Thackrah's initial 1832 report of the new illness of brass ague, however, appears to have gone unnoticed. In 1845, a French investigator named Blandet, apparently unaware of Thackrah's observation, reported to the French Académie des sciences on a febrile reaction among copper founders when zinc is added to the mix. Blandet delineated the syndrome as having an abrupt onset of symptoms the afternoon or evening of exposure, in-cluding headache, muscle aches, vomiting, and chills, with the last punc-tuated at three to four hours with a copious sweat and fever. The total du-ration of illness, Blandet noted, was twenty-four to forty-eight hours. Blandet felt the syndrome was clearly linked to heavy inhalation exposure to zinc oxide fume.[50]

Blandet's detailed report, unlike Thackrah's brief allusion to the syn-drome, at least engendered some response. One Mr. Guérard publicly dis-missed Blandet's claim that zinc oxide was to blame for the condition. The cause, he argued, was more likely due to the overdrinking of fluids in a hot workshop.[51] Even an early American report weighs in on the health of brass founders. In 1848 a New York physician named Augustus Gardner described several cases of urinary and gastrointestinal tract ailments in brass founders. He did not cite Thackrah, however; nothing in the illness described resembles fume fever, and the only causal attribution Gardner made was to the recently opened Croton reservoir that, by centrally sup-plying water, had encouraged the production and sale of brass faucets and other related plumbing supplies in New York City.[52]

It was not until 1862 that Thackrah's original observation was fully re-visited. In a paper entitled "On Brass-Founders' Ague," delivered to the Royal Medical and Chirurgical Society, Edward Greenhow (the same researcher who had worked with John Simon and been so important in documenting the hazards of cotton dust) opened his remarks:

> During a brief holiday visit to Birmingham in the autumn of 1858, I devoted my leisure to visiting the workshops of the various workers in metal, for which that town is famous. . . . While visiting the brass-founders' shops, I learned that this class of operatives are liable to suffer from a well-defined form of ailment, known among themselves by the name of ague, and to which I have therefore applied the term "Brass-founders' Ague" at the head of this paper.[53]

Greenhow is quick to acknowledge his debt to Thackrah. "After completing my own researches I found that Thackrah has mentioned this disease of brass-founders in his admirable [book] published somewhat more than 30 years since" (178).

Greenhow goes on to describe the syndrome of metal fume fever in exacting and correct detail, arguing convincingly that zinc oxide fume inhalation and no other factor is the cause. He also leaves no doubt about the role played by the work conditions he found in leading to such widespread illness in the brass foundries of Birmingham:

> The copper is first placed in the crucible, and as zinc, the other principal ingredient of brass, deflagrates at the temperature at which copper melts, it is only added shortly before the end of the process, when the copper is perfectly molten. When, after the metals are melted, the crucible is uncovered, for the purpose of stirring them together, and more particularly when it is lifted out of the furnace and the molten brass is being poured into moulds, the zinc deflagrates, and a dense, white smoke is formed, which, almost instantaneously, fills the atmosphere in the casting-shop. (185)

BRASS AS A MATTER OF TASTE

Greenhow's account, based on keen observation from firsthand visits to more than thirty brass workshops, authoritatively established metal fume fever as a verifiable entity. Nonetheless, recognition did not translate into safety controls. Far from it. Greenhow presented his paper at precisely the time when a great age of brass was being ushered in. This is epitomized by the brass bed and related decorative accoutrements of the respectable Victorian household. As documented in *Warm and Snug: The History of the Bed* (by Lawrence Wright, author of an earlier history of the bathroom and the water closet), the modern metal bed was originally promoted as a sanitary improvement to reduce bedbug infestation.[54] In France metal beds remained relegated to hospitals and prisons through much of the nineteenth century. But in England it was a different story, with arbiters of middle-class taste responding to the faux elegance of brass beds such as those so prominently displayed in the Great Exhibition, in 1851. The brass bed also called for appropriate brass accessories: brass door handles and fingerplates and, of course, brass bellpulls to call the servants. Moreover, the appeal of brass was not limited to interior furnishings. The professional person, the medical doctor especially, would be sure to have his name engraved on a brass plate placed prominently by the front door.

Throughout the last quarter of the nineteenth century, foundries in Great Britain, on the European continent, and in North America were churning out brass nearly as fast as it could be made. The industry tended to be regionally concentrated: in Birmingham, as Greenhow had noted and Thackrah before him, and in the United States, in Waterbury, Connecticut, and its environs, an area that became known as the Brass Valley. In 1920 over seventy-five thousand brass workers were in the United States, of whom nearly 40 percent were employed in Connecticut.

Given the size of the industry and the high levels of exposure, this period saw no shortage of metal fume fever cases. The condition also came to be called *brass fever, spelter shakes,* and even *spelter bends* among the workers. *Monday morning fever,* the term that had become synonymous with mill fever, also came into use in brass foundries at this time, as it became clear that symptoms were most likely to occur on the first day back to work after a break. The familiarity of the Brass Valley workforce with fume fever is well documented in the oral histories recorded by the Brass Workers History Project. For example, one factory wife reminisced, "I was married one year. One night my husband was shaking. I didn't know what happened. I said, 'I'm going to call a doctor.' He said, 'No. Just get me a lot of blankets.' Their body gets to a certain temperature, and they start shaking. Like a malaria. He told me after about four hours he was all right."[55]

Despite the prevalence of the condition, medical science seemed no closer to understanding how inhaling an otherwise benign and fairly inert substance such as zinc oxide could produce an influenza-like response. Early in the early twentieth century, however, as human medical experimentation began to become a popular avenue of investigation, a series of researchers turned their attention to metal fume fever. In fairly rapid succession, experimental studies were published in the early decades of the twentieth century, originating from Germany, Austria, the USSR, and the United States.[56] The U.S. studies, spearheaded by Dr. Philip Drinker (a Harvard researcher who later helped develop the iron lung), were published as a series of five research articles in the prestigious *Journal of Industrial Hygiene,* which was then the leading U.S. scientific publication on the subject of occupational toxicology.

Like his colleagues in Germany, Austria, and the USSR, Drinker and his team conducted their experimental exposures on their own members. Whereas the earlier studies took the pragmatic approach of using actual brass foundries as their laboratory, exposing themselves during routine operations while quantifying the airborne zinc oxide levels, Drinker took the protocols one step further. Under controlled laboratory conditions, he created experimental atmospheres of pure zinc oxide, in so doing inducing the classic metal fume response. Drinker notes matter-of-factly,

> The first subject was A, aged 32 years, Assistant Professor in the Harvard School of Public Health. . . . The second subject was C, Assistant in the Harvard School of Public Health. . . . Zinc was brought to the boiling point in an electric muffle furnace and a gentle stream of oxygen was blown across the surface. The effluent zinc oxide fumes passed into a 1,600 cubic foot (45 cubic meter) gas cabinet, producing in about ten minutes a cloud of sufficient density to be capable, during the next five hours, of producing fever.[57]

Drinker and the other human experimentalists documented that zinc oxide induced fever in a predictable and reproducible manner. This fever was accompanied not only by standard symptoms of an acute illness, such as aches and chills, but by an increase in the body's white blood cell count as well, another typical indicator of infection. They were not any closer, however, to understanding zinc's mechanism of action. Speculative theories were floated, including the view that zinc inhalation acts as an antiseptic, killing bacteria naturally colonizing the airways, which, having died, stimulate an immune response mimicking that invoked by actual infection. This hypothetical mechanism was not inconsistent with the scientific understanding then emerging of bacterial toxins and their ability to elicit responses, even after the pathogens that produced them were no longer viable. Neither Drinker nor his contemporaries made the link to cotton dust and the parallel Monday morning syndrome of textile workers.

Following the roaring interest in the health of brass foundry workers in the 1920s, there was an abrupt fall-off in further research or other medical writing on the subject. The scientific disinterest parallels the economic decline that brass production began experiencing. Larger negative economic forces combined with other market factors to depress the industry.

Popular tastes had driven the commercial popularity of brass, but popular tastes change. Brass was taking on a tarnish of pomposity, with pejorative connotations reflected in emerging slang, such as *big brass* for top military personnel and, in England, *brass-plater* for someone who ostentatiously displayed his name and petite bourgeoisie job title by the doorbell.

As early as 1913, Elsie de Wolfe dismissively observes in *The House in Good Taste* that

> For the last ten years there has been a dreadful epidemic of brass beds. . . .
> If your house is clean and you intend to keep it so, a wooden bed that has
> some relation to the rest of your furniture is the best bed possible. Otherwise, a white painted metal one. There is never an excuse for a brass one.
> Indeed, I think the three most glaring errors we Americans make are
> rocking-chairs, lace curtains, and brass beds.[58]

GALVANIZED WELDING

Today, it is still possible to find brass foundries here and there, but they are few and far between. Yet despite the decline in brass making, the potential for zinc oxide fume exposure is more widespread than ever because of the intersection of two technologies completely unrelated to each other and having nothing to do with brass. The first is the galvanization of metal, a process invented in the mid-nineteenth century by which iron or steel is dipped into molten zinc, thus providing a thin corrosion-resistant coating. Barring malfunction, the galvanizing process itself is not associated with fume fever, because the zinc that is used is only melted, not heated to near its boiling point. At the turn of the twentieth century, the introduction of pressurized acetylene gas torches and electric arc welding devices provided the second key element for a recrudescence of metal fume fever. Flame cutting, welding, and the related metalworking practice of brazing all provide the ideal conditions for generating zinc oxide fume from galvanized metal. One of the earliest reports of this problem was carried in a brief notice in the *Journal of the American Medical Association* in its 24 January 1914 issue. Dr. Charles Pfender from Washington, D.C., describes a twenty-three-year-old welder and brazier with frequent attacks of fever, which Pfender at first mistook as malaria. The patient himself called the doctor's attention to his brazing work, leading Pfender to conclude, "I would suggest that more care be exercised in inquiring into a patient's occupation and the conditions under which he labors, especially if his disease is refractory to treatment."[59]

In the years that followed, electric welding and acetylene torching became commonplace in industry, but few physicians seemed to heed Pfender's 1914 admonition, at least insofar as these specific work practices were concerned. In a 1935 publication (in the first of a three-part series on electric welding), almost ten years after his seminal work on metal fume fever, Dr. Philip Drinker noted, "The commonest source of metal fume fever used to be the manufacture and casting of brass. In recent years the fever has been reported from time to time among welders of galvanized iron, the causative agent again being zinc oxide which is formed when the zinc of the galvanized coating is boiled off by the welder's torch."[60]

This was still seen at the time as a novel problem, underscored by Drinker's inability to support the link between metal fume fever and welding with the citation of a single published medical case report of the phenomenon in his review article. (He was apparently unaware of Pfender's case report.) In part three of the same series on welding, Drinker points the way to the impending epidemic of welding-related fume fever that would finally force wider medical recognition of the hazard. In describing the special need for local ventilation when welding in enclosed spaces, Drinker remarked, "In constructing the modern light cruiser, destroyer, and the like, great attention by naval architects is given to the reduction in weight so that welding in place of casting and riveting is practiced widely in shipbuilding. Skilled workers are working on both galvanized iron and steel in places and in positions on ships where a few years ago welding was considered impossible and impracticable."[61]

After the outbreak of World War II and through the immediate postwar period, a number of publications began to appear alerting clinicians, especially factory-based medical staff, to the general hazards of welding and metal fume fever among the swelling ranks of shipyard welders. One of the most thorough and illustrative examples of these is a 1946 case series in the *Permanente Foundation Medical Bulletin* (published by the forerunner of the Kaiser health plan) detailing the cases of four of thirteen shipyard welders hospitalized with fume fever over the previous four-year period.[62]

The authors of this paper, Joseph and Clifford Kuh and Morris Cullen, all three physicians at the flagship Permanente Foundation Hospital in Oakland, California, were quite current with the medical literature of their day. Critically, they did indeed make the connection between their clinical experience and the recent NIH investigation of the epidemic fever among rural mattress makers that had been published only four years before. Monday morning fever, whether due to stained cotton in a mill or zinc fume in a foundry or shipyard, appeared to be the same clinical syndrome.

OLD AND NEW JOB FEVER

My colleagues and I carried out our welding experiments more than forty years after the authors of the Kaiser shipyard report had made the first unifying connection among the disparate Monday morning fever syndromes. In our studies, we were able to identify increases in key intercellular chemical messages, called *cytokines,* that correspond to the time course of fume fever and to the exposure levels that induce the response.

In a separate investigation, we were also able to identify the same pattern of cytokines in another febrile condition called *organic dust toxic syndrome.*[63] This syndrome occurs among persons heavily exposed to agricultural dusts and other organic debris. We reproduced the exposure conditions that are known to cause organic dust toxic syndrome simply by having volunteer gardeners shovel a dusty pile of mulch in a public park. One of the best documented outbreaks of this syndrome occurred following a college dormitory party in which the organizers decided to create an *indoor* atmosphere reminiscent of an *outdoor* hayride. They did this by covering a makeshift dance floor with damp and dusty straw. The partygoers danced up a storm and within a few hours nearly all had come down with an abrupt attack of the "flu"—far too many and too close in time to have been acquired as an infectious disease process.[64]

A new term has recently been introduced into the medical lexicon: *inhalation fever.*[65] Few outside the discipline of occupational and environmental health are familiar with it. In concept the term is meant to unite under one heading metal fume fever, mill fever, and organic dust toxic syndrome, along with a growing number of other outbreaks of odd, flulike reactions triggered by differing industrial processes.

In the early 1950s, for example, a new class of synthetic chemicals was commercially introduced, derived from fluorine conjoined to carbon singly or in molecular chains. Technically known as fluorocarbon monomers or polymers, this chemical family includes freon and Teflon. Only after several decades of use did a number of risks from fluorocarbons become known or suspected, ranging from reproductive effects to ozone depletion. In contrast, it became apparent soon after their introduction into the marketplace that some of these substances, especially when overheated, release byproducts that cause fever and flu symptoms. One of the most common sources of what came to be called *polymer fume fever* was the smoke from the tainted cigarettes of workers who had inadvertently contaminated their fingers with workplace chemicals.[66]

A few years later, another new illness began to be reported in factories with large humidifying systems, especially if the humidifiers were run on an industrial scale to keep process materials from becoming too dry. The printing industry has been particularly prone to outbreaks of *humidifier fever.* These outbreaks have been traced to bacterial contamination of recirculating water. The bacteria in these scenarios do not cause actual infection, but their breakdown products, especially endotoxin and related natural feverinducing biological materials, are present in significant concentrations.

An especially noteworthy outbreak of a specific variant of humidifier fever occurred in an office building in Pontiac, Michigan. The precise trigger of the Pontiac fever outbreak went undiscovered for years.[67] Only after the causal microbe of Legionnaire's disease was identified did it become clear, by analyzing blood samples for antibody levels, that the *Legionella* bacterium, in addition to causing outright infection, could induce a form of inhalation fever. More recently, not only humidifiers but also indoor fountains and the other water sculptures so common in enclosed shopping malls have also come to be suspect sources for contaminated aerosols that might be linked to inhalation fever.

The same contamination can also occur in machining lubricants and various metalworking coolants. The natural oils so suspected of being a source of "putrid effluvia" by Dr. Percival and his colleagues in the eighteenth century have almost all been replaced by synthetic, water-based fluids that recycle almost indefinitely in almost any modern factory with moving parts. The natural lubricants had carried at least some inherent antimicrobial power, but the synthetic cooling fluids are wholly dependent on powerful antibiotics and sterilizing agents to keep them from becoming completely overgrown with bacteria. Unfortunately, these additives are often insufficient to the task or may even select for obscure microbes. Not only may they be capable of causing inhalation fever, but also they may induce asthmalike responses and symptoms of bronchitis not unlike the early stages of byssinosis.[68]

Mill fever and byssinosis, in their original forms, have not disappeared. Occasional epidemics of acute mill fever still occur, such as that reported among the peasants in the Yao-Ji commune in Hubei Province, China, in 1983. A flood in October of that year had inundated the mature cotton, which became overgrown with contaminants as a result. A total of 10,258 cases of *cotton fever* were recorded as a result.[69]

But what is far more troubling is the ongoing incubation of future cases of byssinosis in cotton carding rooms and other textile operations around the world. Fifty years of detailed epidemiological study, first in Great Britain, then in the United States, and more recently in China and India, have delineated in exceeding detail the relationship between textile dust exposure and the disease it causes. These studies have relied on refinements of the same breath-size measurements that Thackrah carried out among flax workers more than 150 years ago, only what he called a *pulmometer* to measure breathing capacity is now called a *spirometer*. Moreover, the findings have not been so very different.[70]

Just as there is now a clear and accepted body of scientific knowledge confirming the levels of cotton dust exposure that trigger disease, so too has engineering science yielded technically straightforward control measures that can ensure the prevention of byssinosis. In fact, little about potential engineering controls is different from the simple steps the consumptive Bessy outlined to her sick-caller friend in *North and South*. Even less has changed about the principal obstacle to protection, as Bessy knew too well. "That wheel costs a deal of money . . . and brings in no profit."[71]

One of the first major fights of the U.S. Occupational Safety and Health Administration, newly formed in 1970, was over a proposed standard for cotton dust exposure, intended to prevent byssinosis. At its inception, OSHA put in place a national regulation on cotton dust intended to limit exposure levels to one thousand micrograms of dust per liter of air. By 1974, the National Institute for Occupational Health (OSHA's research arm) recommended reducing that level by 80 percent, to two hundred micrograms. OSHA then opened a period of public comment on this proposal and was petitioned by the Textile Workers Union to promulgate an even more stringent exposure limit of half that value again. After a two-year delay, in late 1976 OSHA went ahead with the two hundred microgram proposal and then proceeded to hold hearings and otherwise review matters for another two years. Finally in 1978, OSHA issued a new standard in which it significantly backed off from the 200 microgram limit, granting most sectors of the industry except yarn making a limit of 500 and some as high as 750 micrograms. OSHA and NIOSH both acknowledged, however, that even at 200 micrograms, more than one out of ten textile yarn workers might develop early-stage byssinosis.

Despite the more lenient standard, OSHA was immediately sued by the American Textile Manufacturers Institute, which charged that *cost-benefit analysis* had not sufficiently driven standard setting. By this they meant that OSHA had not shown how the costs of ill health would outweigh the equipment costs in dollars and cents. In June 1971, the United States Supreme Court sided with OSHA in a landmark decision finding that a cost-benefit rationale was not required by OSHA in promulgating protective standards, as long as those standards were feasible. The Court's five-to-three decision, in an opinion delivered by Justice Brennan, documents that at the time of the new standard, an estimated hundred thousand U.S. active or retired workers suffered from byssinosis, thirty-five thousand of whom had advanced disease. In one of the footnotes to his opinion, Justice Brennan quotes from the testimony of affected workers submitted in evidence,

I suppose I had a breathing problem since 1973. I just kept on getting sick and began losing time at the mill. Every time that I go into the mill I get deathly sick, choking and vomiting losing my breath. It would blow down all that lint and cotton and I have clothes right here where I have wore and they have been washed several times and I would like for you all to see them. That will not come out in washing.[72]

Job fever remains a common problem. To date, neither OSHA nor any other U.S. regulatory agency has developed any protective standard for endotoxin exposure. Even though endotoxin is likely to be responsible for mill fever and many related syndromes, it is unlikely to come up for control any time soon. Maybe, like the worker with byssinosis, everyone has just assumed that it will work itself out in the wash.

Inhalation fever gets relatively little attention, at least from regulators or scientific researchers. "Metal fume fever" did hit the pop charts not long ago in the form of a gritty rock ballad with the chorus, "I got the fever; I got metal fume fever."[73] The chorus is followed by the fatalistic assessment:

You might as well do dope
You're gonna get sick
Of something nasty
Out in the modern world

The findings from our laboratory studies of welders support the theory that zinc oxide stimulates the immune response, somehow causing it to mimic the body's attempts to fight off infection. Any potential benefits of the zinc oxide response, attributes that could hold the promise of therapeutic uses, also remain to be fully explored.

The inhalation fever syndrome on its own may not be dangerous, but it points the way to other, far more threatening exposures with which it is often linked, such as byssinosis in the cotton mills or toxic welding fumes that are less benign than zinc oxide. Even Teflon and related materials may cause polymer fume fever when overheated only to a moderate degree, but at even higher temperatures (such as when a Teflon pan is left on a lighted burner) they can release deadly irritant gases. Indeed, the song "Metal Fume Fever" may have a point.

The most important lesson the story of job fever teaches us is that toxins are not bound to fixed boundaries of specific jobs or avocations. Cotton mills and brass foundries may at least be heavy industries, even if far apart in what they make. But with job fever, a farmer working with grain dust or an office worker inhaling contaminated air from a vent or even a partygoer at a poorly conceived hayride dance can all be at equal risk.

SEVEN

Emerging Toxins

THE NEW TERROR

Fear of contagion induces deep-seated anxieties. The old specter of epidemic allows each of us to tap into artesian sources of angst. These sources may run faster at one time and slower at another, but they never seem to be drained dry. Although this is not a new phenomenon, in these particular times of ever-multiplying dangers, our capacity to worry is near to overflowing. Some of the diseases that cause the most alarm today are truly novel. Others are not new at all; they were once common and close-at-hand killers that have become remote but, as it turns out, have not been banished altogether. This potpourri of pathogens, new and renewed, is conveniently tied together in a neat bundle labeled *emerging pathogens.*

A quick roll call of these new combatants is easily mustered in our longstanding struggle against contagion. Avian flu, SARS, anthrax, monkey pox, and West Nile virus are all fresh enough that they make other relatively recent insurgents such as hantavirus, Lyme disease, multiple-drug-resistant TB, and even HIV seem like seasoned veterans. Emerging pathogens consume an ever-increasing amount of limited public health resources. The Centers for Disease Control have recently invested many millions of dollars in state-of-the-art command centers to track new outbreaks. These pathogen war rooms are intended to address both bioterror threats and spontaneous epidemics of disease, yet these defenses may be little more than a Maginot Line for microbes. Amid all the heightened vigilance against infectious agents, this system ignores *emerging chemical toxins on the home front,* a major strategic oversight.

As these agents slip in under the radar of a public health early warning system geared up almost exclusively to detect contagions, not poisons, workers on the job are the group at greatest risk. Chemical toxins often first become manifest in the workplace, because this can be a highly contaminated environment. Ironically, emerging pathogens, too, often initially strike among specific occupational groups. Health care workers are an obvious example of those who were especially hard-hit by SARS. Another key occupational group in that epidemic was composed of workers who had contact with animals. Indeed, these workers may have been the original source of the outbreak. People who work with animals for a living (including veterinarians and pet shop employees) were also prominently at risk for monkey pox infection.

Deliberate contamination with anthrax may have endangered letter sorters and carriers in the early years of this century, but anthrax has always been an occupational illness. Previously known by the name *wool-sorters' disease,* anthrax was an endemic hazard of the textile industry for many years, until successful prevention and decontamination procedures were adopted early in the twentieth century.[1]

Many of the same basic principles of case detection and follow-up pertain to the control of both biological pathogens and chemical toxins. In fact, it may not be clear at first whether the nature of any new illness outbreak is an unusual infectious syndrome or a novel intoxication. The medical grunt work necessary to determine this is referred to in the trade as *surveillance.* This work can have all the added bells and whistles of the new CDC emerging pathogens program, but its core attribute is systematic, on-the-ground information gathering.

On 3 October 2001, the *New York Times* ran an article in its Living Arts section on the history of popcorn: "An Old-Fashioned, Versatile Treat."[2] On the same day, the *Wall Street Journal* reported an outbreak of lung disease among workers in a Jasper, Missouri, popcorn factory.[3] This outbreak involved no simple pneumonia. The lung condition in question, *bronchiolitis obliterans,* is a rare, life-threatening syndrome of progressive destruction of the airways. Attention was drawn to the Gilster–Mary Lee Corporation factory when several employees all developed this same uncommon syndrome. Of even greater concern, the suspect production process was far from a high-tech operation. Gilster–Mary Lee made microwave popcorn. The causative exposure was to an ingredient called diacetyl, previously presumed to be an innocuous, artificial butter-flavoring agent.[4]

Bronchiolitis obliterans is an *idiopathic* condition, a medical designation for a disease whose initiating cause cannot be determined. Prior to the popcorn-related outbreak, however, other known toxic-chemical links to the disease occurred. Some of the very earliest medical reports on bronchiolitis obliterans documented that it could closely follow the inhalation of nitrogen dioxide, a potent irritant gas. Nitrogen dioxide is a common by-product given off by decaying vegetable matter; agricultural workers can be at especially high risk. Among farmers, nitrogen dioxide poisoning is known as *silo-filler's disease.* Silo-filler's disease came to the fore in the 1950s, with the use of nearly airtight, enclosed metal feed silos for corn silage raised with high nitrogen content fertilizers, conditions highly effective in producing toxic gas.[5] Farmers who unwittingly entered silos in the first few days after filling were sometimes overcome.

In 1997, a few years before the outbreak of *microwave popcorn lung,* another new lung disease was first reported in a Rhode Island–based factory in which textile workers inhaled nylon fibers.[6] Dust levels were high, but the nylon particles were considered little more than an inert nuisance. This proved not to be the case. Technological innovation had allowed the production of exceedingly fine nylon particles to be used for a new synthetic "flock" textile. Additional *flock lung* cases were linked to the same exposure in four different plants in the United Sates and Canada.[7] Recently other synthetics have also caused disease.[8]

Emerging toxins are not limited to factories or farms. In 1992, for example, reports began to emerge of a chemical pneumonia caused by use of Wilson's Leather Protector, an over-the-counter aerosol leather spray. The outbreak was linked to a newly marketed fluorocarbon contained in a revised formulation of the spray. The product was recalled. Less than a year later, a second outbreak occurred in the United States from the use of Magic Guard, another reformulated leather spray. As recently as 2003, sporadic pneumonia cases were still being linked to similar products newly introduced into the European market, and a new U.S. outbreak occurred in 2005–2006.[9]

Another recurring source of emerging toxins arises from alternative medicinal therapies. In 1996, five years before microwave popcorn lung, an outbreak of bronchiolitis obliterans in Taiwan was caused by an herbal diet aid.[10] At about the same time, another herbal weight loss treatment caused more than a hundred cases of severe kidney damage in Belgium. Nearly half of the victims eventually required dialysis or kidney transplant. As more time elapsed, it became clear that these same patients were also developing cancer.[11]

Synthetic chemicals never intended for anything other than industrial use have also found their way into the alternative health marketplace. In the mid-1980s, dinitrophenol was identified as one such emerging toxin—or, more precisely, reemerging. Dinitrophenol blocks one of the body's main metabolic pathways, driving up energy consumption (cyanide acts similarly). In the 1930s, dinitrophenol had first been introduced as a weight loss agent. It was taken off the market because it induced blinding cataracts. Ignoring this history and circumventing FDA interstate jurisdiction by working solely within Texas, a Houston-based physician opened a chain of weight loss clinics prescribing the chemical to more than ten thousand persons. This episode predated the Internet, which is now the main promotion source for chemical self-treatments.[12] Today one can order dinitrophenol (known in bodybuilding circles as DNP) over the Net, with encouragement from informative commentary such as the following: "There are some serious side effects with taking DNP. Most notable is that your body temperature will rise very noticeably. You will be very hot all the time and it is not uncommon to be soaking wet at the end of the day. . . . So why does anyone use DNP then? Quite simply because it works when nothing else does. And it works very well."[13]

Silver, an ancient toxin, has also made something of a comeback recently. Promoted as a naturopathic antibiotic, chronic ingestion of silver permanently turns the skin a deathly blue-gray color, an intoxication called *argyria*. The most famous recent case of argyria was that of Montana's Libertarian Party candidate for the U.S. Senate in 2002. He had taken his silver in preparation for what he anticipated to be Y2K millennial disruptions leading to antibiotic shortages.[14] After the opening of 2000 passed, the anthrax scare proved the next boon to silver loading, as an alternative, preemptive defense against biological terrorism.[15]

As the variety of these new outbreaks of intoxication makes clear, predicting where the next toxic hot zone will be is difficult. In prognosticating microbial threats, infectious disease experts invoke factors such as ease of global travel, sexual practices, and societal disruptions to make educated guesses (but guesses nonetheless) about what may or may not be the nature of the next epidemic. The scope of emerging chemical toxic threats is even harder to gauge with confidence than that of new infectious risks.

A short list of key characteristics, if combined, however, herald the greatest danger of an emerging toxin. These include widespread use in and outside the workplace, the opportunity for broad environmental contamination, insufficient testing of a new product for toxicity, and identification as a substance from a class of materials that have already consistently proved to be especially hazardous. All of the early warning lights on the map board are triggered whenever either of two classes of agent is introduced: chemical preservatives used throughout the wood products industry and additives added ubiquitously to gasoline fuel. The goal of this chapter is to track the homeland trajectories of these two incoming toxins as each hones in on our communities.

DRY ROT

The story of wood preservative treatments provides a compelling case for ongoing vigilance for new toxins. A good place to begin is the summer of 1824, when a mysterious epidemic broke out among the dockyard workers of Plymouth, England. The outbreak was marked by sporadic cases of a rapidly progressive illness with a high death rate. The typical course was marked by a small, localized inflammation quickly spreading to involve an entire limb, accompanied by fever and soon followed by generalized prostration and death. The mysterious illness came to be known as the *Plymouth dock-yard disease.*

Almost all of the victims were shipbuilders in the yard, mechanics who may have known one another but had a variety of specific duties. In most cases the illness began with a small skin wound, sometimes little more than a trivial injury. One such example was the dockyard surgeon, an unfortunate Dr. Bell, who cared for many of the early cases. Performing a postmortem examination on one of the victims, he inadvertently scratched his finger with an autopsy needle. He was dead five days later.

The diagnosticians of the time were perplexed by this unusual illness. It did not have the classic characteristics of tetanus (lockjaw). They also understood that it differed from a number of epidemic diseases, such as typhus, smallpox, and even common skin infections that could sometimes become generalized but were rarely as fulminant as in the dockyard disease.

A modern reading of the case histories strongly suggests that this was an outbreak of a tissue-destroying bacterial infection (the *flesh-eating strep* of tabloid parlance), very likely transmitted in part by contaminated wound dressings provided by the well-meaning and ill-fated attending surgeon, Dr. Bell. What is also striking to a latter-day observer is the thoroughly modern way in which a litany of environmental agents was invoked in a rendition of possible intertwining toxic and infectious threats that might explain the frightening epidemic.

Prominent on the list of suspects was the wood preservative treatment then in use at the shipyard. Dr. John Butter, a physician who investigated the epidemic at the time, highlighted the issue of wood treatments in his detailed report of the outbreak:

> Some people fixed, with no less hesitation, on that particular mixture, called Mineral Tar, with which sheds and the timbers of vessels are painted over. There are two sorts of substances employed in the Dock-yard under the denomination of Tar; the one a vegetable production, is obtained from Fir, *(Pinus Sylvestrus)* and the other a mineral distillation from Coal. The former is considered salutary and remedial, having been recommended for consumptive patients, in the form of vapour, and as a drink *(Tar-water)* in cases of Erysipelas and other cutaneous affections.[16]

Because the second formulation, mineral tar, was relatively new and thus unlikely to be familiar to his readers, Dr. Butter explains, "This last bituminous substance, which is a compound of Asphaltum and Petroleum, probably from its very offensive smell, has been accused of injuring the health of the labourers, and of proving an indirect cause of this disease. But again it is unfortunate for such surmises, that the victims of death had seldom worked immediately within range of its odour."

To underscore his point, Dr. Butter also interviewed the workers who prepared mineral tar at the dockyard, experiencing on his own the effect of its inhalation. "Moreover, the men whom we saw superintending the process of preparing Mineral Tar, had every appearance of health, and never knew any pernicious effects to arise from it. They considered the vapour as a panacea for some pulmonary complaints, particularly the Asthma, and recommended us to try it. The inhalation excited coughing, and a constrictatory sensation in the glettis *[sic]* and bronchial tubes."

Even before the nineteenth century, wood treatment had become central to shipbuilding. Construction with water-resistant wood was routinely combined with water-repellant resins to ensure seaworthy construction. Pitch derived from pine trees (pine tar) was the first principal form of wood treatment in shipbuilding in Europe. Early written resources highlighting pine as a source of pitch and resins date back to the 1600s.[17] The production of pine tar became the major industry in Scandinavia, where the cold climate was understood to be particularly conducive to a resinous growth yielding high-quality pine tar.

Early pine tar treatments of ships were primarily intended for the vessel's outer submerged hull, in part to prevent destruction by marine worm. Many other parts of a ship that were exposed to the elements were not routinely treated. As time went on, degradation of wood both above and below the waterline became an increasingly important economic matter and even a safety concern in the maritime industry. Financial investments were at risk too, not the least part of which was the sheer amount of lumber necessary to produce a single large wooden ship—as much as two hundred acres of old-growth oak forest. Although similar problems of decay in domestic wood construction were not as prominent an issue as in shipbuilding, they did occur and were probably long-standing, particularly for housing stock situated in damp conditions. They accelerated to a considerable degree in the eighteenth century, as old-growth oak, which was relatively resistant to environmental degradation, became an increasingly limited resource.[18]

As early as 1784, the London-based Royal Society for the Encouragement of Arts, Manufactures and Commerce (the Royal Society of Arts) began offering an award to anyone who might discover a method for "preventing the dry rot in timber" (rewarded either with the gold prize or the silver plus ten guineas).[19] The first book devoted entirely to this question was a sixty-five-page text published in 1795 with the title *Some Observations on that Distemper in Timber Called the Dry Rot*. Early on, this text notes wryly, "There is much reason to suspect that the care generally taken to conceal the knowledge of the distemper, when it existed in a house, has been one of the principal causes why we do not at present know more of the dry rot."[20]

The author of *Dry Rot* bases much of his commentary on personal experience with dry rot in his very own house. He chose, perhaps understandably, to remain anonymous. He astutely identifies critical factors predisposing to dry rot, especially poor soil drainage with constant dampness and construction that seals in humidity rather than allowing it to dissipate. He addresses the common links between dry rot in ships and that in domestic architecture. He also recognizes that mold infestation is a common denominator of dry rot, going so far as to discuss whether molds are best classified as animal or vegetable.

The final pages of *Dry Rot* describe various preventive options. For house posts, this included dipping damp-exposed parts of the wood in melted pitch, coating them with tar, or scorching the ends with fire. The *Dry Rot* book also describes a technique used in shipbuilding wherein green timber oak was dried and then soaked in a mixture of mineral coal and turf. In another treatment for marine worm, wood was treated using an iron sulfate solution. Both techniques are of particular note because they are harbingers of other more industrialized methods of wood treatment that were to come.

The next major publication on the subject of dry rot, Ambrose Bowden's 1815 work *A Treatise on Dry Rot,* is based less on personal experience but contains an extensive review of all of the various wood preservative options then extant.[21] These ranged from boiling lumber in water (suitable for smaller items such as "wood nails") to treatment with alkali or gallic acid and iron or even soaking timber in a solution of water and common salt. As an example of the last method, Bowden cites "the ship *Florida* lately captured from the Americans," whose salted timbers were found to be impressively free of dry rot.

In the first several decades of the nineteenth century, various wood treatments were promoted, although none was particularly successful. It was during this period that mineral tar became as commonly used as pine tar to protect naval timber. The most reliable approach to dry rot prevention seemed to be felling trees for ship timber in cold winter months, using the best old oak that could be obtained.

Contemporaneous with the dockyard fever outbreak, another book appeared—*An Essay Addressed to Captains of the Royal Navy, and those of the Merchant's Service; on the Means of Preserving the Health of their Crews: with Directions for the Preservation of Dry Rot in Ships.* It gives explicit attention to the health benefits of controlling dry rot. "A ship's crew cannot remain long in a healthy state, when the martial walls of their habitation are quickly mouldering into dust."[22]

KYANIZATION

The precise turning point in wood treatment can be fixed to 22 February 1833. It was on that date that Michael Faraday, the leading chemist of his day, giving his first public lecture at the Royal Institution as the new Fullerian Professor of Chemistry, addressed the topic through a presentation titled "On the Practical Prevention of Dry Rot in Timber."[23] Faraday's lecture was not so much a general review of the topic (although he certainly emphasized the overall importance of the problem of dry rot in ships) as a presentation entirely focused on a newly patented process for wood preservation that came to be called *Kyanization.* Invented by John Howard Kyan, this method employed the toxin mercuric chloride as its key ingredient.

Mercuric chloride, also known as *corrosive sublimate,* had long been employed as a pharmaceutical agent.[24] Indeed, corrosive sublimate was well known to be a medicinal poison. What was new in Kyan's process was not simply the application of corrosive sublimate to timber rather than to people but also the use of a specialized tank in which the treated wood was submerged in mercuric chloride solution for at least one week.

Faraday himself had been personally present as a witness to a key demonstration of the success of Kyan's process. Specimens of wood, both treated and untreated, were removed from the Fungus Pit at the Woolwich shipyard after several months of potential moldering. The untreated wood had virtually disintegrated; the Kyanized wood was intact and undamaged!

Faraday brought the near miraculous specimen with him to the Royal Institution, displaying it to his audience along with a model of a Kyanization treatment tank. In his brief manuscript notes for the lecture, preserved in the Royal Institution archives, Faraday noted to himself, "What is elaborate in nature quickest runs to decay—My subject a case of such decay."[25]

In his lecture that evening, Faraday recounted an experience from years earlier when his mentor, Sir Humphry Davy, was approached with a plan to use corrosive sublimate as a fumigant to eradicate pest infestation in the Earl of Spencer's library. Davy, rejecting the idea, noted that the treatment "might possibly be more hurtful to those beings who were more worthy of attention than the maggots in the books."[26]

Despite Davy's doubts, Faraday voiced no personal concern over any potential toxicity to those applying corrosive sublimate or using the Kyanized timber afterward. In laudatory terms, Faraday praised Kyan's invention as a great improvement that justified extensive application. Overall, Faraday's uncritical approach that October evening in 1833 bears a strong resemblance to a celebrity hosting a modern television infomercial.

The following year, a similarly promotional public lecture was given by George Birkbeck at the London Society of Arts. Unlike Faraday, Birkbeck took head-on the question of possible ill effects, noting that the shipwrights who recently built a Kyanized vessel were unusually healthy and concluding with a dismissive commentary aimed at naysayers to the new process. "Recently, some very ingenious gentlemen have chosen to believe that, in the application of timber thus prepared for ships, the crews might be effected injuriously by the exhalation or evaporation of the corrosive sublimate, forgetting, or not knowing, that the corrosive sublimate is decomposed, and it will not sublime at any such temperature as ever takes place in the hold of a ship."[27]

In addition to ship and building construction, other uses of Kyanized timber highlighted by Birkbeck included poles for raising hops in the beer industry (extending their agricultural life from an average of six years to at least thirty) and the Southampton railway's recent application of the Kyanizing process to wooden railroad sleepers (track ties). Hop poles were soon overshadowed by telegraph poles as a major market for wood treatment. Yet as large as this latter use came to be, it was a relatively minor sales niche compared with the market for railroad track ties. This use quickly expanded to become the driving economic force for wood preservative treatment throughout the nineteenth century and much of the twentieth as well.

For six years Kyanization was the only patented process on the market.[28] Kyan was even praised, if not immortalized, in the following song:

Have you heard, have you heard
Anti–dry Rot's the word?
Wood will never wear out, thanks to Kyan, to Kyan!
He dips in a tank any rafter or plank,
And makes it immortal as Dian, as Dian![29]

Despite this early success, all was not smooth sailing for Kyanization. Its introduction into the U.S. railroad market ran into a snag in its first tryout in Maryland in 1838, although it was only documented years afterward when General T. J. Cram reported on the experience to a committee of the American Society of Civil Engineers. "This experiment of Kyanizing timber was the first, I believe, ever practiced in our country. . . . The process, however, was so unhealthy, salivating all the men, it had to be abandoned."[30]

Hypersalivation to the point of drooling is one of the classic symptoms of mercury poisoning, a hazard that would be anticipated when using corrosive sublimate. Kyanization is one of the few work-related hazards to be specifically highlighted in Chadwick's landmark report of 1842, even if the root of the problem is attributed to the victims themselves:

Some workmen employed in "Kyanizing" wood become frequently ill from the fumes created in the process, to which fumes they unnecessarily exposed themselves. Admonitions to care were found to be of no avail, and the employer at length gave notice that he would discharge entirely from employment the first that was attacked with the peculiar illness produced by the fumes of the metal. This threat was acted upon, and no other cases of illness afterwards occurred.[31]

Or at least if any illness occurred, no cases were reported for fear of job loss. It was, however, neither rumor of salivating workers from distant shores nor report of poisoned if feckless laborers closer to home that brought an end to the brief dynasty of Kyan. Rather, it was a sudden burst of competition from a variety of newly patented alternatives. Each was argued to be as effective as corrosive sublimate or more so in preserving wood (although this remained to be established); none was argued to be any more or less safe to use. Effectiveness, however, was beside the point. The writing was on the wall: tested in the balance, Kyanization was found to be more expensive than the other competitors.

By this time John Howard Kyan had already sold his invention for a tidy sum that had been raised through an act of Parliament acquiring his patent rights. He continued inventing and, at the time of his death in 1850, was in New York working on a new filtration system for the Croton aqueduct.

ALTERNATIVES TO CORROSIVE SUBLIMATE

One popular alternative to Kyanization was called *Burnettizing*, a process based on the use of zinc chloride. Its inventor, William Burnett, was physician general of the Royal Navy, and he had a lot of expertise in dry rot. Burnett also was a booster for the use of zinc chloride in other applications, including as a disinfectant fluid and as a preservative for anatomic specimens. When he retired from the navy, he set up his own patent manufacturing company.[32]

Burnettizing came to be more popular in the United States than in Britain.[33] In the States, Burnettizing's binding capacity was increased through an American technique known as the *Wellhouse process*. Separately, the French promoted a related, but chemically distinct, wood treatment using copper sulfate. Yet another metal-based wood preservative method, *Payne's patent process,* relied on pressure treatment with an iron sulfate solution.[34] This process was touted not only as a means of preventing rot but also as a flame retardant.

Compared with wood treatments using mercury, treatments based on simple zinc, copper, or iron salts or sulfates carry considerably less toxic risk for applicators, consumers, and the environment. Unfortunately, none of these safer treatments is used any longer on a significant commercial scale in the United States or even worldwide. Zinc chloride treatment, which was by far the most successful in its time, largely disappeared by the 1920s.

Today, few have ever heard of any of these extinct wood preservative methods. The one group that is well versed in these matters is a small cadre of avid hobbyists who collect railroad track tie nails, dated by the year they were spiked. *Date nails* were introduced by the railroad industry in order to monitor the life span of track ties and thus evaluate the effectiveness of various preservative strategies. My own education on the arcana of wood preservatives is deeply indebted to Jeff Oaks's *Date Nails and Railroad Tie Preservation,* now in its fifth printing.[35] It lists all of the various preservatives that were attempted over the years and specifies when they fell in and out of favor.

CREOSOTE

As soon as the ultimate method of wood treatment was first patented, it became clear that it would dominate the industry. Even the skeptics who questioned whether any wood preservative was of benefit were soon won over. One well-placed critic, Sir John "Let our ships be built of good sound English oak" Barrow, wrote in 1838:

> While on this subject, it is to be hoped that we shall have no more tampering with dry-rot doctors and their nostrums for the preservation of Her Majesty's ships. The steeping of large logs of timber in solutions of any kind is perfectly useless. . . . The only plausible and promising preservative of timber is the gas of the kerasote *[sic]*, procured from the distillation of coal or vegetable tar, which, when driven off in the shape of gas, will penetrate every part of the largest logs.[36]

Barrow may be allowed some confusion in terminology. Unlike the processes patented by Kyan and Burnett, creosote (Barrow's *kerasote*) was not named after a person, although it was, like *Kyanizing* and *Burnettizing,* a newly coined term, meant to convey the sense of "flesh preserving" from its original Greek root. Creosote was first discovered in 1830 by a German chemist sorting a group of substances he had isolated through a laborious, stepwise distillation of beech wood.

Creosote was touted to have great medicinal value, in line with an ancient tradition holding that the tarry essence of mummies, derived from Egyptian burials, also carried great health-giving powers.[37] By 1836, an entire treatise on the subject of creosote had been published.[38] It was written by a twenty-one-year-old medical student named John (later Sir John) Rose Cormack. Much convinced of creosote's potential value as a treatment, he cautions on quality and points out that high-grade, medicinal creosote should be prepared from wood. He warns that much of the product on the market was obtained from the tar of coal gasworks.

Creosote, the medicine, started out as a therapy of questionable efficacy but was soon transformed into creosote, the trusty wood preservative. A promotional brochure from 1858 summarizes the creosoting process and touts some of its virtues:

> The antiseptic properties of tar applied externally, are so well known that they need not be enlarged upon; and inasmuch as the invention consists in charging the pores of the wood, by exhaustion and pressure, at a high degree of temperature, (when the oil becomes extremely volatile and penetrating) with the oil of tar and certain bituminous matters containing creosote, there can be no doubt of the advantage of preparing timber, not exposed to fire, and where appearance is of no importance, by this menstruum; it being a great preventative against worms.[39]

Because creosote could be distilled from coal tar, a low-value residue left over from illuminating-gas manufacture, the product had obvious economic advantages. Because it was patented as an application performed in large, high-pressure tanks, it was efficient for large boards and small railroad ties alike. On top of all that, creosote still carried with it some of the cachet of a new pharmaceutical. What could be healthier than that?

For the next hundred years down to our own time, creosote was to remain the dominant wood preservative worldwide. Wherever tracks were laid, moorings sunk, or poles raised, creosote was sure to be. It was a relatively expensive product (advantageously so for the Germans and British, who controlled the coal tar industry), but it was also effective and persistent. From the perspective of wood fiber, the flesh was indeed preserved. The effect on human flesh, unfortunately, was not so salutary.

Well before creosote was first patented, the coal by-products from which it was later derived were known to cause cancer following prolonged skin contact. The prototypical at-risk occupation, chimney sweeping, was first linked to cancer of the scrotum in 1775.[40] Cases continued to be reported again and again throughout the ensuing century. The key factors causing disease were the nature of the soot given off by burning hard coal in open grates and the accumulation of soot on an area of skin particularly vulnerable to cancer-causing coal by-products.

After a century of the smoldering scrotal cancer epidemic, the problem still had not gone away. True, childhood chimney sweeping had been curtailed through a series of legal restrictions. From adolescence on, however, little had changed since the eighteenth century. In 1892, a series of three lectures on the subject was delivered by Dr. Henry Butlin to the Royal College of Surgeons.[41] His first two lectures reviewed classic chimney sweeps' cancer, describing the cases that Butlin and his colleagues were continuing to see. It was clear that these Victorian chimney sweeps were far from happy-as-happy-can-be.

Butlin's third and final lecture was even more disturbing. Butlin turned his focus to scrotal cancer cases occurring in "predisposing occupations" *other than chimney sweeping.* Three cases were among barge and boat builders exposed to gas tar used to coat wood. This new cancer link should not have come as a surprise. Creosote and related extracts of gas tar are simply essence of chimney soot. Evidence continued to accumulate. A brief report published in the *British Journal of Dermatology* in 1898 presented a case of *tar eruption.* "The patient, a man aged 60, had been employed for thirty years in dipping railway sleepers in liquid creosote, in an air-tight chamber. His arms and hands only came in contact with the dripping planks. His arms have, he says, been in their present condition for years. The forearms, front and back, and the backs of the hands and fingers, have the mouths of the hair-follicles plugged by a black crust."[42]

This patient also had other ominous skin lesions, including scrotal involvement that appeared alarmingly precancerous. Ten years later, a 1908 textbook documented a case of coal tar skin cancer, although not specifically in a creosote worker.[43] In an attempt to stop the cancer, the victim's arm was amputated, but it soon became clear that the disease had already spread and was terminal. He was twenty-seven years old, remarkably young for this type of cancer. Because his father was employed in the same coal tar trade, he might have been exposed as a boy at home or as a very young apprentice. The father, age fifty-eight, despite thirty years on the job, had escaped only with early coal tar eruptions.

The link to cancer was reinforced through an in-depth investigation of the gasworks pitch industry in Britain, carried out just before World War I. This industry manufactured patented fuel briquettes used for home heating. These were manufactured by adding coal pitch to coal dust, a production process that involved many of the same exposures as might be found in making or using creosote. The briquette industry was not large, but it was geographically concentrated in Swansea and Cardiff, South Wales. It was also an industry with an organized labor force. The Dockers' Union demanded an investigation of the growing reports of skin cancer among its members. Their call was taken up by a Swansea alderman, a briquette worker who himself was stricken by skin cancer.

The study that resulted, published in 1912, confirmed conclusively an excess of skin cancer cases. Moreover, this solid epidemiological investigation was matched with an elegant set of animal experiments duplicating the same cancer link, some of the earliest laboratory work ever done in the field of chemical carcinogenesis.[44] The Swansea alderman succumbed to his disease before the investigation was complete, and he was long dead by 1 January 1920, the year that Great Britain added skin cancer from coal tar to an official list of diseases that must be reported to the governmental factory health inspector.[45] Making or applying creosote was clearly an occupation linked to this reporting requirement. In the summer of that year, a description was published in two parts describing a series of skin cancer cases in coal tar workers unrelated to briquette production; four of the sixteen reported cases involved creosote workers. But distinctions within the coal tar trades were somewhat arbitrary. "Tar distilling and creosoting plants are often associated; in the latter process the articles to be treated, e.g., railway-sleepers, are piled by hand on trolleys and run into large tanks into which hot creosote is driven at great pressure. The men who attend this process are generally bespattered with evidence of their calling, their clothes are soaked and their faces and hands browned by long exposure."[46]

The 1920 medical publication is somewhat equivocal about the outcomes of all of the patients it describes, although "J. R.," a sixty-four-year-old who had worked forty years creosoting timber and had noticed various skin warts for at least seven years, is described as having cancer of the scrotum considered "inoperable."

By 1924, a thoroughly documented case report of a fatal skin cancer in a creosote worker appeared in the *British Medical Journal,* replete with a dramatic antemortem photograph of the man's right hand being eaten away by a tumor.[47] This was no mere tar eruption or wart, although it had started out that way.

Even in the face of mounting medical evidence, creosote use was not curtailed. Indeed, it not only continued unabated; it actually expanded. As had occurred in England two centuries before, by 1900 lumber was becoming a more limited resource in the United States. Pretreating railroad ties, rather than simply replacing them more frequently, became appealingly cost effective. At the same time, a technological innovation called the *empty cell process* markedly reduced the amount of creosote required for effective wood preservative treatment, thus reducing costs. In 1923, the U.S. Southern Pacific adopted creosote over zinc chloride as its wood preservative of choice; in 1927 the Union Pacific, the last major Burnettizing holdout, followed suit.[48]

The induction period for cancer from a chemical toxic trigger is twenty to thirty years. In 1956, the *New England Journal of Medicine* reported the first U.S. case of creosote-related carcinoma.[49] In 1956, Peyton Rous, a preeminent cancer researcher, confirmed that commercial wood preservatives cause cancer in laboratory mice, although he did so not as the result of an intentional experiment.[50] Rather, Rous's observations involved mice bred from a new strain, selected for their cancer susceptibility, and raised in standard (for that time) preservative-treated wooden boxes; they developed multiple types of cancer. Despite this evidence, it took another thirty years for regulatory bodies, in the United States and internationally, to officially designate creosote as a cancer-causing agent.

QUERIES AND MINOR NOTES

In 1993, an elderly physician wrote in with a personal query to the longstanding Questions and Answers section of the *Journal of the American Medical Association:* Why couldn't he find a painter willing to apply creosote to his house? He knew creosote's use was restricted, but wondered, "Is there a medical reason for its ban? When I began my practice in 1929, I used to prescribe creosote in the form of drops on a lump of sugar to treat lung conditions."[51]

Creosote for cough (variants of the old beech wood remedy, including chaparral or "creosote bush" tea) had disappeared from the standard pharmacopoeia, having come to be considered inferior to the products of a newer pharmaceutical biochemistry. Creosote wood treatment also came to fall out of favor, at least for some types of application. It was not regulatory restriction and certainly not concern generated by the delayed U.S. medical notice of its link to skin cancer that put a crimp in creosote sales. It was the effective marketing of novel agrochemical products created through technological innovations in petroleum by-products.

One does not have to delve into the archives of obscure trade journals to trace these changes. Past question-and-answer columns in *JAMA* reveal sufficient indications of creosote's emerging competition. In the pages of the June 1936 Queries and Minor Notes section, for example, a physician writes in from Mississippi, "In recent years since the virgin yellow pine timber has been exhausted in this section of the country, sawmills have been cutting second growth or sappy pine and, in order to prevent it mildewing or turning blue, various chemicals are being used as a dip." The same physician goes on to note:

> I saw a patient who has come in contact daily with lumber so treated and his body gets damp with this solution. As a result his arms, legs, and body have broken out in a raised eruption, from the size of a small shot to larger than a split buckshot; most of these places develop a pustule at the crest or peak. The solution being used in this case, I am told, is called Dowicide. . . . I thought possibly that you might know what chemicals are in this solution and what may be the injurious element and the treatment for the condition. Please omit name.[52]

The anonymous doctor from Mississippi was informed in the column's response section that Dowicide referred not to a single substance but to a group of substances made by the Dow Chemical Company of Midland, Michigan. All of the substances in the group shared a chemical structure in which chlorine is linked to phenol, a carbon-based ring structure with an alcohol-like appendage. The skin lesion was a likely result of Dowicide, although the lack of "personal cleanliness may have been a contributory factor." Without continued exposure, the querying physician was assured, the rash should go away.

Less than two years later, in January 1938, a second letter came in to *JAMA*. It was briefer than the first and went directly to the point. "Are you able to give me any information concerning the water soluble salt of pentachlorphenol, an agent which was used as a fungicide in the preparation of lumber and other forest products? I am especially interested in knowing the effects of this agent on the skin and a suitable means of prevention of skin irritation." The respondent to this query was less reassuring. He did not assume that the problem would simply go away:

> Answer.—Published material on the toxicity of the sodium salt of pentachlorphenol (C_6Cl_5ONa) is most meager. . . . In view of the highly toxic properties of chlorinated naphthalenes, it is desirable to regard all chlorinated phenols with apprehension until greater experience may make this concern unnecessary. It is predictable that two types of dermatitis may be produced by chlorinated phenols, one the usual diffuse chemical rash and the second "chlor-acne."[53]

If the health risks from the new wood preservatives were already a gamble, invoking the specter of *chloracne* raised the stakes considerably. Chloracne is exclusively a man-made skin disease. It is the equivalent of an industrial leprosy that can profoundly scar its victims, especially their faces. Worse yet, chloracne progresses years after the cessation of any further exposure. Until the 1930s, this rare, disfiguring condition was virtually unknown in America.

The first outbreak of chloracne in human history occurred in Germany at the turn of the twentieth century. The condition was limited to a specialized workforce exposed to spent carbon rods used up in a recently introduced electrolytic process to manufacture chlorine; other cases occurred when chlorine in these manufacturing plants was stored in tanks lined with coal tar. Soon after the German reports, additional outbreaks were noted in France.

Chloracne was a new disease that resembled common acne but was far more pernicious. The name *chloracne* was coined by Dr. Karl Herxheimer in 1899.[54] He was a leading dermatologist of his day and an astute medical observer. He had also been the first to describe an important manifestation of treatment for syphilis, still known as the *Herxheimer reaction.*

For many years, the nature of the precise chemical trigger of chloracne was debated. The mechanism became clearer in the 1920s, when another new industry emerged using chlorine to convert coal-derived naphthalene oil into a dense waxlike material, much as cooking oil is converted to Crisco. The chloronaphthalene coating material was applied as an insulator in electrical equipment, filling a growing technological demand in an expanding industry.

The new outbreak caused by this insulating wax was reported in 1927 by Dr. Ludwig Teleky, an industrial physician in Germany.[55] He initially named this particular form of chloracne *Perna disease*. Perna was a trade name for the product derived from the German *Perchlornaphthalin*. Fortunately (or unfortunately), this new German corner on the chloracne market did not last. By the 1930s, production was up and running in the United States, led by Halowax Corporation (a division of Bakelite).[56]

Chloronaphthalene and pentachlorophenol are indeed related chemicals; the 1938 *JAMA* respondent was right to be cautious. By November 1939, a new outbreak of disease was documented. Dr. Karl O. Stingily of Meridian, Mississippi, presented the paper "A New Industrial Chemical Dermatitis" to the Southern Medical Association. All of those afflicted shared a common exposure to chlorinated phenols used to prevent fungus attacks in green lumber. Dr. Stingily had seen his first case in 1936 (one suspects that he may have been the very name-omitted physician who first wrote the query to *JAMA* in that year). He was not basing his report on a single lumber worker, however, or even a score of afflicted persons; he had treated far more than that.

> There have been called to my attention some three or four hundred cases affected with this particular type of dermatitis among workers.
>
> The persons most commonly affected are those who come in direct contact with the material in solution. The parts affected are those exposed and those which are contacted by clothing which has been subjected to splashing of the solution. Negro help is chiefly employed in this procedure, therefore most of the cases seen by the writer were negroes *[sic]*.[57]

The skin disease Dr. Stingily observed seemed peculiar to him on several counts. It was pustular, evolving into hard lesions in a process that seemed to spread locally (in fact, like a bad acne, although Stingily never uses that descriptor or the specific medical term, *comedones,* for a blackhead pimple). Even more unusual, in his experience, the skin eruptions seemed capable of continuing for months or even years.

Stingily, who apparently had not read any European descriptions of chloracne, was baffled. "Nowhere in the literature have I found any case of caustic or chemical burn which lasted over a period of years unless the patient was in constant contact with the agent" (1270).

Stingily, lacking any better explanation, suspected that fungal infection might be playing a role in the strange, persistent skin disease that he was observing. In the discussion that followed the delivery of his paper and was published along with it, a colleague from Florida agreed with Stingily's suspicion, suggesting one might attempt more aggressive antifungal treatment. Finally, Dr. M. Toulmin Gaines of Mobile, Alabama, spoke up. He told the story of a man who was sent to him by a lumber company. When he came for the doctor's visit, the patient was accompanied by his two children:

> He had acne . . . with comedones all over his face and back and shoulders and arms and thighs. His two children were a girl about five years old and a little boy about three. They had comedones all over their faces. They had a typical acne on the face. The boy had an indurated acne on the back of his neck such as you would see on a man about thirty years old. . . . I diagnosed it as chlorine acne and the children got it from the patient's clothing. He said that when he came home with his overalls on, the children would grab him around the legs and hug him and he would take them up in his lap. (1272)

The discussion ended. So, too, did any follow-up on pentachlorophenol or related chlorine-containing wood preservatives. Not long after Stringily's report there was a war on, after all. The health problems of workers and their families down south, most of them black, were of low priority. The U.S. Public Health Service's 1943 *Manual of Industrial Hygiene and Medical Service in War Industries* pays no attention to this issue, even though it was certainly relevant to the war effort. (There is passing mention of Halowax-related chloracne, and it does warn also of the remote potential for chloracne from contaminated metal-cutting oils.)[58] The medical press also falls silent on the subject, although a brief notice in a 1942 issue of *Industrial Medicine* reports an outbreak of irritant dermatitis (far more benign than chloracne) among war-industry workers, attributed to newly creosoted wooden floors in several armaments factories.[59] Ludwig Teleky, dismissed from his German post in 1933 and fleeing from Austria in 1939, was by this time also contributing work to *Industrial Medicine* and related publications, although not on the subject of Perna disease. Dr. Karl Herxheimer, in his eighty-third year, was starving to death in the concentration camp Theresienstadt.

The silence on pentachlorophenol was finally broken only after the war, when a 1948 outbreak of chloracne occurred in a rehabilitated factory operation in Germany. Underscoring how little attention had been paid to the problem in the previous decade, the researchers reporting the cases in 1951 believed that theirs was the very first report of this hazard's link to pentachlorophenol.[60]

Medical case reports from a foreign factory would have been little more than a distraction, if noticed at all. The post–World War II petrochemical industry boom was a busy time for Dow and for its corporate colleagues, such as Monsanto. All were knee-deep in similar agrochemical manufacturing lines. Pentachlorophenol was a big-ticket item, part of a growing family of related materials. For example, the extension from a wood mildew killer (a mildewcide) to a leafy plant–killing substance (an herbicide) wasn't much of stretch. Cut down the chlorine atoms from five to three, modify the phenol attachment modestly and, voilà: trichlorophenoxyacetic acid (2,4,5-T).

Back in 1940, Dr. M. Toumlin Gaines of Mobile could have known little about the structural subtleties of chlorine-containing agricultural chemicals. More than twenty years later, had Dr. Gaines been following the story closely, he might have come to worry that the same toxins that had covered the father and his children with blackheads might also cause profound damage to the liver and impair other bodily functions. This story, too, played itself out in the pages of *JAMA*'s Questions and Answers section (the now renamed Queries and Minor Notes section).

In April 1964, a doctor from Nevada wrote in to ask whether the fifty-eight-year-old man he had treated for acne might have contracted his skin condition as a driver of a disinfectant truck, a task that required him to handle both pesticides and herbicides. The responding consultant went through each pesticide, suggesting that theoretically three of them might have caused the problem, but not the weed killers. In his conclusion, he reassured, "The other compounds noted by the inquiring physician I do not believe need be considered as possible causative agents for the acneform lesions."[61]

Two physicians from New Jersey read the exchange and realized that the consultant had made a dangerous error. They quickly wrote to the *JAMA* editor in follow-up, indicating that they had already treated more than forty cases of chloracne in workers manufacturing an herbicide (weed killer) called 2,4,5-T.[62] They also felt one additional case was worthy of note. A consulting federal public health physician involved in assessing the outbreak had applied a drop of the herbicide to his own skin. He too developed a focal case of chloracne shortly thereafter.[63]

In the spring of 1964, production of the herbicide 2,4,5-T was on the upswing. Following its liberal application to the fields and forests of Vietnam, the herbicide came to be better known as Agent Orange, originally a military code name matching the color band around the fifty-five-gallon drums in which it was shipped for application in Vietnam.[64] The letter reporting the New Jersey outbreak of chloracne was published in the 6 July 1964 issue of *JAMA*. A month and a day later, the U.S. Congress approved the Gulf of Tonkin Resolution, authorizing the Vietnam War's escalation.[65]

The physicians who wrote to *JAMA* also published a more complete report of their work in a dermatology specialty journal.[66] That article contained even more disturbing information. Many of the same workers with chloracne also suffered from an otherwise rare liver disease called *porphyria*. This condition is marked by severe metabolic dysfunction that can be manifest in a variety of symptoms, including pain and mental disturbance. One of the more bizarre findings about porphyria can involve abnormal hair growth; one of the victims was described in the medical publication as having hair growth on his eyelids as thick as normal eyebrows.

Although detailed in clinical terms, the official medical report left much out as well.[67] Workers from the factory who would show up for treatment at the dermatologist's private office reeked so badly of chemicals that other patients in the waiting room began to complain. To address this, office visits were scheduled for 6:00 A.M. so that the poisoned workers could come in directly from their night shift and be gone before the practice opened for regular patients. The number of cases increased so much, however, that eventually the dermatologists simply set up a dispensary on the factory grounds, a Diamond Shamrock facility in Newark, New Jersey.[68]

The medical publication did call attention to the fact that many chemical intermediates were generated in the herbicide manufacturing process. The treating physicians presumed that one of these chemicals was causing the disease they observed. They were particularly suspicious that the culprit might be a chlorine-containing *ether* derivative by-product of the herbicide.

An etherlike compound is so named because of the fundamental structure of the anesthetic ether. This includes two molecular groups, each containing a carbon atom attached to the same oxygen atom, which serves as the bridge linking the carbons, like a macramé construction centered on an O ring that designates the oxygen. This particular herbicide was of a phenol type. Phenol is a hybrid of the aromatic compound benzene and an alcohol. Thus, the treating doctors suspected a chemical by-product that consisted of phenol molecules linked by ether bridges. This arrangement is very similar to a key structural chemical attribute of a dioxin molecule.

Dioxin had already been discovered before the Newark outbreak of chloracne and porphyria, but it had not been connected directly to 2,4,5-T. Dr. W. Sandermann, working at the Institute for Wood Chemistry in Hamburg, reported the first synthesis of the chemical in 1957, describing a two-ringed molecule containing four chlorine atoms. The complicated designation for this compound, according to standard chemical nomenclature, is abbreviated by the initials TCDD. Dioxin, its common name, has stuck better, but by any name it is a potent toxin. Sandermann's unlucky laboratory assistant developed chloracne when some of the newly synthesized experimental material accidentally blew into his face.[69]

By the time the Vietnam War was in full swing in the latter part of the 1960s, the serious nature of dioxin contamination from the herbicide 2,4,5,-T was well understood. Dioxin also turned out to be the same contaminant accounting for chloracne due to pentachlorophenol. The industrial manufacture of both pentachlorophenol and 2,4,5-T has a distinct propensity to be contaminated by dioxin as an unintended by-product. In the normal course of chemical engineering, such by-products are little more than an annoying negative value that must be factored into projected output yields. The negative impact of dioxin, however, has taken years to estimate, complicated by the confirmation of many of its additional and terrible effects in the aftermath of the Vietnam War. Some of these include cancer, immune system abnormalities, and birth defects in the offspring of those contaminated.

Dioxin exposure almost always occurs through trace contamination; in concentrated, pure form, dioxin has no commercial applications. This point was underscored by the campaign poisoning of Viktor Yushchenko in the run-up to the Ukrainian presidential elections in 2004.[70] The only treatment, insofar as it helps the body to clear dioxin, appears to be the consumption of large amounts of potato chips that have been cooked in the fat substitute olestra, which draws out the toxin from the body's fat, in which dioxin is otherwise stored long-term.[71]

ARSENIC, CREOSOTE, AND PENTACHLOROPHENOL

In the 1970s, just as an expanding list of dioxin-related dangers was being fully cataloged and initial steps were taken to consider restrictions for pentachlorophenol, yet another wood preservative began vying successfully for an increasing share of the commercial market. This wood preservative was especially well suited to applications in pressure heat–treated lumber in-tended for outdoor use. It, too, was related to a major Vietnam-era toxic herbicide, *cacodylic acid,* or *Agent Blue.*

Agent Blue is chlorine-free. Instead of chlorine, it is based on arsenic, a mineral poison long recognized to be injurious to plant and animal life alike. For hundreds of years, arsenic was known to be the agent that fouled the air from metal smelters, defoliating all growth in the vicinity. Even as far back as 1815, Bowden's *Treatise on Dry Rot* had recommended boiling wood in a solution made with a mineral called *mundic* as one preservative option. *Mundic* is a Cornish term for a locally mined arsenic ore. Bowden noted enthusiastically, "A garden walk where there are some pieces of mundic never has any weeds growing."[72]

Despite this early praise, arsenic never seemed to catch on as a wood pre-servative. For example, the annals of railroad date nails record only two brief periods of arsenic use, one in 1871 and another in the late 1920s. Ar-senic never caught on until recently, that is. The recent arsenic renaissance, in the form of chromated copper arsenate (CCA), is a relatively new phe-nomenon. Over the last twenty years, the blue-green-tinged arsenic-treated wood has become nearly ubiquitous, such as in children's wooden playground installations, welcomed as a relatively safe alternative to the perceived hard-edged dangers of a metal apparatus, for example, a jungle gym. CCA has also become common in many other applications.[73]

On 18 October 1978, the U.S. Environmental Protection Agency first initiated a special review of the trinity of toxic wood preservatives: cre-osote, pentachlorophenol, and chromated copper arsenate. It was the eightieth anniversary of the first reports of cancerous creosote skin lesions and the fortieth anniversary of the initial large-scale chloracne outbreak from pentachlorophenol.[74]

The 1978 EPA review initiative was supposed to be on a fast track. Six years later, in 1984, the EPA tentatively proposed moderate restrictions. The agency's proposals were immediately enjoined by industry trade groups. In response, the EPA proposed an even more limited approach, re-stricting sales to certified applicators, instituting a mandatory consumer awareness program, and reducing (but not eliminating) dioxin contami-nation in pentachlorophenol.

When even the consumer awareness program appeared to be too con-troversial for industry, the EPA backed off this proposal too, deferring in-stead to the American Wood Preservers Institute and the Society of Amer-ican Wood Preservers to run a voluntary public education program as opposed to any required controls. The two major manufacturers of pentachlorophenol objected to the proposed reduction in dioxin contamination put forward by the EPA. The EPA further modified its proposal, increasing the allowed amount of dioxin by 100 percent overall and by 400 percent in any one batch of the preservative.

In backing off the issue of pentachlorophenol, the EPA appears not to have been keeping track of the findings of OSHA inspections. In the early 1980s, OSHA investigated two separate plants where pentachlorophenol misuse was rampant. Typical of the industry, they were small wood treatment operations. In one of them, two out of four employees examined by OSHA had chloracne. On top of that, a series of workers had experienced direct poisoning from pentachlorophenol independent of any dioxin contamination. The principal manifestation of the poisoning was uncontrolled fever, usually misdiagnosed by physicians who did not suspect an unusual toxic syndrome. The wood treatment plant was more savvy in making a diagnosis; its managers routinely fired the affected employees once they were released from the hospital. One twenty-two-year-old worker spared them the trouble of firing him: he died after reaching a peak body temperature of more than 109 degrees. This factory was not an isolated "bad player" in the industry. At roughly the same time at another facility OSHA inspected in follow-up, a twenty-two-year-old worker died of hyperthermia. He'd been on the job for only about three weeks. It is surprising he lasted that long. His assignment was breaking up huge blocks of pure pentachlorophenol with a jackhammer, extremely dusty work, which he carried out in a poorly ventilated shed.[75]

To this day, the EPA has never proposed an outright ban on the use of any one of the three wood preservatives, even though many other countries have done so, especially in the case of pentachlorophenol. Creosote is still widely used in the United States, with many thousands exposed on the job, and creosote cancer continues to be reported.[76] Pentachlorophenol use is restricted but not banned. Along with the effects of dioxin contamination and direct immediate toxicity caused by heavy exposure, the possibility of chronic bone marrow effects related to pentachlorophenol, similar to the effects of benzene, has also been raised.[77]

The failure to effectively ban the use of arsenical preservatives in structural wood destined for human habitations is no less an ongoing threat. Until fairly recently, arsenate-treated lumber has been freely available in every home supply store across the country. Warning labels, spawned by the voluntary system of industry-supervised consumer education, have proven to be no guarantee that every hapless Bob Villa wannabe can't convert "this old house" into a split-level toxic waste dump.

Arsenic contamination of children's playgrounds became sufficiently high profile that even the slow-moving Consumer Product Safety Commission was finally compelled to take up the issue. It had not yet reached a decision on the matter when in 2003 the EPA, under increasing pressure, announced an industry "accord" to halt the availability of arsenic-treated wood for most consumer uses. This allowed the EPA to sidestep any formal regulation; in response the CPSC delayed any rule making it might have been considering in the matter.

TOXINS IN WOOD TREATMENT

What will emerge next out of the hot zone of wood preservatives is far from clear. A variety of other chemical treatments are brewing. Each is touted to be a safe alternative to the existing toxins of creosote, pentachlorophenol, and especially CCA, which has been more in the spotlight recently. As one trade publication rued, "The clock's run out for CCA pressure-treated lumber. The potent brew of three biocides—copper, chromium, and arsenic—ran afoul of bad publicity, and the chemical industry opted to switch to safer substitutes rather than keep fighting the public relations battle."[78]

Non-arsenic-based treatments are becoming popular. One example is copper azole (also know as CA). In some markets outside the United States, this is combined with boric acid (copper boron azole, or CBA). Another copper-based preservative, alkaline copper quaternary, is a major competitor of CA and CBA. Trade names for wood impregnated with these chemicals, such as Wolmanized Natural Select Treated Wood and Lumber and Naturewood Amine Base Treated Wood, give the vague impression of being green-friendly products.[79] For outdoor uses, wood composites of sawdust bound with various polymers are meant to serve a similar rot-resistant purpose. Such composites also have reassuring neutral product names such as Fiberon and TREX.[80]

For each and every one of these supposed *advances,* a healthy dose of skepticism is in order. From corrosive sublimate to creosote and from pentachlorophenol down through chromated copper arsenate, a narrow, technologically driven chemical-manufacturing sector has managed to introduce new health hazards with each wood treatment innovation that it markets. If we are to learn a lesson from the past and recent history of wood preservatives, it is clearly one that teaches us to be vigilant going forward. Chemicals toxic to one form of life are likely to cause human health problems too, one way or another. These problems are unlikely to be missed unless scientific-medical recognition is obscured by misplaced priorities of public health surveillance or economically driven counterspin in the chemical industry's ongoing public relations battle.

The paean to Kyan had promised us that wood doused with his patented anti–dry rot mercurial would never decay; it would be as immortal as the forest goddess Diana. Woody Guthrie's ballad "Deportee" serves as a fitting counterpoint to the song praising Kyan. Guthrie's lyrics describe a time when wood preservatives were intentionally used as a human poison. During the Depression, farmers applied creosote to spoil surplus fruit rather than have it make its way to market at reduced cost or, having been discarded, let it be gleaned for food by hungry migrants. As "Deportee (Plane Wreck at Los Gatos)" describes it, "The crops are all in and the peaches are rott'ning / the oranges are piled in their creosote dumps."[81]

PARKINSON'S DISEASE

Gasoline fuel additives have proved themselves to be toxins every bit as threatening as wood preservatives, even though these gas-pump toxins manifest their effects in quite a different way. Wood preservatives have shown themselves to be inconsistent in their behavior, exerting their toxic effects in a variety of ways that change with each new substance marketed. In contrast, gasoline fuel additives, in particular antiknock agents, have behaved more discretely if, ultimately, more insidiously. Indeed, the ongoing liaison between antiknock additives and gasoline has proven to be an especially dangerous partnership.

The prime concern in the case of fuel additives is an emerging toxin that causes neither cancer nor damage to any of the body's internal organs, such as the heart, lungs, or liver. The vulnerable target in this case is the brain. The impairments that result can touch many of the central nervous system's key functions of physical control and can compromise consciousness itself. The syndrome in question is *Parkinson's disease.* A small technological innovation, if its proposed introduction goes forward on a mass scale, could lead to an epidemic of Parkinsonism dwarfing any incidence seen before. Parkinsonism is a devastating neurological condition. It is not a rare disease; chances are most of us have been personally acquainted with someone with it. All the same, Parkinsonism does not occur frequently, even among people at the ages most often affected, those being fifty to seventy years.[82]

One of the hallmarks of the disease is difficulty walking, marked by a shuffling gait and a tendency to keep going in the same direction, even if this means falling face forward. It's as if the person so afflicted is always starting off as a novice skater, with skates that are broken and feet that are weighed down with lead. Other distinctive features of Parkinsonism include an uncontrollable shaking of the hands and, as the condition progresses, a loss of the ability to make normal facial expressions, down to the smallest smile or frown. This is often described in medical jargon as being *masklike,* but if the description is apt, these masks are without any caricature, either comedic or even tragic, despite the tragedy that is inherent in such loss of functional humanity. Dr. James Parkinson described this disease, now eponymously named, in his *Essay on the Shaking Palsy,* first published in 1817. Of the afflicted persons described in this thin volume, Parkinson seems to have recruited at least two as passersby on the street after noticing their abnormal posture and gait. One of these (Case III) Parkinson describes as

a man of about sixty-five years of age, of a remarkable athletic frame. The agitation of the limbs, and indeed of the head and of the whole body, was too vehement to allow it to be designated as trembling. He was entirely unable to walk; the body being so bowed, and the head so thrown forward as to oblige him to go on a continued run, and to employ his stick every five or six steps to force him more into an upright posture, by projecting the point of it with great force against the pavement.[83]

Even in so brief an essay, Parkinson takes pains to provide the social and occupational background of this case, continuing in the following sentence: "He stated, that he had been a sailor, and attributed his complaints to having been for several months confined in a Spanish prison, where he had, during the whole period of his confinement, lain upon the bare damp earth." Another (Case I) is described as having "industriously followed the business of a gardener," and one other (Case II) as having been "an attendant to a magistrate." Provision of these details may reflect, in part, Parkinson's larger worldview. Although remembered now only by reference to the disease that bears his name, James Parkinson was a remarkable physician–natural scientist–social reformer, prototypical of his time and place.

Years before his *Essay on the Shaking Palsy*, Parkinson had authored a number of radical political pamphlets (most under the pseudonym "Old Hubert") bearing titles such as *An Address to the Hon. Edmund Burke from the Swinish Multitude* and *Whilst the Honest Poor are Wanting Bread—a Sketch*. Parkinson was particularly attuned to the plight of the working man. In *Revolutions without Bloodshed; or, Reformation Preferable to Revolt*, he wrote, "Workmen might no longer be punished with imprisonment for uniting to obtain an increase in wages, whilst their masters are allowed to conspire against them with impunity."[84]

Parkinson even published an essay on work-related hernias *(Hints for the Improvement of Trusses . . . for the Use of Labouring Poor)*.[85] Yet Dr. Parkinson's notice of his patients' trade does not merely reflect the interests of a political reformer. It also reflects good basic medical practice. Parkinson observed and then noted down many of the key features of the condition he reported, but he could not claim to understand either its root causes or its neurological underpinnings.

In Parkinson's time, other nerve palsies were recognized as illnesses caused by workplace toxins such as mercury and lead. For Parkinson, the important link among an afflicted gardener, clerk, and sailor would have been their lack of any connection at all. These are not occupations that would have suggested the mischief of lead or mercury or any other shared insidious poison. To this day, the majority of Parkinsonism cases are labeled idiopathic; that is, their specific cause is unknown.

Even though the cause may not be known, the pathological process involved in Parkinsonism is well understood. In key areas of the brain, nerve cells simply die out. The interrupted nerve cell pathways lead to disruption: some signals don't go out at all, and others, which would normally be damped down through elaborate internal control mechanisms, are let loose when they shouldn't be.

All of these signals, in the final analysis, are electrical in nature, but many are mediated by chemical agents. These agents, or *neurotransmitters*, traffic back and forth among the nerve cells. Modern medicine has taken advantage of this trafficking to supply the body with synthetic neurotransmitters. The goal of such therapy is to try to supply the messages lost from missing nerve cells and thus override the interrupted pathways. The most well known of these synthetic neurotransmitters, L-dopa, was the first major advance in the drug treatment of Parkinson's and was the focus of Oliver Sacks's popular account *Awakenings* (later portrayed on film by Robin Williams as the exuberant neurologist).

Most, but not *all,* cases of Parkinsonism are idiopathic. In fact, quite a number of different and distinct occupational and environmental factors, physical and chemical, have been linked to this specific debilitating condition.[86] As was noted in an earlier chapter, carbon disulfide is one such factor. One of the strongest job-related Parkinson's links is among professional boxers, for whom repeated blows to the head can lead to a form of diffuse neurological damage in which Parkinsonism is a predominant feature. Muhammad Ali is the most famous victim of this condition, known by the lofty diagnostic label of *dementia pugilistica.*[87]

Two other examples are also important, not because they are widespread, but because they show how insidious the chemical triggers of Parkinsonism can be. In the western Pacific a number of mysterious hot spots of Parkinsonism began to appear in the years following World War II. The epicenter of this outbreak was focused in the Mariana Islands of Guam and Rota, where Parkinsonism rates at their peak were a hundred times greater than those of the United States, although the rates have fallen off since. At first, the cause of this rise and fall in Parkinsonism was completely obscure. An infectious agent was initially suspected, but the pattern of disease argued against that theory. Moreover, not all groups seemed equally susceptible; the most traditional, least "Westernized" Chamorro natives of the islands were the ones with the highest rates of Parkinsonism.

The link in the cases turned out to be dietary. A plant native to the Marianas, the false sago palm, or cycad, contains a potent but slow-working natural toxin. Scientists called attention to this source, noting that during the Japanese occupation of Guam (1941–44), food shortages, especially of the staple rice, led to a major dependence on *fadang* seed flour, as the cycad foodstuff was called. In the 1980s, in further support of this link, laboratory primates fed the purified cycad toxin, known by its initials BMAA, seemed to develop features of Parkinsonism, displaying "periods of immobility with an expressionless face and a blank stare, a crouched posture and a bradykinetic, shuffling bipedal gait."[88]

Other scientists rejected the cycad theory, arguing that *fadang* flour contains relatively low levels of BMAA. Although there was no compelling alternative theory, the potential role of the cycad toxin was discounted. By the mid-1990s, scientists were bemoaning the decline in the Guam Parkinsonism epidemic, given that its original trigger might never be identified.[89]

Finally, a scientist from the Institute for Ethnobotany at the National Tropical Botanical Garden in Hawaii, who is an expert on bats, came to a startling insight. Although the BMAA levels in cycad flour are indeed low, this flour was not the only dietary exposure to cycad on Guam. It turned out that the meat of the flying fox bat was a prized Chamorro delicacy, so much so that the local animal population was hunted to the point of extinction in the years preceding the decline in the Parkinsonism epidemic. Cycad served as a key natural food source for the Guam flying fox; furthermore, BMAA toxin bio-accumulated in the animal's flesh.[90] This accumulation occurred without apparent harm to the bat but seemed to explain the dire consequences for humans higher up the food chain.

Around the same time as the first BMAA primate studies, another group was experimenting with what turned out to be a chemical unfortunately similar to the cycad toxin: a narcotic derivative and heroin substitute called MPTP. During May and June 1982, intravenous drug abusers in Northern California became abruptly ill after using a street drug sold as China White.[91] The exact number of persons affected has never been established with certainty but is estimated to be near four hundred. Users reported that immediately upon self-injection, they experienced an unusual burning, followed by a disorienting "high." It was unlike heroin and was accompanied by jerking of the arms and legs and muscle stiffness. In the months that followed, even more ominous symptoms evolved, including difficulty speaking or even getting out of a chair, drooling, and loss of facial expressions. Those affected were younger and experienced a far more rapid progression of disease than is usually the case with idiopathic Parkinson's disease. Yet without question, all were victims of a syndrome that in any other context would be diagnosed as that condition. In the end, MPTP proved to be the neurotoxin most clearly linked to the condition, establishing beyond any lingering doubt that toxins can induce the manifestations of Parkinsonism.

MANGANESE AS A NUTRIENT

The preeminent distinction of being the oldest and most widespread cause of Parkinsonism, however, can be claimed by neither BMAA nor MPTP. This distinction is rightfully awarded to another toxin altogether: the metallic element manganese.

Manganese is not an inherently poisonous metal, differing fundamentally from lead or mercury in this way. Neither lead nor mercury has any role in normal biological functions. If they were ever tried out somewhere on the evolutionary path, they were rejected very early along the way, because they just don't work. Simply put, these metallic poisons screw everything up. Enzymes, the delicate protein tools that biological systems depend on both to construct and to take down the building blocks of life, are essentially gummed up by lead and mercury. Vital work grinds to a halt.

Manganese does not have that effect. Certain enzymes not only don't mind having this metal around but indeed have to have it in order to function properly. Not much manganese is required for the performance of this critical set of enzymatic functions in the body—just enough to place it on a short list of *essential* mineral nutrients. This is not to say that too much manganese is not a problem. The overactivation of key enzymes can cause damage. For example, manganese-responsive enzymes in the brain tightly control the production of key neurotransmitters. The overproduction and release of such neurotransmitters can lead to the overstimulation of nerve cells. This overstimulation, in turn, appears to be a key factor in wiping out pivotal brain centers, the very brain centers tied to Parkinson's disease. Indeed, this mechanism of overstimulation may be shared among manganese, cycad toxin, and the heroin analogue MPTP.

Manganese is not the only metal that can be essential for life and yet at the same time can paradoxically act as a poison when present in too high a concentration. Copper, for example, also serves as a cofactor for important enzymes, but high levels are toxic to both the brain and the liver. Iron, too, can poison the liver as well as the heart when too much is present.

For essential nutrients, for which a balance between not too much and not too little is so critical, the body tries to avoid problems of overload and deficiency through an elaborate system of checks and balances. This system is meant to control how much of these metals comes in, principally from natural dietary sources, and how much is eliminated. Only under extraordinary circumstances do these natural controls break down. Devastating inherited diseases can occur with the overaccumulation of both copper *(Wilson's disease)* and iron *(hemochromatosis)*. Because the buildup takes years to develop, these genetic diseases usually manifest themselves only in adolescence or adulthood.[92]

No known similar human genetic disorder occurs with the overaccumulation of manganese from natural sources. Similarly, no inherited human syndrome of manganese deficiency exists, although a genetic defect related to manganese does ravage certain inbred animal strains. The most notable victim of natural manganese deficiency is the screw-neck mink, so named because the key manifestation of the syndrome is a severe inner-ear failure of balance. Because of this, the unfortunate animals go about with tilted necks, exhibiting an uncoordinated gait and, when put into water (usually a favorite haunt for minks), an inability to paddle horizontally or even float successfully. The manganese-deficient minks were initially bred for a mutation linked to an unusual and highly marketable pastel shade of fur, trademarked as Autumn Haze.[93]

The reason that dietary manganese is not a problem in humans may be simple. Inorganic metallic manganese, the form that exists in the environment, is fairly abundant and yet is very poorly absorbed from the stomach and intestines. Enough can get into the body without any complicated system to facilitate its entry; too little gets into the system to cause harm.

THE NEW MANGANESE CHEMISTRY

The rules of the manganese game were changed by the new chemistry of the late eighteenth and early nineteenth centuries. Manganese, which had been identified as an elemental metal unique unto itself in the eighteenth century, was found to be a critical metal catalyst in experimental synthesis. As chemistry moved from the laboratory to small-scale workshops and then to full-blown factories, manganese was applied on an ever-increasing scale.

No matter how intensely manganese was used in manufacturing, its toxic effects could not have occurred had the route of exposure been limited to ingestion. But when manganese dust or fume gains entry to the body through the respiratory tract, it does not pass through unabsorbed.

In 1837, only twenty years after Parkinson's seminal description of the disease that came to be named for him, a fascinating report was published in a British medical journal. It described a strange neurological illness that attacked five workmen from one chemical factory. Their job was grinding manganese dioxide to be used as a catalyst in chlorine bleach manufacture. The workers labored under the poor hygienic conditions typical of the time. "The surface of their bodies is of course constantly covered with the manganese; the air which they breathe is loaded with it in the form of fine powder." The neurological illness from which the men suffered was characterized by several different impairments:

> The loss of power is most apparent in the lower extremities. . . . The patient staggers, and inclines to run forward when he attempts to walk. . . . The pa-

tient complains that in speaking he cannot make himself heard by persons at a moderate distance, as formerly. . . . There is an obvious expression of vacancy in the countenance. . . . The saliva is apt to escape from the mouth, especially during speaking.[94]

We can recognize today that this description is wholly consistent with Parkinsonism, especially the telltale gait so much like the ex-sailor's in the *Essay on the Shaking Palsy.* It is not surprising that the connection between the two conditions could not be made at the time. Despite Parkinson's detailed case histories in 1817, his classic case description did not become generally appreciated as a distinct medical syndrome until much later in the nineteenth century, well after the initial 1837 occupational report of manganese disease.

Without any specific disease with which to link this isolated outbreak, the first report of occupational manganese poisoning fell into obscurity. Manganese, on the other hand, continued to enjoy a modest amount of industrial popularity throughout the years of the mid-nineteenth century. In fact, it was argued to have a beneficial effect on miners of the ore by curing them of scabies, which at one point provoked a rationale for manganese's use as a medicinal agent.

During this time, manganese even entered into the literary canon through a minor subplot in George Eliot's *Middlemarch.* In the novel, the hypocritical banker, Bullstrode, and the miserly invalid, Mr. Featherstone, make a financial killing from a new manganese-based dye for calico. Unfortunately, the dye destroys the fabric and brings financial ruin to others. Eliot, who was meticulous in her research for *Middlemarch,* kept a preparatory notebook for the novel, which she called her *quarry.* The notebook (which surfaced when the poet Amy Lowell purchased it in 1923 and donated it to Harvard University) includes the following brief entry: "*Uses of Manganese;* In dyeing & calico printing: in the colouring of glass and enamel; in furnishing oxygen & chlorine. It supplies the cheapest oxygen. Also, it is used in making bleaching powder."[95]

MANGANESE STEEL

Despite the diverse commercial applications of manganese, three-quarters of a century elapsed before any further published medical reports appeared recognizing its toxicity. Manganese toxicity, however, could not be ignored indefinitely. A twenty-three-year-old industrial inventor in Sheffield, England, Robert Hadfield (later Sir Robert), saw to a revived interest.[96] Hadfield was trying to meet a key technological challenge in steelmaking. This was an industry that was vital to the booming Victorian infrastructure, and Sheffield was at its manufacturing heart. The beams and pistons and tracks and metal plates that were so much in demand required a steel alloy that was strong yet not brittle. In addressing this challenge, metallurgists achieved a number of technological improvements in the early decades of steel manufacturing, producing different steel alloys by including a variety of metal additives in the basic iron and coal mix.

In all this tinkering, the addition of manganese had already been attempted before the time of Hadfield's efforts, but this approach was abandoned because the increased proportion of manganese had produced a steel alloy that was a brittle failure. In 1882, however, Hadfield discovered a paradox: if the proportion of manganese was increased higher still, not only did the problem resolve itself, but the steel alloy produced was very much superior in its tensile strength.

Worldwide mining, milling, and purification of manganese exploded in response to the sudden demands of the steel industry. This increased demand was intensified by other new industrial applications for manganese (particularly the invention of the dry cell battery). Then, the twentieth-century birth of reinforced steel armaments of modern warfare gave manganese a final extra push.

In 1901, the first renewed scientific notice of manganese-related Parkinsonism appeared in two separate reports; in the following twelve years at least six additional articles on the subject were published, documenting various similar cases. All were in the German medical literature. The first case involved an unfortunate nineteen-year-old, initialed simply "M. J." He was exposed to high levels of manganese dust through a job that required his wearing wooden clogs and stomping on cakes of ground metal oxide heated to 220 degrees on metal plates. M. J. started working in March 1909. By the week before Christmas of the same year, he already had a tremor and difficulty walking.[97]

In 1913, the first nine American cases of manganese Parkinsonism, all from one manganese mill, were reported in the *Journal of the American Medical Association*. The operation employed a relatively new technology, using powerful electromagnets to separate manganese and iron from finely crushed metal ore. It was an extremely dusty process. The paper begins on this optimistic note: "A certain indication of the humanitarian trend of modern times is the ever-increasing interest in the accidents, intoxications and diseases coincident with various trades."[98]

The humanitarian impulse noted in 1913 was apparently not all that it might have been. By 1919, the number of cases at the same factory had climbed to thirty-eight, "driven to extreme intensity of production as a result of the war." The complaints of the mill hands were movingly quoted in their own terse words and sad phrasings such as "My legs—I can't feel good." Another stated simply that he "walks bad."[99] The one new clinical feature of manganese poisoning that began to emerge from these new cases was a tendency among the most heavily exposed to display peculiar mental disturbances such as uncontrolled laughter and weeping.

To the public health hygienists who investigated this World War I industry outbreak, it was self-evident that even rudimentary dust control measures might prevent the worst manifestations of disease. To this was added the "urgent hope . . . that industrial physicians having opportunities to observe men handling manganese compounds will be on the alert for poisoning and see that their observations reach the literature upon the subject."[100]

MANGANESE MADNESS

Over the next fifty years, industrial physicians more than fulfilled the hope for reported observations, often documenting cases from far-flung mining sites where manganese ore was extracted and processed. Their accumulating scientific papers, from Cuba and Japan and Chile among other sites, served to establish beyond any doubt the cause and effect of manganese overexposure, showing how it later leads to the onset of Parkinsonism.[101] Newer studies indicate that welders also may be at risk of Parkinsonism with an early age of onset, especially those who have worked on manganese-rich steel in close quarters. The diagnosis of manganese-related illness in such cases has been made possible by refinements in imaging techniques that allow detection by MRI of subtle signals given off by metal deposits in the brain.[102]

Clinical observation has also shown that manganese can induce psychiatric illness. Moreover, when this illness occurs, it usually precedes the later development of the Parkinsonian features of chronic poisoning. The term *manganese mania* was coined as the descriptor of this psychiatric phenomenon. Signs of manganese mania have been documented to include aggressive behavior, incoherent speech, sleep disturbance, euphoria, and even frank hallucinations.

This bizarre pattern of illness, marked by a form of madness evolving into Parkinsonism, remained inexplicable until the development of antipsychotic medications that were first introduced in the 1950s. The prototype drug of this class, Thorazine, proved potent in its ability to dampen the manifestations of psychiatric illness, such as aggressive behavior, incoherent speech, and hallucinations. A terrible side effect, however, became evident in some of these patients: a syndrome very much like Parkinson's disease. This peculiar adverse effect of Thorazine was linked with other, related neurological symptoms, all of which are tied to excesses or shortfalls of various neurotransmitters. This pattern of toxicity has lent support to a unifying hypothesis of biochemical imbalance linking such disparate conditions as schizophrenia and Parkinsonism.

Manganese is an ideal toxin for illustrating this effect: first, neurotransmitters overload, leading to madness; then, with time, the cells driven to overproduce the neurotransmitter die out, allowing Parkinsonism to become manifest. Indeed, the first laboratory primate study of manganese-induced neurological damage was published in 1924, establishing one of the earliest experimental models of Parkinsonism.[103]

ORGANIC MANGANESE

Until the late 1980s, all of the world's scientific literature on manganese-caused Parkinsonism was limited to observations of the inorganic forms of the metal, simple oxides and salts that are processed and used routinely in industrial applications. Then, in 1988, a disturbing study reported illness in agricultural workers exposed to a newly introduced chemical designed to kill fungus. It was called Maneb, the trade name for a chemical known as *manganese ethylene-bis-dithiocarbamate.* Two young workers with heavy exposure developed Parkinsonism. Other exposed workers were screened and were also found to have subtle manifestations of neurological disease that could be consistent with changes leading to Parkinsonism.[104] The cases were intriguing but inconclusive. Then, in 1994, a second report confirmed the findings of the first. It documented Parkinsonism in a man who had spent two years daily treating barley seed with Maneb fungicide. Two years later he developed Parkinsonism. He was only thirty-seven years old.[105]

Maneb has never been banned, only restricted. A related fungicide, Mancozeb, is also in use. Together their sales amount to more than eleven million pounds annually. As with most industrial chemicals, even pesticides, the premarket testing required for Maneb was limited. It did not include testing on monkeys, for example. Chronic experimental exposure testing in nonhuman primates, the only kind of research study likely to be sensitive enough to detect an effect such as chemically induced Parkinsonism, is expensive and time consuming. Such evaluations are almost never performed routinely for industrial chemicals.

Nonetheless, suspicious environmental toxicologists—and many have learned to be suspicious—were not surprised to learn of Maneb's link to Parkinsonism. The key limiting step (often referred to as the rate-limiting step by analogy to chemical reactions) in manganese toxicity is its poor absorption from the gut. Without that block, we would all be adversely affected merely from the natural manganese in our own diets.

Human manganese poisoning came into existence only when technological change introduced a new variable into the equation—sufficient airborne manganese dust to bypass the intestinal tract. The most obvious path to this means of poisoning is via direct absorption into the bloodstream through the many small vessels that line the lungs. Recent research into metallic manganese has found that this peculiar toxin may have an even more insidious route of entry. Olfactory nerve cells, those responsible for our sense of smell, appear able to take up manganese from the nose and transport it directly into brain centers, where it can do the greatest damage.[106] Other experiments suggest that the body has no specific mechanism to clear manganese away once it has gained entry into the brain, further magnifying the risk of accumulating the toxin.[107]

These characteristics of absorption and accumulation are relevant only to *inorganic* forms of manganese, that is, metallic manganese and related compounds. This is the principal state of manganese that exists in nature or has been exploited by industry, but, luckily for us, it is relatively difficult to achieve toxic exposures, barring the specific industrial scenarios already described. At least that was the case up until recently. Maneb represents a form of manganese linked to carbon, thus transformed into an *organic* molecule, like carbon dioxide and ethanol or, as more apt examples, like benzene and carbon disulfide. Maneb and chemicals like it have the potential to break all the rules when it comes to manganese toxicity.

Modern industrial chemistry has become increasing intrigued with the marketplace possibilities of manganese linked to carbon, as it is in Maneb, even though the potential human health impacts of such manipulations are unknown. Through the allure of such compounds, bleach became another key commercial application of organic products containing manganese. In 1995 the title of an American Chemical Society publication cheerfully pronounced "'Green' Detergent Catalysts Herald Cleaner, Brighter 21st Century."[108] The purported environmentally friendly laundry bleach in question contained a complex organic chemical (derived from *1,4,7-trimethyl-1,4,7-triazacyclononane* and linked to metallic manganese). The novel manganese catalyst was a highly sophisticated chemical hybrid in which manganese is not firmly bound to carbon but rather fits into place. The catalyst was announced with due fanfare, accompanied by publication of the breakthrough chemical structure in *Nature* (the journal where Watson and Crick first presented the structure of DNA).[109] Patented by Unilever, the European arm of the Lever Brothers detergent company, the product was marketed as Omo Power in the Netherlands and Persil Power in the United Kingdom.

The new manganese bleach catalyst did not make it to the U.S. market for reasons that had nothing to do with either human health or the environment. The advantage of manganese bleach was purported to be its effectiveness at low water temperatures, the preferred laundry practice in Europe. Unfortunately, at higher water temperatures, such as those typically used in American washing machines, the same catalyst that worked so well in the United Kingdom and the Netherlands bore right through the clothes being washed. In a plot twist reminiscent of *Middlemarch*, archrival Proctor and Gamble pounced quickly, seizing on the trouble and creating a public relations fiasco for Lever. This was followed by a fiscally painful recall. The organic manganese bleach catalysts were put aside indefinitely.[110]

ORGANIC LEAD

The technical limitations of manganese bleach, not its potential for adverse health effects, drove corporate decision making, thus sparing us all. To date, disease linked to this specific formulation has not been reported. We still have ample reason to be concerned, however, whenever inorganic metals known to be toxic are converted into carbon-linked forms. Not only do such molecules pass into the body much more efficiently than those of inorganic metals, but once inside the system they tend to move into the brain far more rapidly as well.

The best example of this danger is what happens when the toxic metal lead is transformed from its natural inorganic state into an organic, carbon-linked form. Inorganic lead, of course, is toxic in and of itself, even without this modification. Its native inorganic form is toxic because, unlike manganese, it is well absorbed through the intestinal tract. This occurs because the body mistakes lead for nutrients it needs, such as calcium and iron. Nonetheless, when lead is converted into an organic form such as tetraethyl lead, absorption is far greater and the toxin is more potently delivered directly to the brain.

What makes tetraethyl lead particularly hazardous is twofold. First and foremost is its ubiquitous dissemination as a fine, postcombustion inorganic metal dust that can be inhaled and thus absorbed rapidly through the lungs. Second, the parent tetraethyl organic compound is more potentially toxic at even lower levels of exposure than the inorganic toxin from which it is derived.

The controversy over tetraethyl lead goes back to the administration of President Harding. Dr. Alice Hamilton, writing about events that had taken place twenty years earlier, had this to say about tetraethyl lead in her 1944 autobiography, *Exploring the Dangerous Trades:* "This is a very dangerous form of lead, it is more quickly absorbed than any of those ordinarily used in industry and concentrates in the central nervous system, causing insomnia, excitement, twitching muscles, hallucinations like those of delirium tremens, even maniacal attacks and convulsions, and death." Hamilton goes on to describe the publicity surrounding the new toxin:

> In 1923–1924 . . . newspapers carried stories of a number of cases of severe poisoning among chemists and workmen who had been exposed to a new poison, tetraethyl lead, which was being produced by *one large company.* . . . The New York World took up the crusade against this dangerous poison; there was widespread panic lest the use of the blended gasoline involve risk to the public; several states hastily prohibited the sale of "ethyl gasoline" and foreign countries threatened to forbid its import. . . . [At] a conference in May 1925 . . . industrialists, chemists, labor representatives, and physicians agreed to entrust the problem to a small group of experts. . . . The committee found that the hazard to producers and blenders could be wholly prevented by mechanical devices and the danger to garage workers was slight and to users none at all. (italics added)[111]

In fact, the users were actually in danger after all. The reassuring experts were all proved to be very much wrong, as the ultimate folly of leaded gasoline amply showed us. The lesson of the misguided consultants is particularly instructive on this score.[112] Low-level exposure to lead, introduced in the environment through tetraethyl lead added to gasoline, has been implicated as a cause of widespread, subtle neurological damage for millions of people around the globe. Those most at risk have been children, whose developing nervous systems are particularly prone to damage from toxins that affect the brain.

In the United States, the relatively recent elimination of leaded gasoline has been one of the greatest single environmental accomplishments of the last fifty years.[113] The European Community and other industrialized countries have also been phasing out tetraethyl lead. Even these progressive, albeit halting, steps have been taken only after a vociferous regulatory debate and a long delay.

There is, however, another aspect to this story: an important unanswered question. Whatever became of that discreetly unnamed *one large company* noted by Alice Hamilton as championing tetraethyl lead back in 1924? *"Together we're making the world run smoother"* announces the motto emblazoned on an annual report cover of Ethyl Corporation—the corporate equivalent of the veteran stage hoofer belting out a lyric to insist that she's still here.[114]

This tagline about making the world run smoother was meant to give prominence to Ethyl's acquisitions in the lubricant additives business. In fact, a hefty component of corporate cash flow (total annual sales in the range of three-quarters of a billion dollars) still comes from none other than tetraethyl lead. This fact is hard to tease out, because around three hundred million dollars in lead sales is funneled through offshore marketing agreements that do not appear directly as Ethyl income.

Nonetheless, the leaded gasoline market is, undeniably, in a long-term decline. Ethyl's R&D folks believe they have a solution to the looming economic problem of a fall in tetraethyl lead sales as environmental controls spread, inevitably, on a global basis. They call their solution HiTec 3000, a lead-free(!), octane-booster gasoline additive. HiTec 3000 also goes by the initials MMT, which, in turn, stand for *methylcyclopentadienyl manganese tricarbonyl.* Remarkably, PaineWebber even described MMT at one point as an "environmentally friendly gasoline additive," but, in general, the stock market has not been that bullish on Ethyl. The defunct newspaper the *New York World* may not be on the scene to crusade anymore, but the *Wall Street Journal* has given fairly close attention to the ups and downs of HiTec 3000.

MMT was developed initially by Ethyl in the mid-1950s. Canada was the first country to be sold in a big way on this organo-manganese fuel additive. MMT has been fully marketed there since 1976, with an annual price tag of thirty-six million dollars. Surprisingly, relatively little study of MMT's environmental impact has been pursued, even in Canada, despite this huge human experiment.

Among the few research projects that have been carried out, one examined air levels of manganese in garage workers with those of blue-collar employees of the University of Montreal. The study investigators were comforted in finding that although the garage mechanics they examined experienced airborne manganese exposures ten times greater than those of the university workers, their blood levels of the metal were only 10 percent higher. A follow-up study of gas station and freeway exposures by the same research group came to similar conclusions. These are the same sort of findings (and shortsightedness) that falsely reassured scientists studying tetraethyl lead in the garage workers sixty years previously. This disturbing parallel was apparently lost on the new generation of technical experts.[115]

Canada, at least at first, was reassured by this research and went on buying HiTec. For Ethyl Corporation, the U.S. marketing nut has proved a bit harder to crack. Ethyl has had its small successes, to be sure. Selling MMT under the name *Combustion Improver No. 2,* Ethyl convinced the U.S. Navy to use the additive to reduce "telltale exhaust" from its fighter and attack aircraft. The same approach has also been used to market MMT as a turbine fuel combustion improver. Still, these uses represent only a fraction of the potential market for automotive fuel additive.

In the United States, MMT has run into unexpected problems from a surprisingly vigilant EPA. In response, Ethyl Corporation has played hardball every inch of the way. Ethyl's single U.S. MMT manufacturing facility, in Orangeburg, South Carolina, may not have been producing at full capacity, but the corporate lights have been burning late in its Richmond, Virginia, headquarters.

To Ethyl, the EPA actions must have come as something of a betrayal, because back in the early 1970s, the EPA had briefly promoted the use of MMT. But the EPA reversed its early pro-MMT stand as a result of concern over hydrocarbon exhaust pollution caused by MMT, not through alarm over manganese health effects. In 1977, the U.S. Congress specifically legislated that MMT could be marketed as an automotive fuel additive only if the EPA granted a formal "waiver," which required a conclusive finding that the manganese additive did not worsen fuel emissions. In

1978, Ethyl sought such a waiver, and the EPA turned the corporation down.

The EPA reevaluated MMT in the mid-1980s and again in 1990, 1991, and 1994.[116] By this time, the agency allowed that hydrocarbon exhaust might not be the major problem with MMT, finding that the principal stumbling block to its approval was the potential adverse health effects of manganese itself. While the EPA continued to consider the matter, Ethyl promoted a series of studies that have come out in academic publications such as the *Journal of Toxicology and Environmental Health*, the *American Industrial Hygiene Association Journal*, and the all-encompassing *Science of the Total Environment*. The thrust of these reports has been: Since most of the population's exposure to manganese is in the diet, not in the air, why worry? Admittedly, an Ethyl-sponsored study of monkeys inhaling high levels of MMT did show "a slight vacuolation of some types of brain tissue" (i.e., brain cells pockmarked by many empty spaces).[117] Remarkably, this study was actually interpreted as being somehow reassuring to the public, ratcheting up the "What, me worry?" approach to a level that even *Mad* magazine might have trouble parodying.

INVITATION TO AN EPIDEMIC

Despite these efforts, Ethyl Corporation was frustrated in obtaining the necessary waiver. Unlike in the tetraethyl lead controversy so many years earlier, dispassionate science alone did not seem to do the trick. So Ethyl Corporation went to court to get its way. In October 1995 the corporation won the most important in a string of legal challenges to the EPA, arguing that the agency had gone beyond its statutory authority in invoking "potential" health risks to block MMT, absent any dead bodies. The federal courts agreed, saying to the EPA, in essence, "show us the smoking tailpipe." The waiver was finally obtained.

The way now appeared to be open to start shipping MMT to U.S. gasoline formulators. Criticism was likely, certainly, and that would call for a firm response. A leading environmental group, the Environmental Defense Fund (EDF), began to take on MMT as a major public policy issue. The group would have to be dealt with. Ethyl was prepared. A full-page advertisement in the *New York Times* in March 1996 opened its public relations blitzkrieg. "Ethyl Corporation wants to remove millions of pounds of smog-related pollutants per year from the environment," read the lead line, followed in the second line by *"The Environmental Defense Fund prefers that we don't."*[118]

While the first sentence was in bold type in the original advertisement, the jab at the EDF below it was printed in a slightly smaller, soothing italic typeface. The Ethyl advertising consultant may have chosen this latter print style to make the form seem less aggressive than the words themselves, subliminally suggesting a friendly social invitation, perhaps.

It was not the EDF but the EPA that responded to the "invitation." In a hastily called news conference, Carol Browner, then administrator of the EPA, attacked Ethyl's advertisement as misleading, bluntly stating, "The EPA believes that the American public should not be used as a laboratory to test the safety of MMT."[119] The agency went so far as to support the EDF's campaign for warning labels on gas station pumps should any fuels containing MMT actually come on the market. Of note, this highly unusual public stance by a federal regulatory agency coincided with the Democratic Party's political offensive concentrating on environmental issues during the presidential campaign in the spring of 1996.

Ethyl countered briskly. One week after the EPA news conference, it distributed a heavily technical, twenty-one-page single-spaced set of briefing materials entitled "MMT and Public Health: *Separating Fact from Fiction.*" This document is a tour de force of scientific spin control (the monkeys with holes in their brain cells were conveniently put aside). It waxes fully polemical on its final page. "While it is apparent that EDF has chosen to focus on MMT for purposes of its fund-raising, how is the 'public interest,' as opposed to EDF's private interests, served through the spread of incomplete information and misinformation about MMT?"[120]

Surely, Ethyl must have felt on the eve of the ultimate victory. The corporation, however, did not realize that inside the fortress of corporate America, a dangerous fifth column was already in place. It seems that the automotive industry was never truly keen on MMT. Ford and General Motors may not have been particularly concerned about the electrical signals transmitted between nerve cells, but they have been worried about the potential degeneration of spark plugs caused by long-term exposure to this chemical. Reportedly in response to the urging of the automobile industry, the major gasoline formulators in the United States, who would have had to purchase MMT from Ethyl, agreed to a de facto moratorium on the use of the additive.

As if this was not bad enough, even Ethyl's old ally north of the border began to get cold feet. In December 1996, Canada's Lower House of Parliament voted to ban MMT, and in April 1997, Canada's Senate followed suit. Needless to say, Ethyl sued, creatively invoking clauses of the North American Free Trade Agreement and claiming 250 million dollars in damages. By July 1998, faced with a costly legal battle, Canada backed off, rescinding its ban. Ethyl stock jumped by more than 6 percent. MMT is still pumping in Canada—with a concentration of up to eighteen milligrams of metallic manganese equivalent per liter of gasoline.[121] In South America, China, and Europe, MMT use is also widespread.

Despite the EPA's waiver, the status of MMT in the United States has been in something of a limbo.[122] In addition to lingering reluctance in the auto industry to accept MMT, another factor delaying its use has been the evolving air pollution control standards for gasoline mandated by the Clean Air Act. Specific regulations promulgated by the EPA define how much oxygenation capacity gasoline must have when it is marketed in areas of high ozone pollution. Although MMT is an effective antiknock agent (like lead), it provides no substantive oxygenation value. Fuel that is modified through additive mixes intended to achieve targeted oxygenation levels is referred to as *reformulated* gasoline. The specifications for reformulated gasoline (which accounts for about a third of the U.S. market) were not changed by the EPA waiver for MMT. To date, the EPA has not allowed MMT use in any reformulated gasoline sold in forty-nine of the fifty states. The State of California, acting independently of the EPA, simply banned MMT altogether, thus blunting potential sales even further.

Needless to say, the story is not over yet. Ethyl Corporation still sees itself as the fat lady waiting to sing. Its hopes have been buoyed by the spectacular failure of methyl tertiary butyl ether (MTBE), a carcinogenic chemical that was widely introduced as the oxygenation additive of choice in reformulated gasoline. MTBE, a persistent chemical that imparts a foul taste and odor to water even at low levels of contamination, was withdrawn after discovery of its widespread seepage into ground and surface water across the United States. The potential cleanup bill may be staggering, a prospect that prompted Tom DeLay, then House Republican majority leader, to promote a 2003 legislative loophole protecting the MTBE reformulators (mostly based in Texas) from any legal indemnity for their product. The DeLay get-out-of-jail-free card was widely credited for the failure to pass the 2003 energy policy bill to which it was appended; a renewed attempt to insert protections for the MTBE manufacturers into an omnibus energy bill also failed in 2005.[123]

Ethyl may have imagined that any review of reformulation policy triggered by MTBE would only be to the corporation's benefit. Such a Machiavellian assessment could be correct. On 11 May 2000 the EPA wrote a letter to Donald R. Lynam, vice president for air conservation at Ethyl Corporation. The letter contained the EPA's formal notification of the detailed safety testing requirements that, if met by Ethyl, could help to clear the way to MMT's wider introduction.[124]

In 2004, Ethyl Corporation restructured. Its petroleum additives operations, including those involving both MMT and the old standby tetraethyl lead, were transformed into Afton Chemical. Afton and the remaining parts of Ethyl Corporation were subsumed under the name NewMarket Corporation. The state-of-the-art Web site for Afton, with a streaming video option, is headed with the new logo "A Passion for Solutions." This is embedded in an azure graphic of water, presumably meant to reinforce the reassuring connotations of the Afton moniker, which plays on Robert Burns's idyllic "Flow gently, sweet Afton, disturb not her dream."[125] Ethyl/Afton was originally scheduled to transmit new data on MMT to the EPA in late 2004; although a first phase report was completed more than a year after that, further studies that are required are not expected until 2008 or later, with additional EPA review and possibly further testing beyond that.[126]

In a 1996 op-ed piece on MMT in the *New York Times,* entitled "Toxins at the Pump," two leading experts commented on the environmental effects of lead in children on the basis of their long experience. Herbert Needleman of the University of Pittsburgh and Philip Landrigan of the Mt. Sinai School of Medicine in New York stated their concerns, expressing a view still shared by fellow scientists and clinicians around the country. "Children are more vulnerable than adults to most neurotoxins. They live and play close to the ground, where fumes from tailpipes settle. The nerve cells in young brains continually change, laying down connections and pruning back others. The effects of such a noxious influence—learning disabilities and behavioral problems—could show up years later."[127]

These very same points can also be made about the potential risks to children using playground equipment tainted with the wood preservative chromated copper arsenate. Moreover, such children are vulnerable to the long-term cancer-causing effects of arsenic in addition to nervous system damage. It is difficult to imagine any more efficient ways of indiscriminately distributing dangerous, long-acting toxins than these: an organic form of manganese employed as a common gasoline additive with ubiquitous airborne spread, and arsenic or other poisonous chemical treatments applied ad libitum to wood products and set out to disperse slowly into a contaminated landscape.

When it comes to wood preservatives, the forces of regulatory control seem to have gone AWOL altogether. They may have been a bit more vigilant in the case of MMT. But in spite of this, regulators can be thwarted even in their best efforts, not only through their own slow-moving rule-making apparatus, but also by being outflanked by legal maneuvering or directly reversed by executive order.

For the most toxic agents, such as MMT and wood preservatives, any legislative remedy short of an outright ban presents an uncertain prospect. Exerting public pressure for protection can be effective in achieving such controls, but such broad-based efforts are difficult to mobilize. One only wishes that James Parkinson, both as the scientist and as the radical polemicist, were still around writing pamphlets and haranguing.

Each of us has been offered an invitation to a future epidemic easily made possible by emerging toxins. Manganese is one example of these. The latest wood preservative waiting to be promoted could be another. The invitation we have received comes printed in an elegant script such as the typeface used in Ethyl's publicity campaign. Embossed with the finest reassurances that public relations experts can manufacture, this invitation obscures the true nature of the threat. It is an invitation that must be declined—we would be foolhardy to do otherwise.

CONCLUSION

THIS IS A TIME OF PARTICULARLY intense political struggles over occupational and environmental health and safety in the United States. Examples of old yet new issues are emerging all the time. I began this book with the description of a case of mercury ingestion as a folk-medicine treatment and juxtaposed that case with an episode of public exposure to mercury through the inhalation of contaminated paint. As this manuscript was nearing completion, a major environmental public policy debate emerged with the proposal of the U.S. Environmental Protection Agency to weaken its air pollution emission standards for mercury, to the benefit of the utilities industry. In a highly controversial action, White House staffers had personally edited the EPA's rule-making proposal, systematically softening the agency's findings of mercury-associated risk in order to justify better the relaxed controls being proposed.[1]

The EPA is not the only regulator in the political crosshairs. The Occupational Safety and Health Administration and its related scientific research agency, the National Institute for Occupational Safety and Health, are also on the defensive now more than ever. For some time at OSHA the trend has been to downgrade penalties and forgo prosecutions, even for the most egregious offenders. In the current political climate, this formerly ad hoc practice has been elevated to the status of de facto policy.

A three-part *New York Times* exposé in late 2003, "When Workers Die," documented this pattern of inaction, both with national statistics and with individual examples.[2] One of the downgraded OSHA cases involved the 2002 death of a twenty-two-year-old plumber's apprentice in Cincinnati, Ohio, buried alive in a trench cave-in that could have been easily prevented. Although of limited means, the surviving family felt compelled to lay out the added expenses required for interment in a mausoleum rather than witness the victim's reburial.

NIOSH, for most of its history since its establishment more than thirty years ago, always held the status of a freestanding health-related institute. Even though titularly a part of the federal Centers for Disease Control (CDC), NIOSH was sufficiently independent to pursue its own research agenda until several years ago. Since then, the CDC has reined in NIOSH, including such detailed requirements as the replacement of its building signage to embolden the CDC logo. The final stricture came in 2004, when the CDC announced a reorganization plan that effectively reduced NIOSH to a CDC department reporting to a midlevel administrator. The response at NIOSH to its marginalization has been to hunker down and promote the most nonthreatening research projects possible. For example, NIOSH has diverted limited resources to the matter of potential attacks by chemical terrorists, a prioritization that is unlikely to make the institute politically vulnerable.[3]

Perhaps the most symbolic representation of NIOSH's new agenda over the last several years is a study that it released to much fanfare in October 2002. This particular study received wide press coverage, including a feature in the health column of the *Wall Street Journal*.[4] The NIOSH report was formally titled *Health Hazard Evaluation Report HETA 2000–0305–2848; City of Long Beach Police Department; Long Beach, California, May 2001*.[5] The NIOSH press release had a pithier header: "Prolonged Riding Linked to Decrease in Erectile Measure in Bicycle Patrol Officers."[6] This was based on a study that was highly unlikely to arouse the wrath of any entrenched power group. Ironically, it is merely a variant of one of the oldest yet new vocational health issues of all time: Hippocrates argued that horseback riding was associated with impotence and sterility, whereas Aristotle held that it augmented sex drive.[7]

The Consumer Product Safety Commission seems to be striving for new benchmarks for ineffectiveness and then congratulating itself on reaching them. In 2003, after a four-year-old child in Oregon wound up in the intensive care unit with severe poisoning from swallowing a vending machine–dispensed toy necklace made of lead, the CPSC orchestrated "voluntary" recalls of over a million similar items.[8] It then relied on importers to carry out their own testing of products in order to determine what constitutes a safe threshold of lead in an easily swallowed toy. By the summer of 2004, the CPSC acknowledged that 150 million additional pieces of leaded toy jewelry had been sold in the interval. Only then did it order a more comprehensive recall. The CPSC chairman Hal Stratton, in announcing the recall, stated, "There is actually a lot of success in this story. . . . We've caught the problem before any known significant damage, and the companies have agreed to the heartburn of a recall and have cooperated fully."[9] Nancy Steorts, a past head of the CPSC during the Reagan administration, served as an adviser to the lead toy jewelry importers in negotiations with her former agency.

In April 2005, the U.S. Senate approved the latest commissioner for the CPSC, Nancy Nord. At one time president of the Republican National Lawyers Association, Nord stated in her confirmation testimony, "The commission should encourage product manufacturers, working cooperatively with consumer and standard setting groups in appropriate situations, to design safety into products so that regulatory action by the commission is a rare occurrence."[10]

The FDA seems to be on a trajectory parallel to those of the EPA, OSHA-NIOSH, and the CPSC and equally off target. The FDA, compromised by leadership gaps, has been criticized in the debacle over aspirin-like drugs causing heart attack and for its failure to gauge accurately the potential risk of adolescent suicide following antidepressant use.[11] This scrutiny is consistent with the FDA's primary jurisdictional responsibility for medications, but its recent track record hasn't indicated any better control of other substances in our environment that we are liable to ingest, such as herbal supplements and chemical additives.

The story of ephedra serves as one example of another such substance. Widely marketed in consumer goods, especially in herbal teas marketed as asthma self-treatments (as the Chinese remedy "ma-huang") and in over-the-counter stimulant aids, ephedra is a product over which the FDA claimed it had no jurisdiction. It was not until Steve Bechler, a twenty-three-year-old pitcher for the Baltimore Orioles who had been using ephedra, collapsed and died at 2003 spring training that the FDA was goaded into action.[12]

Even more dramatic is the tragic case of a toxic chemical dye called FD&C Blue no. 1. With the full approval of the FDA as a relatively harmless coloring agent, this chemical was used until recently in hospitals across the United States. The chemical was added to feeding tube solutions in intensive care units with the intent to trace the flow of material to guarantee that none was passing inadvertently into a patient's respiratory tract. Administration of the dye was permitted at high levels on the basis of animal studies indicating that little of the chemical toxin was absorbed through an intact gastrointestinal tract. Unfortunately, the intestines of an acutely ill person are often not as impervious as those of a healthy lab rat. Beginning in 1999, a series of reports began to appear, all indicating that FD&C blue no. 1 could pass across the digestive tract and into the bloodstream, often with disastrous consequences.[13] It was not until September 2003 that the FDA finally issued an advisory against the practice of using the test dye in feeding tubes.[14]

In the end, it seems that the lessons that pharmaceuticals, industrial materials, and potentially toxic household consumer products have to teach us are not all that different from one another. A new family of calcium-lowering cancer treatment drugs, it turns out, is causing an upsurge in cases of osteonecrosis of the jaw, which hasn't been seen since the days of phossy jaw in the nineteenth-century match industry.[15] A novel agricultural chemical growth regulator, hydrogen cyanamide, is responsible for outbreaks of illness, in part because it acts just like the old alcohol abstinence drug disulfiram (Antabuse), blocking the body's breakdown of ethanol and leading to the buildup of a toxin causing nausea, vomiting, and, in severe cases, heart rhythm irregularities.[16] "Sculpted" fingernails, a product whose application and removal require dangerous household toxins, also turn out to be such a breeding ground for bacterial infection that several hospital epidemics have been traced to the artificial nails of health care personnel.[17]

Regulatory battles are ongoing or looming on the horizon over issues that range from limiting pesticide residues to controlling greenhouse air pollution emissions to reining in diesel truck exhaust (in regard to which the European Union is even more reluctant to take action than the United States is) to banning persistent chemicals such as bromine-containing flame retardants.[18] Detailing each and every one of these examples is not necessary. The general principles that have been elucidated in this book are also applicable to these issues. First and foremost, when a new or reintroduced exposure is at hand, we must determine what history has taught us from other, comparable hazards. We must ask ourselves and, more important, our legislators and regulators, What are the hidden costs of a novel source of profit? Has the price tag for those who will ultimately "foot the bill"—the future cases of injury and illness, the victims of accidents waiting to happen—been factored into these costs?

In parts of the world beyond the United States and Europe, the salient issues are the same and appear in even sharper contrast against a backdrop of inaction and indifference. Apologists for toxic pollution, lax consumer protection, and poor industrial working conditions often claim that the degradation related to these issues is a relative *improvement* in the Third World within the context of expanded industry and economic gain. Laissez-faire economic excuses such as these echo from an earlier time. They rang just as hollow then as they do now.

For example, in many rural Asian and Pacific sites, pesticides are a major cause of death that could be easily prevented.[19] The fatalities, ranging into the hundreds of thousands annually, are almost entirely due to suicides facilitated by easy access to widely disseminated, potent toxins. As in the West, the scenario of grabbing what is most easily available often characterizes self-harm ingestions (especially among adolescents), but the nature of these poisons converts what might have been little more than a gesture (as in taking an over-the-counter painkiller in the United States) to a successful suicide (as in guzzling a poorly regulated organophosphate pesticide in Sri Lanka). Some of these pesticides, the bulk of which can be manufactured only under license from multinational corporations, are banned altogether in the United States; at a minimum they are severely restricted in their sales and their application.

The statistics from the coal industry in China tell a grim story too—213 killed in a single mine explosion in February 2005, 166 in November 2004, 148 the month before.[20] The Chinese have officially estimated that, over the last twenty to thirty years, more than a hundred thousand deaths have occurred as a result of black lung disease from coal dust, with ten thousand new cases appearing every year. Yet nothing is inevitable in all this. Safety data from the largest coal mines of China are similar to those of the United States; it is often the smaller, and in many cases illegal, operations in which conditions resemble those of the West a century or more ago.

One of the most telling international episodes of poor industrial working conditions involves an outbreak of silicosis in Turkey. Silicosis, a progressive scarring of the lung, is a well-recognized hazard in sandblasting, because the dust generated is copious and pernicious. Sandblasting is usu-ally carried out in construction to clean metal before painting it. In Turkey, sandblasting jeans has become an important manufacturing niche in sup-plying an international market hungry for a stylish "distressed" denim look. The small Istanbul workshops in which this work is carried out offer little, if any, protection from the dust. Some workers begin in the trade at age fourteen or fifteen. Their silicosis is already advanced when they are still in their teens.[21]

As important as it is to see the larger societal and even global picture of regulation and public policy, also critical is the appreciation of another re-ality that can be discerned only at a finer level of resolution, in which one can actually make out the faces of the individuals involved. One element is invariably missing from a story such as the one told in these pages: a full and consistent retelling of the experience of industrial disease and environmen-tal illness in the victims' own words. Most of the time, we don't even know the victims' full names. Even in fictional renderings, a victim can be trivi-alized by a nickname or given such conveniently simple specifics as to be little more than a John Doe. Thus, in a broadside the eighteenth-century moralizer Hannah More asks:

Have you heard of a Collier of honest renown,
Who dwelt on the boarders of Newcastle Town?
His name it was Joseph—you better may know
If I tell you he always was called patient Joe.

Although Joe is a good Christian, his workmate Tim Jenkins is a jester and profaner. Jenkins, heading into the mine, ridicules patient Joe, who has had to chase after a dog that ran off with his lunch.

When Joseph came back, he expected a sneer,
But the face of each Collier spoke horror and fear;
What a narrow escape hast thou had, they all said,
The pit is fall'n in, and Tim Jenkins is dead![22]

More recently, we can be edified by the cautionary tale told in Li Yang's Chinese film noir *Blind Shaft (Mang jing)*.[23] In it, the miner-grifters Tang and Song have an ongoing scam in which they counterfeit a coworker's identification, kill the mark underground, and then falsely claim a sur-vivor's compensation benefits while extracting payoffs from the equally corrupt mine owners. It has taken us more than two hundred years and globalization to go from "Joe and Tim" to "Tang and Song."

The stories we are told are not always about fictional inventions such as Joe and Tim. Sometimes snippets of real personal detail come to us through a clinical report or from the transcript of an official commission of inquiry. For example, a pivotal twentieth-century industrial research experiment gives us considerable personal details of one the workers who was a key participant, although we are not told her first or last name:

> No. 2, of Italian origin, was undoubtedly the leading member of the group. She was the fastest worker, showed the highest score in an intelligence test, and possessed the most forceful character in the room. This girl was ambitious and at times hoped to obtain a secretarial post, but circumstances had prevented this. At the date in question, April, 1928, her mother and sister had recently died, and No. 2 ran her father's house, looked after her younger brothers, and was the principal wage-earner of the family. In the main shop, No. 2 had found little scope for satisfaction, but the test room seemed to offer a greater outlet for her ambitions and energies, and she threw herself into the new situation with vigor.[24]

The "test room" was a separate work area for assembling telephone relays off the main factory floor of the Hawthorne Plant of the Western Electric Company (AT&T). The "Hawthorne effect" has since come to mean any change in behavior induced by the mere fact of being part of an experiment, although No. 2's experience could equally be interpreted as the impact of a stifling job and the improvement induced by the opportunity for personal empowerment.

We know both the full name and something of the personal details of Antonio Udina, an old man who was killed in an industrial explosion while road building near the Adriatic coast on 10 June 1898. Notice of his death was printed several days later in a Trieste newspaper. "At 6:30 in the morning on the road being renovated, leading directly to the fields in the a rural area, a mine being activated suddenly exploded, instantly killing Antonio Udina, a good elder of 77 years, who was holding the plunger of the detonator."[25] Antonio Udina, also known as Tuone Udaina, was, as it turns out, the last native speaker of a Romance language called Dalmation (or Vegliote), a language that officially became extinct at his death. Thus, this single event was memorialized while so many other deaths through industrial trauma or occupational illness have remained anonymous, even though each ended a personal voice, if not an entire language.

Only rarely before the modern era did the fine arts provide us with any images of workingmen or women going about their tasks. Ambrogio Lorenzetti's fourteenth-century fresco series, *Allegory of Good Government, Effects of Good Government on the City Life,* and *Effects of Good Government in the Countryside,* gives us a glimpse of laborers in the city and countryside; two centuries later, the mannerist artist Giovanni Moroni's full portrait *The Tailor,* depicting the subject with scissors in hand and looking straight at us, is exceptional not only in its choice of subject but also in the dignity it affords him. An eighteenth-century engraving is the earliest picture we have illustrating a specific work injury. The image, printed on the cusp of the Industrial Revolution, identifies the victim by name: *Samuel Wood, Whose Arm with the Shoulder blade was torn off by a Mill ye 15th of Aug: 1737.*[26]

Novelists, playwrights, and poets sometimes speak for otherwise silent and unnamed witnesses. At its most concrete, this phenomenon is exemplified in Franz Kafka's nonfiction writing: the official industrial safety reports that he filed as a functionary in the Workers Accident Insurance Institute in Prague, which constitute an apt corollary to his fictional account of the individual trapped in a social apparatus beyond his control.[27] Kafka's theme is echoed, with an explicit allusion to the victims of occupational disease, in W. G. Sebald's *Austerlitz.* At one point early in the novel, as part of a longer architectural monologue, its eponymous protagonist comments on the large nineteenth-century mirrors in the room in which he is seated. His digression serves as a kind of verbal footnote, dispassionate and disconnected from the main point he is making. "How many of the workers perished while making such mirrors, as a result of fatal effects from inhaling the vapors of mercury and cyanide?"[28]

George Bernard Shaw is more emphatic when, speaking through Mrs. Warren, he rails against the hypocrisy of a society that can revile a house of prostitution but ignore the exploitation that poisoned his protagonist's sister. "One of them worked in a whitelead factory twelve hours a day for nine shillings a week until she died of lead poisoning. She only expected to get her little hands paralyzed; but she died."[29]

William Dodd lends another powerful voice from an even earlier time. On the basis of his own experiences as a child laborer, he agitated for factory reform. In 1847 Dodd, also known as the Factory Cripple because of a disabling industrial accident that he had suffered when but a youth, published a slim volume titled *A Voice from the Factories.* Although the book is in prose form, it concludes with a heartfelt poem written by the author. It includes this verse:

What is it to be a slave? Is't not to spend
A life bowed down beneath a grinding ill?—
To labor on to serve another's end,—
To give up leisure, health, and strength, and skill—
And give up each of these *against your will*?[30]

In her 1938 work "Book of the Dead," the American poet Muriel Rukeyser wrote the following lines, echoing Dodd's words of the previous century:

these carrying light for safety on their foreheads
descended deeper for richer faults of ore,
    drilling their death.
These touching radium and the luminous poison,
carried their death on their lips and with their warning
    glow in their graves.
These weave and their eyes water and rust away,
these stand at wheels until their brains corrode,
    these farm and starve,
all these men cry their doom across the world,
meeting avoidable death, fight against madness,
    find every war.[31]

These writers' words remind us of our deep responsibility to the voiceless of our own time. It is to them that this work is dedicated.

NOTES

INTRODUCTION

1. "Industrial Disease" by Mark Knopfler, © 1982 by Chariscourt Ltd. All rights in the United States administered by Almo Music Corp./ASCAP. Used by permission. All rights reserved.

2. In *An Enemy of the People,* the protagonist, Dr. Stockmann, pinpoints the source of contamination as effluent from the town's tanneries, pollution of "decomposing organic matter" (presumably from the processing of animal skins). Stockmann identifies the contamination as being "infusoria" (*infusorier* in the original Norwegian). In a modern technical sense, infusoria refers to a specific family of single-celled organisms, but in nineteenth-century usage this term was more generally applied to microorganisms found in decaying animal or vegetable matter. In fact, the metallic toxin chromium is a more likely threat from tannery runoff because of its use in treating animal hides.

3. The history of the 1976 Legionnaire's disease outbreak at the Bellevue-Stratford Hotel was reviewed in 2005 by one of the main protagonists in the episode. See David W. Fraser, "The Challenges Were Legion," *Lancet Infectious Disease* 5 (2005): 237–241. It is interesting to note that although the print article was illustrated with a photograph of the hotel, rights were not granted to include the image in the electronically accessible version of the article.

4. Additional background on the West Virginia silicosis episode can be found in Martin Cherniack, *The Hawk's Nest Incident: America's Worst Industrial Disaster* (New Haven, CT: Yale University Press, 1986).

5. "Silicosis Blues," Josh White ©. Used with permission. The song was originally issued under the name of Pinewood Tom in 1936. See also Josh White, *The Josh White Song Book* (Chicago: Quadrangle Books, 1963), 104–105.

6. The Hebrew reads: "בנפשו יביא לחמו" (translation by the author; all other translations, unless specified otherwise, are also by the author). This can lead to cumbersome translation, for example, as "His sustenance is obtained at the constant expense of his life," found in A. de Sola, *The Festival Prayers* (London: P. Valentine, 1901), 192. The prayer in which the phrase appears, "U-Netanneh Tokef" (ונתנה תוקף), was introduced in its current form in the eleventh century and is attributed to Kalonymus ben Meshullam Kalonymus, but its origins are probably far older. See Rachel Posner, Uri Kaploun, Shalom Cohen, eds., *Jewish Liturgy: Prayer and Synagogue Service through the Ages* (Jerusalem: Keter Publishing, 1975), 170–171.

I. THE FORGOTTEN HISTORIES OF "MODERN" HAZARDS

1. For a similar case report of a mercury-impacted appendix and a review of the literature, see Patrick E. McKinney, "Elemental Mercury in the Appendix: An Unusual Complication of a Mexican-American Folk Remedy," *Journal of Toxicology Clinical Toxicology* 37 (1999): 103–107.

2. The *Morbidity and Mortality Weekly Report* (hereafter cited as *MMWR*) first documented the latex paint source in 1990 on the basis of a family poisoned in 1990. See "Mercury Exposure from Interior Latex Paint—Michigan," *MMWR* 39 (2 March 1990): 125–126. A follow-up survey by the Centers for Disease Control found potentially hazardous mercury levels in nineteen homes painted with the same latex paint brand. See Mary M. Agocs et al., "Mercury Exposure from Interior Latex Paint," *New England Journal of Medicine* 323 (1990): 1096–1101. A single student's recent liquid mercury misadventure—of a sort that might have been completely ignored a generation ago—became a major environmental event. The student's school was closed for cleanup, fifteen school buses also required testing, and the contamination of the family's mobile home was so extensive that it and the possessions in it were deemed irremediable. The mercury had been obtained from a storage area in a dentist's office that also served as a patient restroom. See "Mercury Exposure—Kentucky, 2004," *MMWR* 54 (19 August 2005): 797–799.

3. The history of mercury hazards has been well documented. See M. Buckell, D. Hunter, R. Milton, and K. M. Perry, "Chronic Mercury Poisoning," *British Journal of Industrial Medicine* 3 (1946): 44–63; or, for mercury mining specifically, see George Rosen, *The History of Miners' Diseases* (New York: Schuman's, 1943). The medicinal uses of mercury through the eighteenth and early nineteenth centuries are well documented in such contemporary reports as Henry Bradley, *A Treatise on Mercury; Shewing the Danger of Taking it Crude for*

all Manner of Disorders . . . (London: J. Roberts, 1733); and George Alley, *Observations on the Hydrargyria; or that Vesicular Disease Arising from the Exhibition of Mercury* (London: Longman, Hurst, Rees, and Orme, 1810). The history of lead is reviewed in Richard P. Wedeen, *Poison in the Pot: The Legacy of Lead* (Carbondale: Southern Illinois University Press, 1984); and in Jerome O. Nriagu, *Lead and Lead Poisoning in Antiquity* (New York: John Wiley and Sons, 1983).

4. The *revisionist* label has been applied to environmental commentaries with differing and sometimes contradictory meanings. My usage of this term is intended to be consistent with the critique of Paul Ehrlich and Anne Ehrlich, *Betrayal of Science and Reason* (Washington DC: Island Press, 1996). In that publication, they label rhetorical efforts to downplay or minimize environmental threats as "brownlash." See also Kevin Carmody, "It's a Jungle out There; Environmental Journalism in an Age of Backlash," *Columbia Journalism Review* (May–June 1995): 40–45. An example of an op-ed piece with an environmental revisionist thrust can be found in Nicholas D. Kristoff's promotion of an Internet-based tract, *The Death of Environmentalism.* (See Kristoff's "I Have a Nightmare," *New York Times,* 12 March 2005. Kristoff writes: "The fundamental problem, as I see it, is that environmental groups are too often alarmists. They've lost credibility with the public.")

5. Randall Lutter, *Valuing Children's Health: A Reassessment of the Benefits of Lower Lead Levels* (Washington DC: American Enterprise Institute—Brookings Joint Center for Regulatory Studies [Working Paper 00–2], March 2000). The body of the report is ten pages with three additional pages of references. The quoted text is from the report's executive summary.

6. It is now clear that the modern revisionist effort itself dates at least as far back as the Manufacturing Chemists' Association's efforts to orchestrate a response to Rachel Carson's *Silent Spring* in 1963, soon after its publication. See John H. Cushman Jr., "After 'Silent Spring,' Industry Put Spin on All It Brewed," *New York Times,* 26 March 2001; and Gerald Markowitz and David Rosner, *Deceit and Denial: The Deadly Politics of Industrial Pollution* (Berkeley: University of California Press, 2002).

7. Confusion over the time line and substance of environmental history is underscored by Joyce Carol Oates in her 2005 novel *The Falls,* in which, for fictional purposes, she moves the community struggle over Love Canal back in time to the early 1960s (before the publication of *Silent Spring*) and even adds in a subplot borrowed from the nuclear industry story of Karen Silkwood. An excellent contemporaneous chronology of Love Canal events can be found in John Elliott, "Lessons from Love Canal," *Journal of the American Medical Association* (hereafter cited as *JAMA*) 240 (1978): 2033–2034, 2040.

8. Neil Kensington Adam, *The Pollution of the Sea and Shore by Oil: A Report Submitted to the Council of the Royal Society: For Private Circulation Only* (London: Harrison and Sons, December 1936); the quotations that follow in the text

are from page 6. The only copies that I have identified in public collections are at the University College London and the London School of Economics.

9. Fisheries Preservation Association, *On the Pollution of the Rivers of the Kingdom* ([London]: Fisheries Preservation Association, 1868). See also a somewhat later publication: Vincent B. Barrington-Kennett, *River Pollution By Refuse from Manufactuties and Mines Together with Some Remedies Proposed* (London: William Clowes and Sons, Limited, 1883).

10. An early scientific report on the Donora, Pennsylvania, episode can be found in H. H. Schrenk, "Causes, Constituents, and Physical Effects of Smog Involved in Specific Dramatic Episodes," *Archives of Industrial Hygiene and Occupational Medicine* 1 (1950): 189–194. The Donora episode was also a focus of Devra Davis, *When Smoke Ran Like Water* (New York: Basic Books, 2002).

11. Benoit Nemery has written an excellent review of the Meuse episode based on the primary Belgian reports of the time. See Benoit Nemery, Peter H. M. Hoet, and Abderrahim Nemmar, "The Meuse Valley Fog of 1930: An Air Pollution Disaster," *Lancet* 357 (3 March 2001): 704–708.

12. Philip Drinker, "Atmospheric Pollution," *Industrial and Engineering Chemistry* 31 (1939): 1316–1320, quotation from 1318.

13. W. P. D. Logan published one of the first reports of the 1952 London Fog: Logan, "Mortality in the London Fog Incident, 1952," *Lancet* (14 February 1953): 336–338.

14. Three years before 1952 Logan had reported another similar but less extreme episode: W. P. D. Logan, "Fog and Mortality," *Lancet* (8 January 1949): 78.

15. The London School of Hygiene and Tropical Medicine hosted the anniversary conference on the London Fog on 9–10 December 2002 and has produced a Web-based Smog Witness Seminar transcript of some of the personal reminiscences presented at that meeting: www.lshtm.ac.uk/history/bigsmoke .html. The Greater London Authority also produced a thirty-four-page glossy pamphlet in commemoration of the event: *50 Years on: The Struggle for Air Quality in London since the Great Smog of December 1952* (London: Greater London Authority, 2002).

16. Jean Firket, "Fog along the Meuse Valley," *Transactions of the Faraday Society* 32 (1936): 1192–1197.

17. A number of nineteenth-century reports linked acute air pollution episodes to patterns of increased mortality. See, for example: George Blundell Longstaff, *Studies in Statistics* (London: Edward Stanford, 1891), 376–377, plate XXIV; Frances Alberto Rollo Russell, *The Atmosphere in Relation to Human Life and Health*, Smithsonian Miscellaneous Collections 1073 (Washington DC: Government Printing Office, 1896), 32–33; and J. B. Cohen, *The Air of Towns*, Smithsonian Miscellaneous Collections 1073 (Washington DC: Government Printing Office, 1896), 29.

18. Jonathan Ribner, "The Politics of Pollution," in *Turner Whistler Monet: Impressionist Visions*, ed. Katharine Jordan Lochnan, contr. Luce Abéles et al. (London: Tate Publishing, 2004), 51–63, 236–238.

19. The recent scholarly work of Stephen Mosley, *Chimney of the World* (Cambridge: White Horse Press, 2001), provides a detailed account of air pollution in Manchester, England, in the Victorian and Edwardian periods. See also Stephen Mosley, "Fresh Air and Foul: The Role of the Open Fireplace in Ventilating the British Home, 1837–1910," *Planning Perspectives* 18 (2003): 1–21.

20. Dr. Thomas Scattergood, quoted from a manuscript text of a public lecture, "The Air We Breathe in Large Towns," given 22 November 1886 at the Working Man's Institute (presumably in Leeds) (Wellcome Institute Collection, London). The term *acid rain* appears to have been first introduced in R. Angus Smith, "The Air in Towns," *Quarterly Journal of the Chemical Society* 11 (1859): 196–235. On page 232, Smith states: "It has often been observed that the stones and bricks of buildings, especially under projecting parts, crumble more readily in large towns where much coal is burnt than elsewhere *[sic]*. Although it is not sufficient to prove an evil of the highest magnitude, it is still worthy of observation, first as a fact, and next as affecting the value of property. I was led to attribute this effect to the slow but constant action of the acid rain."

21. The early history of air pollution is covered in Peter Brimblecombe, *The Big Smoke: A History of Air Pollution in London since Medieval Times* (London: Methuen, 1987). See also Paul D. Blanc and Jay A. Nadel, "Clearing the Air: The Links between Occupational and Environmental Air Pollution Control," *Public Health Revues* 22 (1994): 251–270.

22. John Evelyn, *Fumifugium: or, the Inconvenience of the Aer, and Smoake of London Dissipated*, 2nd ed. (London: B. White, 1772). The first edition of 1661 was printed by W. Godbid for the publishers Gabriel Bedel and Thomas Collins.

23. John Evelyn, *Memoirs, Illustrative of the Life and Writings of John Evelyn, ESQ. F.R.S.* (London: Henry Colburn, 1818), vol. 2, 66 (diary entry for 25 November 1699).

24. Evelyn, *Fumifugium*, 19.

25. For an early promotion of the virtues of asbestos, see Giovanni Aldini, *A Short Account of Experiments Made in Italy and Recently Repeated in Geneva and Paris, for Preserving Human Life and Objects from Destruction by Fire* (London: P. Rolandi, 1830). For the earliest treatise on asbestos, see Giovanni Ciampini, *De Incombustibili Lino, Sive Lapida Amianto, Deque Illius Filandi Modo* (Rome: Typis Rev. Camerae Apostolicae, 1691).

26. "H. W. Johns' Patent Asbestos Materials," printed full-page advertisement, *Godey's Lady's Book Magazine*, 1878 (collection of the author).

27. W. E. Cooke, "Pulmonary Asbestosis," *British Medical Journal* (3 December 1927): 1024–1025 (with special plate). In this 1927 publication, in addi-

tion to expanded details of an earlier 1924 case, Cooke also reports the 1900 death on the basis of notes on the case, to which he was given access by the Home Office (the death was given brief notice in the *Charing Cross Hospital Gazette* in 1900). Apparently Cooke was unaware of this case at the time of his initial 1924 publication (see following note). For a summary of the chief inspector of factories data and other early asbestos reports, see Morris Greenberg, "The British Approach to Asbestos Standard Setting: 1898–2000," *American Journal of Industrial Medicine* 46 (2004): 534–541.

28. W. E. Cooke, "Fibrosis of the Lungs Due to the Inhalation of Asbestos Dust," *British Medical Journal* (28 July 1924): 127 (with a special plate).

29. "Section of Preventive Medicine," *British Medical Journal* (6 August 1927): 216–217. The British Medical Association meeting took place on 21 July 1927 in Edinburgh, Scotland.

30. The three papers published as a series by the *British Medical Journal* were: W. E. Cooke, "Pulmonary Asbestosis"; Stuart McDonald, "Histology of Pulmonary Asbestosis"; and Thomas Oliver, "Clinical Aspects of Asbestosis," *British Medical Journal* (3 December 1927): 1024–1025 (with special plate); 1025–1026 (with special plate); 1026–1027. Although the *Oxford English Dictionary* (2nd ed., 1989) (s.v. "asbestosis") cites these December publications as the earliest printed appearance of the medical term, the August announcement (see n. 29) clearly takes precedence. Moreover, Thomas Oliver published another version of his paper one month prior to the December *British Medical Journal* appearance (Thomas Oliver, "Pulmonary Asbestosis in Its Clinical Aspects," *Journal of Industrial Hygiene* 11 [November 1927]: 483–485). Earlier in 1927, Cooke presented a paper that overlaps considerably with the material he presented to the British Medical Association, but this paper refers to the lung fibrosis of asbestos solely as a pneumoconiosis—the word *asbestosis* does not appear: W. E. Cook and C. F. Hill, "Pneumokoniosis Due to Asbestos Dust," *Journal of the Royal Microscopical Society* 47, ser. 3 (1927): 232–238. Remarkably, in the same year, an M.D. thesis entitled "Asbestosis" was also presented (Ian Martin Donaldson Grieve, "Asbestosis," M.D. thesis, University of Edinburgh, September 1927. These medical reports (and that of Cooke in 1924 as well) were preceded by an interesting 1918 U.S. medical publication describing both a series of chest X-rays and some on-site workplace inspections for 137 dust-exposed workers from a variety of occupations. This group included fifteen asbestos workers. Although the authors noted that typical pneumoconiosis did indeed occur in asbestos workers (albeit somewhat later than in coal miners and certain metal grinders) and also stated that the asbestos mills were among the dirtiest buildings they had inspected, they provide no clinical information on any specific case among the fifteen workers exposed to asbestos. See Henry K. Pancoast et al., "A Roentgenologic Study of the Effects of Dust Inhalation upon the Lungs," *American Journal of Roentgenology* 5 (1918): 129–138.

31. Theodore Dreiser, *Tragic America* (New York: Horace Liveright, 1931). Occupational diseases, including asbestosis, are discussed on pages 19 and 196.

32. The *Index Medicus* first began listing asbestosis in its July–December 1927 volume, but only as a cross-reference to the index heading "pneumoconiosis." It was not until 1960 that a separate full index entry appeared.

33. Paul Brodeur, *Expendable Americans* (New York: Viking Press, 1974).

34. Barry Castleman has done extensive work on the issue of the international export of asbestos. See Barry Castleman, "RE: Call for an International Ban on Asbestos: Why Not Ban Asbestos?" *American Journal of Industrial Medicine* 37 (2000): 239–240. Castleman's proposal was later endorsed by Collegium Ramazzini, an international occupational health professional society. See Philip J. Landrigan and Morando Soffritti, "Collegium Ramazzini Call for an International Ban on Asbestos," *American Journal of Industrial Medicine* 47 (2005): 471–475.

35. An excellent review and bibliography on the current and historical aspects of the medical literature regarding cumulative trauma disorders are provided in Allard Denbe, *Occupation and Disease: How Social Factors Affect the Conception of Work-Related Disorders* (New Haven, CT: Yale University Press, 1996).

36. Ralph Barnes Grindrod, *The Slaves of the Needle; an Exposure of the Distressed Condition, Moral and Physical, of Dress-Makers, Milliners, Embroiderers, Slop Workers, &c.* (London: William Britain and Charles Gilpin, 1845). The pamphlet cites in full Thomas Hood's poem "Song of the Shirt."

37. The weaver's lament is quoted in Kate Fitz Gibbon, *Ikat: Splendid Silks of Central Asia from the Guido Goldman Collection* (London: Laurence King Publishing, 1999), 89, citing, in turn, Viktor M. Beliaev, *Central Asian Music* (Middletown, CT: Wesleyan University Press, 1975), 179. The symptoms described are consistent with "tarsal tunnel syndrome," the ankle-related equivalent of carpal tunnel wrist injury.

38. For additional details of the nosology of trade disorders, such as chauffeur's knee, see Martin G. Cherniack, "Diseases of Unusual Occupations: An Historical Perspective," in *Unusual Occupational Diseases, Occupational Medicine State of the Art Reviews,* ed. Dennis J. Shusterman and Paul D. Blanc (Philadelphia: Hanley and Belfus, 1992), vol. 7, 369–384.

39. The earliest English-language report of repetitive-use nerve injury (trade palsies) is in Christopher Robert Pemberton, *A Practical Treatise on Various Diseases of the Abdominal Viscera* (London: W. Bulmer and Co., 1806), 157–158.

40. On Neolithic period cumulative trauma, see Theya Molleson, "The Eloquent Bones of Abu Hureyra: The Daily Grind in an Early Near Eastern Agricultural Community Left Revealing Marks on the Skeletons of the Inhabitants," *Scientific American* (August 1994): 70–75.

41. Henry E. Sigerist, "The Wesley M. Carpenter Lecture: Historical Background of Industrial and Occupational Diseases," *Bulletin of the New York*

Academy of Medicine 12, ser. 2 (1936): 597–609. Sigerist is quoting Papyrus Sallier II (also known as the Satire of Trades), column VI, lines 1–3, and column VII, lines 2–4. For a complete variant translation, see www.digitalegypt.ucl.ac .uk/literature/satiretransl.html (14 January 2006).

42. The National Institute of Occupational Safety and Health and the National Academy of Sciences (Institute of Medicine) scientific reviews of carpal tunnel syndrome are documented in U.S. Department of Health and Human Services, National Institute for Occupational Safety and Health, *Musculoskeletal Disorders and Workplace Factors,* DHHS (NIOSH) Pub. no. 97–141 (Cincinnati, OH: NIOSH, 1997); and Panel on Musculoskeletal Disorders in the Workplace (National Research Council and Institute of Medicine), *Musculoskeletal Disorders and the Workplace* (Washington DC: National Academy Press, 2001).

43. Bruce Bernard, editor of the NIOSH document, and Anne Mavor, study director for the Institute of Medicine report, also provided me with additional background information on the political context of these projects.

44. The U.S. Chamber of Commerce counsel was quoted in a newswire story: Associated Press, "Workplace Controls Could Cost Billions; Industry Groups Say They Lack Scientific Basis," 14 November 2000. A Chamber of Commerce press release dated 13 November 2000 was entitled "Chamber Files Suit to Block OSHA Ergo Rule as Unconstitutional, Unscientific and Unworkable," www.uschamber.com/press/releases/2000/november (7 October 2005). The Chamber of Commerce followed this in January 2001 with a Web-based editorial by Thomas Donohue (chamber president and CEO), "The Mother of All Regulations," www.uschamber.com/press/opeds/0101donohueergo.htm (7 October 2005). This editorial attacked the standard and invoked prominently the recently released National Academy of Sciences (Institute of Medicine) report because it acknowledged that other factors besides workplace overuse were *also* linked to strain injury syndromes, suggesting that this devalued the clear workplace causes.

45. "Senate Joint Resolution 6," providing for congressional disapproval and thus voiding the ergonomics standard, was passed on 6 March 2001 on a roll call vote of 56 to 44. The House of Representative introduced the same text as "Resolution 79" on 6 March 2001, passing it one day later on a role call vote of 223 to 206 (*Congressional Record,* vol. 147). The Office of Management and Budget, announcing Executive Office support for the resolution, noted, "In addition, a recent report by the National Academy of Sciences found that none of the common musculoskeletal disorders are uniquely caused by work exposures" www.whitehouse.gov/omb/legislative/sap/107-1/SJR6-s.html (7 October 2005). The resolution became Public Law 107–5 on 20 March 2001.

46. These numbers are based on a review of the PubMed (National Library of Medicine) database.

47. Antonio Gazio (Antonius Gazius), *Aerarium Sanitatis* (Padua, Italy: J. Fabrianus, 1549). The Latin text cited in the original reads: "Pectori et pulmonaria contraria: Aer omnis malus, borealis, fumosus, pulverulentus, locus inclusus cavernosis, praefertim, qui juxta fornaces, inquibus metallica sunt, & exercentur opera. Fumus carbonum, loga apud ignem mora & converfatio. Incessus sub lunae radiis. Exhalatio, que ex horreis diu primu et mox apertis occurrit."

48. Andrew Wynter, "Mortality in Trades and Professions," in *Curiosities of Civilization Reprinted from the "Quarterly" & "Edinburgh" Reviews*, 2nd ed. (London: Robert Hardwicke, 1860), 499–535 (article reprinted from *Edinburgh Review* [January 1860]).

49. Lewis W. Leeds, *Lectures on Ventilation: Being a Course Delivered in the Franklin Institute, of Philadelphia, During the Winter of 1866–67* (New York: John Wiley and Son, 1868).

50. The connection between outdoor air pollution and indoor air quality was also a matter of concern. See Robert Stuart Meikleham, *The Theory and Practice of Warming and Ventilating Public Buildings, Dwelling-Houses, and Conservatories . . . by an Engineer* (London: Thomas and George Underwood, 1825), 93–94: "Cleanliness is therefore not only a private but a public duty. And although the peculiar processes or manufactures carried on in many of our great towns cannot altogether be suspended on any consideration of public health or the public convenience, yet the nuisance or inconvenience might be in many instances mitigated, if proper measures for preventing the disengagement of noxious matter in the atmosphere, or else arresting its progress were so engaged instead of allowing it to incorporate with the air, and insinuate itself into the dwellings and even the chambers of the inhabitants of such towns and districts."

51. George T. Palmer, "What Fifty Years Have Done for Ventilation," in *A Half Century of Public Health: Jubilee Historical Volume of the American Public Health Association, in Commemoration of the Fiftieth Anniversary Celebration of its Foundation, New York City, November 14–18, 1921*, ed. Mazÿck P. Ravenel (New York: American Public Health Association, 1921), 335–360, quotations from 359–360.

52. K. Nishiyama and J. V. Johnson, "Karoshi—Death from Overwork: Occupational Health Consequences of Japanese Production Management," *International Journal of Health Services* 27 (1997): 625–641.

53. In 1993, the National Institute for Occupational Safety and Health put out a special "alert," acknowledging that "some homicides are caused by disgruntled workers," although it emphasized the more frequent phenomenon of robbery-related homicides. NIOSH, *Preventing Homicide in the Workplace*, DHHS (NIOSH) Pub. no. 93–109 (Cincinnati, OH: NIOSH, 1993).

54. Guglielmo Gratarolo (Guilelmus Gratarolus), *A Direction for the Health of Magistrates and Studentes* (London: William How for Abraham Veale, 1574).

The original Latin edition was titled *De Literatorum & Eorum qui Magistratibus Funguntur Conservanda Praeservandaque Valetudine* (Basil: Henrichum Petri, 1555).

55. Vopiscus Fortunatus Plemp, *De Togatorum Valetudine Tuenda Commentatio* (Brussels: Francisci Foppens, 1670). Bernardino Ramazzini cites this in relation to the indoor air hazards of tallow wax candle fumes. See Ramazzini, *Diseases of Workers: The Latin Text of 1713 Revised, with Translation and Notes by Wilmer Cave Wright* (Chicago: University of Chicago Press, 1940), 402–405.

56. Aside from mental strain, the ill effects of indoor air were also invoked as an argument against sedentary occupations. See W. A. Pearkes, *Popular Observations on the Diseases of Literary and Sedentary Persons* (London: W. Pearman, 1819), 32: "The confined air which men shut up in studies, counting-houses, manufactories &c. are continually breathing may be reckoned as another cause of disease, and to which too little attention is paid."

57. S. A. Tissot, *An Essay on the Disorders of People of Fashion; and a Treatise on the Diseases Incident to Literary and Sedentary Persons,* trans. James Kirkpatrick (Edinburgh: A. Donaldson, 1772).

58. Ramazzini, *Diseases of Workers,* 381.

59. S. Weir Mitchell, *Wear and Tear, or Hints for the Overworked* (Philadelphia: J. B. Lippincott, 1871), 47.

60. Ibid., 38–39.

61. Charlotte Perkins Gilman's story "The Yellow Wallpaper" was published years after her treatment by Mitchell. See Charlotte Perkins Stetson, "The Yellow Wall-paper," *New England Magazine* 5, n.s. (January 1892): 647–656. See also Elaine R. Hedges, afterword to *The Yellow Wallpaper,* by Charlotte Perkins Gilman (Old Westbury, NY: Feminist Press, 1973), 37–63; and Kenneth Levin, "S. Weir Mitchell: Investigations and Insights into Neurasthenia and Hysteria," *Transactions and Studies of the College of Physicians of Philadelphia* 38, ser. 4 (1970–71): 168–173. The view that literary pursuits posed an occupational hazard was not universally shared. In discussing work-related diseases, Benjamin Ward Richardson, a leading British figure in the Victorian public health movement, noted, "Concerning those who follow poetry as an art, we have heard much said,—a vast deal more, I take it, than was ever true,—as to their sufferings." See Richardson, *Diseases of Modern Life* (London: Macmillan and Co., 1876), 410.

62. Rachel Carson, *Silent Spring* (Cambridge, MA: Houghton Mifflin, 1962), 6.

2. THE SHADOW OF SMOKE

1. Bernardino Ramazzini, *Diseases of Workers: The Latin Text of 1713 Revised, with Translation and Notes by Wilmer Cave Wright* (Chicago: University of

Chicago Press, 1940), 50–51; see also fn. 499. The original Latin text referring to the "shadow of smoke" is "in quibis acriter de fumi umbra disputatum est."

2. Karl Marx, "Debatten über das Holzdiebstahlsgesetz" (On the law on the theft of wood), *Rheinische Zeitung* 298 (supplement) (25 October 1842).

3. Marx cites Ramazzini in a footnote to *Capital,* vol. 1, chapter 14, in the section "Capitalistic Character of Manufacture," along with a number of items related to industrial disease. Among the other sources listed by Marx is a catalog of the "Twickenham Economic Museum." This annotated resource list of printed materials related to public health included approximately thirty different titles, including works in German and French. See Twickenham Museum, *Handbook of Economic Literature. Being a Descriptive Catalogue of the Library of the Twickenham Economic Museum or Repository of Useful Knowledge for Every-Day Life,* Part 1: "Domestic and Sanitary Economy" (London: T. Twining, 1861). See also I. V. Vengrova, "Publications Used by K. Marx on Occupational Pathology from B. Ramazzini to English Medical Officers of Health," *Atti del XXI Congresso Internazionale di Storia della Medicina Sienna Italy* (conference proceedings) 1 (1968): 678–680.

4. Harriet Martineau, *The Factory Controversy; A Warning Against Meddling Legislation . . . Issued by the National Association of Factory Occupiers, 13, Corporation Street, Manchester* (Manchester, England: A. Ireland and Co., 1855), 25.

5. For Charles Dickens's critique of Martineau on worker safety, see *Household Words* 11: 14 April 1855 (no. 264), 12 May 1855 (no. 268), 23 June 1855 (no. 274), and 28 July 1855 (no. 279). Of note, Florence Nightingale, on whom Martineau was an important influence, breaks with her worldview when it comes to occupational health and comes closer to Dickens (if not to Clifford Odets in *Waiting for Lefty*). In the 1861 revision of her classic *Notes on Nursing* (retitled *Notes on Nursing for the Labouring Classes*), Nightingale inserted, among other changes, additional comments on the air of workrooms and health: "Workpeople should remember that health is their only capital, and they should come to an understanding among themselves to secure pure air in their places of work, which is one of the prime agents of health. This would be worth a 'Trades' Union,' almost worth a 'strike.'" See *Florence Nightingale's Notes on Nursing,* ed. with Introduction, Notes, and Guide to Identification by Victor Skretkowicz (London: Scutari Press, 1992), 27.

6. Martineau, *The Factory Controversy,* 29.

7. A. J. Lanza and Joseph H. White, *How a Miner Can Avoid Some Dangerous Diseases,* Miners' Circular 20 (Washington, DC: U.S. Department of the Interior, 1916); "Rock Dust," 24–25; quoted passage, 25.

8. Samuel Roberts, *Tom and Charles, or, the Grinders; Being the History of Two Boys, Educated in the Charity-School at Sheffield: Faithfully Delineating Personages and Scenery Peculiar to that Neighbourhood, By a Trustee of that Institution* (Sheffield: J. Montgomery, 1823). Although published anonymously in its first

edition, the British Library copy is signed by Roberts. The book went through at least seven editions by 1868, with a modified title, *Tom and Charles, or, the Two Grinders*. A copy of the second edition (1835) in the Stanford University library notes that it was presented to George W. Pinder, along with one shilling, on leaving the Sheffield Charity School. An inscription by his son documents that Pinder, who entered the school at age six, went on to become a metalworker in Sheffield, eventually working as a "hammer man." George Pinder died in 1873 at age forty-three, older than the majority of his contemporaries in the trade. All page citations, which are given parenthetically in the text, pertain to the second edition.

9. For the life expectancy of grinders, see Andrew Wynter, "Mortality in trades and professions," *Curiosities of Civilization Reprinted from the "Quarterly" & "Edinburgh" Reviews,* 2nd ed. (London: Robert Hardwick, 1860), 499–535.

10. Andrew Wynter, "Special Diseases of Artisans, &c.," *Curiosities of Toil and Other Papers* (London: Chapman and Hall, 1870), 278–279. This book was a follow-up to *Curiosities of Civilization.* In commenting on a recent report of the Commissioners for the Employment of Children (for more on the commissioners, see n. 15), Wynter notes: "The fact that one of the last Reports issued by the Commissioners for the Employment of Children treats mainly of the evil conditions under which a large class of the adult artisans of Sheffield labour is significant. It must indeed have been a very serious case that could have induced them to transfer their own proper sphere of inquiry to another quarter; but, in truth, the case of the Sheffield knife-grinders has been so long notorious that we are by no means surprised they have brought the matter officially before the Government. Indeed, there seems to be no reason why Government should delay turning their attention far more than they have done to the conditions under which adult artisans labour. They are supposed, it is true, to be free agents, but, practically, they are little more so than the children Government has so properly taken under its protection. Artisans working in factories, mines, &c., are, to a certain extent, subordinate to conditions over which in many cases they have but little control. They are but part of a great machine, the human cogs in a system of labour employed for the production of certain articles. When, indeed, they possess the means of obviating the adverse conditions under which they labour, they are often so ignorant or so indifferent to the evils which affect them that, to all intents and purposes, they are no better than children with no wills at all."

11. The general history of phosphorous-related bone destruction in the match industry has been covered by Jean Spencer Felton, "Classical Syndromes in Occupational Medicine: Phosphorous Necrosis—a Classical Occupational Disease," *American Journal of Industrial Medicine* 3 (1982): 77–120; and Jeffrey Nemhauser, "Phosphorous Necrosis of the Jaw in Matchmakers: An Extinct Occupational Disease," *Mithradata* 12 (2002): 11–12. A popular general history

of phosphorous also includes an account of the disease: John Emsley, *The 13th Element* (New York: John Wiley and Sons, 2000).

12. Henry J. Bigelow, "Necrosis of the Maxillary Bones; of the Nasal Plates; and of the Sella Turcica, resulting from the Fumes of Phosphorous," reported in W. W. Morland, "Extracts from the Records of the (Boston) Society for Medical Improvement from its January 26, 1852 Meeting," *American Journal of Medical Sciences* 24, n.s. (1852): 82–83.

13. Anton Chekhov, *The Steppe and Other Stories,* trans. Ronald Hingley (Oxford: Oxford University Press, 1998), 40. "The Steppe: The Story of a Journey" was first published in 1888. In the same year the Russian Ministry of Finance put in place a special excise tax on the match industry in an effort to control the yellow phosphorous problem. Russia produced more than a hundred million yellow phosphorous matches per annum at this time. See also G. P. Shul'tsev, "[Observation of the Physician and Talent of the Writer (On the Novel by A. P. Chekhov 'The Steppe')]" (original in Russian), *Klinical Med (Mosk)* 68 (1990): 150–152. According to Shul'tsev, the first phosphorous match factory in Russia was founded in 1837 in St. Petersburg.

14. Kirtley Ryland, "Phosphoric Necrosis of the Maxillary Bones—Peculiar to Lucifer Match-Makers, Its Pathology and Hygienic Treatment," *Saint Louis Medical and Surgical Journal* 12 (1854): 28–35. Although an 1856 report (James R. Wood, "Necrosis of Inferior Maxilla from the Vapor of Phosphorous—Removal of the Entire Lower Jaw—Recovery—Remarks upon Phosphorus Disease," *New York Journal of Medicine* 16 [1856]: 301–308) is usually cited as the earliest U.S. notice of the disease, both Ryland's 1854 report and Bigelow's 1852 cases (cited above, n. 12) predate this.

15. Dr. Henry Letheby's testimony was taken on 5 April 1862 by the Commissioners Appointed to Inquire into the Employment of Children and Young Persons in Trades and Manufactures Not Already Regulated by Law. See their *First Report of the Commissioners with Appendix* (London: Eyre and Spottiswoode for Her Majesty's Stationery Office, 1863), 46, 54. This report also documents the practice of wearing cans of turpentine around the neck as a supposed protective device. Letheby (1816–76) was an important figure in British public health, taking over from John Simon as the author of the annual *Report on the Sanitary Condition of the City of London* in 1856. See also William Arthur Jobson Archbold, "Letheby, Henry," *Dictionary of National Biography,* ed. Leslie Stephen and Sidney Lee (Oxford: Oxford University Press, 1959–60), vol. 11, 1010.

16. "Phossy Jaw; Messrs. Bryant and May at Worship Street, Seventeen Cases of Phosphorous Poisoning Reported, The Full Penalty Inflicted," *Daily Chronicle* (London), 2 June 1898. For the related commission report, see T. E. Thorpe, Thomas Oliver, and George Cunningham, *Reports to the Secretary of State for the Home Department on the Use of Phosphorus in the Manufacture of Lu-*

cifer Matches (London: Her Majesty's Stationery Office, 1899). (This source also provides the data for Russian match production and its 1888 excise tax mentioned in n. 13 above, pages 76–77.)

17. The history of British regulations related to phosphorous leading up to international treaty controls is summarized in Thomas Oliver, *Diseases of Occupation from the Legislative, Social, and Medical Points of View* (London: Methuen and Co., 1908). The effectiveness of the British regulations in practice has been recently reviewed in P. W. J. Bartrip, *The Home Office and the Dangerous Trades: Regulating Occupational Diseases in Victorian and Edwardian Britain* (Amsterdam: Rodopi, 2002). The international context of phosphorous control in the early part of the twentieth century is documented in Ludwig Teleky, *History of Factory and Mine Hygiene* (New York: Columbia University Press, 1948), 28, 43, 88–89, 113; and in two articles: L. Ferrannini, "Phosphorous (Amorphous Red)" and "Matches (Lucifer)," *International Labour Office, Occupational Health: An Encyclopedia of Hygiene Pathology and Social Welfare* (Geneva, Switzerland: International Labor Organization, 1934), vol. 2, 161–167, 635–637.

18. John B. Andrews, "Phosphorous Poisoning in the Match Industry in the United States," *United States Bureau of Labor Statistics Bulletin* 86 (January 1910): 31–146.

19. House Committee on Ways and Means, *Hearings on Bill (61), HR 26540, 29469, 30022,* 61st Cong., 3rd sess., 16 December 1910 and 20 January 1911; *Hearings on Bill (62), HR 22896,* 62nd Cong., 2nd sess., 10 January 1912.

20. For a prime (but by no means isolated) example of the upbeat interpretation given to the long-delayed control over yellow phosphorous that finally came into effect in the first decades of the twentieth century, see Alice Hamilton, *Exploring the Dangerous Trades* (Boston: Little, Brown, 1943), 116–118. A more recent reiteration of this view can be found in Melvin L. Myers and James D. McGlothlin, "Matchmakers' 'Phossy Jaw' Eradicated," *American Industrial Hygiene Association Journal* 57 (1996): 330–332.

21. As late as the mid-1920s, occupational phosphorous poisoning from match manufacture and nonindustrial poisoning from accidental and intentional ingestion of matches remained a public health problem in China, which signed the control convention only in 1923, with a five-year grace period on top of that. See Charles T. Maitland, "Health and Industrial Conditions in China," *China Medical Journal* 39 (1925): 1089–1099; and Peter C. Kiang, "Studies in Acute Phosphorous Poisoning," *China Medical Journal* 40 (1926): 1091–1100.

22. Herbert Spencer, *Social Statics, or, The Conditions Essential to Human Happiness Specified, and the First of them Developed* (London: John Chapman, 1851).

23. John Tierney, "Best Incentive to Make Sure Workers Don't Get Hurt: Money," *New York Times,* 9 March 2001.

24. The summary of events is based on my own experience with the Film Recovery Systems case. See Paul D. Blanc et al., "Cyanide Intoxication among Silver-Reclaiming Workers," *JAMA* 253 (1985): 367–371.

25. The story of Bessie Gabrilowich Cohen is based on her obituary. See Michael T. Kaufman, "Bessie Cohen, 107, Survivor of 1911 Shirtwaist Fire, Dies," *New York Times,* 24 February 1999. See also the obituary of Rose Freedman, the last Triangle fire survivor, who also died at the age of 107: Douglas Marin, "Rose Freedman, Last Survivor of Triangle Fire, Dies at 107," *New York Times,* 17 February 2001.

26. A new history of the fire was published in 2003. See David Von Drehle, *Triangle: The Fire That Changed America* (New York: Atlantic Monthly Press, 2003). As a reflection of the importance of the Triangle fire among the immigrant groups most affected, the event was even a subject of Yiddish songwriters of the day. See A. Schorr and J. M. Rumshinsky, *"Mameinu" or the Triangle Victims* (מאמעניו אדער דאד טדויד אויף די טדייעגל קדבנות) (New York: Hebrew Publishing Co., 1911).

27. Kaufman, "Bessie Cohen."

28. OSHA's gift of the charred doors from Imperial Food Products was reported in "Work Week: OSHA's Quarter-Century Inspires a Poignant Gift to a Museum," *Wall Street Journal,* 30 April 1996.

3. GOOD GLUE, BETTER GLUE, SUPERGLUE

1. The nitropropane sealant death is reported in Robert Harrison, Gideon Letz, Gary Pasternak, and Paul D. Blanc, "Fulminant Hepatic Failure after Occupational Exposure to 2-Nitropropane," *Annals of Internal Medicine* 107 (1987): 466–468.

2. Cyril Aldred, "Fine Wood-Work," in *A History of Technology,* vol. 1: *From Early Times to the Fall of Empires,* ed. Charles Singer et al. (Oxford: Clarendon Press, 1954), 695, 696.

3. The Egyptian use of glue is covered in far greater detail in the very first chapter ("Adhesives") of Alfred Lucas, *Ancient Egyptian Materials and Industries,* rev. by J. E. Harris, 4th ed. (London: Histories and Mysteries of Man, Ltd., 1989), 1–9.

4. The instructions on medieval glue making are quested from Robert Hendrie, *An Essay Upon Various Arts in Three Books, by Theophilus, Called also Rugerus, Priest and Monk, Forming an Encyclopaedia of Christian Art of the Eleventh Century* (London: John Murray, 1847), 23, 43.

5. Charles Turner Thackrah, *The Effects of Arts, Trades, and Professions, and of Civic States and Habits of Living on Health and Longevity,* 2nd ed. (London: Longman, Rees, Orme, Brown, Green, and Longman, 1832), 59–60.

6. For technical background on gums, resins, and latex, see "Gums and mu-cilages," "Resins (natural)," and "Rubber (natural)," in *Van Nostrand's Scientific Encyclopedia,* ed. Douglas M. Considine and Glenn D. Considine, 7th ed. (New York: Van Nostrand Reinhold, 1989), 1389–1391, 2426–2428, 2486–2488, respectively.

7. The early technical history of the dyestuffs industry has been covered extensively elsewhere. See J. Holmyard, "Dyestuffs in the Nineteenth Century," in *A History of Technology,* vol. 5: *The Late Nineteenth Century,* ed. Charles Singer et al. (Oxford: Clarendon Press, 1958), 257–283. For an early account of early synthetic dyestuffs, see M. Reiman, *On Aniline and its Derivatives: A Treatise on the Manufacture of Aniline and Aniline Colors* (New York: John Wiley and Son, 1868).

8. A recent popular biography of William Perkin also provides useful context. See Simon Garfield, *Mauve: How One Man Invented a Colour That Changed the World* (London: Faber and Faber, 2000).

9. A recent social and technical history of coal by Barbara Freese puts a positive ecological spin on the development of coal gas: "These fossil light sources [coal gas and kerosene] thus helped save the whales, just as coal had for centuries helped save the remaining forests." See Barbara Freese, *Coal: A Human History* (Cambridge, MA: Perseus Books, 2003), 147.

10. L. Snelling, "A Preliminary Report of Some Cases of Purpura Haemorrhagica Due to Benzol Poisoning," *Bulletin of the Johns Hopkins Hospital* 21 (February 1910): 33–37, quotation from 34.

11. Carl Gustaf Santesson, "Ueber chronische Vergiftungen mit Steinkohlentheerbenzin; vire Todesfälle," *Archiv für Hygiene* 31 (1897): 336–376. Dr. Santesson drafted this paper in "June 1897," but it was not published until later in that year. He presented his findings before publication, however, at the 12th International Medical Congress, Moscow, 19–26 August 1897; presentation made on 20 August under the auspices of the section "Pharmacology, Balanology, and Climatology"; *Programme, 12th International Medical Conference* (Moscow, 1897), section 4B. Contemporaneous with Santesson's, another report of benzene anemia appeared, of which Snelling was apparently unaware at the time of his 1910 U.S. investigation: [P.] Le Noir and [H.] Claude, "Sur un case de purpura attribué a l'intoxication par la benzine," *Bulletins et Mémoires de la Société Médicale des Hôpitaux de Paris* 14, ser. 30 (1897): 1251–1260. This case involved exposure to benzene in a textile dyeing operation. Le Noir, who presented the case at the 29 October 1897 meeting of the Medical Society, cites Santesson's recent report, at that point available only as a brief abstract of the Moscow meetings noticed in the *Gazette Hebdomadaire de Médecine et de Chirurgie,* 26 August 1897.

12. Snelling, "A Preliminary Report of Some Cases of Purpura Haemorrhagica Due to Benzol Poisoning," 37 (both text quotation and footnote).

13. The remarkably close timing of the first benzene-related blood disease and notice of radiation effects is notable. In early 1897 the *Bulletin of the Johns Hopkins Hospital* published the first medical reports documenting a problem that was anything more serious than a superficial skin effect from X-ray exposure: T. C. Gilchrest, "A Case of Dermatitis Due to the X Rays," *Bulletin of the Johns Hopkins Hospital* 8 (January 1897): 17–23; and T. C. Gilchrest, "Additional Cases of Dermatitis Due to the X Rays," *Bulletin of the Johns Hopkins Hospital* 8 (March 1897): 72. Despite the titles indicating dermatitis, these reports also documented bone lesions, a deeper tissue effect from radiation overexposure.

14. The industrial use of benzene (benzol) had become so widespread that by 1910 a general review of the subject was presented at the 2nd International Congress of Occupational Diseases in Brussels (Joseph Rambousek, "Die gewerbliche Benzolvergiftung," conference proceedings). Another participant at the Brussels congress, a leading British occupational medicine figure named Robert Prosser White, was so impressed by Rambousek's paper that he modified his own presentation (on a fatal exposure to aniline in a twenty-two-year-old dye worker), noting in part: "Dr. Rambousek has presented a most instructive paper on the dangerous properties of benzol. . . . The object of this Congress is not to cure the workers, nor bury them when they are dead, but rather to study ways and means to prevent illnesses. Cannot this Congress impress upon the government of each country represented here, the necessity of investigating thoroughly and scientifically by experiment any new ingredient used in any of the industrial processes unless it be certainly known to be harmless?" (Robert Prosser White, manuscript notes for his presentation as part of the 2nd International Congress of Occupational Diseases, Brussels, 1910, author's collection).

15. V. H. Veley, "An Examination of the Physical and Physiological Properties of Tetrachlorethane and Trichlorethylene," *Proceedings of the Royal Society of London. Series B, Containing Papers of a Biological Character* 82 (1910): 217–225, quotation from 217.

16. Karl B. Lehmann, "Expirementelle Studien über den Einfluss technisch und hygienisch wichtiger Gas und Dampfe auf den Organismus (XVI–XXIII)," *Archiv für Hygiene* 74 (1911): 1–60.

17. Anonymous, "A Fatal Case of Poisoning by Tetrachloride of Ethane," *Lancet* (26 December 1914): 1489–1491, quotation from 1489. See also, by the treating physician who testified at the inquest, William Henry Willcox, "An Outbreak of Toxic Jaundice Due to Tetrachlorethane Poisoning," *Lancet* (13 March 1915): 544–547. The terms *tetrachlorethane* and *tetrachloroethane* were both used for the same compound; the latter is the preferred modern term.

18. Anonymous, "A Fatal Case of Poisoning by Tetrachloride of Ethane," 1491.

19. Alice Hamilton, "Industrial Poisoning in Aircraft Manufacture," *JAMA* 69 (15 December 1917): 2037–2039. This report also summarizes the earlier German literature on the subject. An unsigned editorial accompanies the publica-

tion: "Trinitrotoluene (T.N.T.) Poisoning among Munitions Workers," *JAMA* 69 (15 December 1917): 2041–2042. See also Alice Hamilton, "Dope Poisoning in the Manufacture of Airplane Wings," *Monthly Review of the U.S. Bureau of Labor Statistics* 5 (July–December 1917): 18–25 (Washington, DC: Government Printing Office); and New York State Division of Industrial Hygiene (Lester Ross and Rosalie Bell), "The Aeroplane Industry," *Bulletin of the New York State Industrial Commission* 2 (June 1917): 185–189.

20. P. Delore and [C.] Borgomano, "Leucémie aiguë au cours de l'intoxication benzénique: Sur l'origine toxique de certaines leucémies aiguës et leurs relations avec le anémies graves," *Journal de Médecine de Lyon* 9 (1928): 227–233, quotation from 233, "cette possibilité est bien connue por la radiothérapie."

21. Prior case reports of leukemia due to benzene include P. E. Weill, "La leucémie post-benzolique," *Bulletins et Mémoires de la Société de Médecine des Hôpitaux de Paris* 46 (1932): 750–752; and Ernst Falconer, "An Instance of Lymphatic Leukemia following Benzol Poisoning," *American Journal of the Medical Sciences* 186, n.s. (1933): 353–361. In the latter report, the treating physician at the University of California San Francisco recognized the initial presentation as acute benzol toxicity; as he notes, "The author has seen 4 cases of typical benzol poisoning from the same plant during the previous year" (354).

22. Manfred Bowditch and Hervey B. Elkins, "Chronic Exposure to Benzene (Benzol). 1. The Industrial Aspects," *Journal of Industrial Hygiene and Toxicology* 21 (1939): 321–330; Francis T. Hunter. "Chronic Exposure to Benzene (Benzol). 2. The Clinical Effects," *Journal of Industrial Hygiene and Toxicology* 21 (1939): 331–354; Tracey B. Mallory, Edward A. Gall, and William J. Brickley, "Chronic Exposure to Benzene (Benzol). 3. The Pathological Results," *Journal of Industrial Hygiene and Toxicology* 21 (1939): 355–377. Despite the systematic review, the authors overlooked the 1928 case of F. M., a twenty-two-year-old Mexican American with aplastic anemia who had worked with benzene since age sixteen. His Los Angeles factory job, like those of the Baltimore girls a generation before, was sealing cans with benzene-laced rubber. John Martin Askey, "Aplastic Anemia Due to Benzol Poisoning," *California and Western Medicine* 29 (1928): 262–263.

23. Aldous Huxley, *Brave New World* (London: Chato and Windus, 1932), 17. The initial reference to acetate silk occurs in chapter 1; Huxley comes back to acetate silk (as well as rayon) as a symbol of modernity in chapter 7, when a character exclaims, "A civilized face. Yes, and civilized clothes. Because I thought I should never see a piece of real acetate silk again. . . . And those adorable viscose velveteen shorts!"

24. "Gutta Percha," *Van Nostrand's Scientific Encyclopedia,* ed. Douglas M. Considine and Glenn D. Considine, 7th ed. (New York: Van Nostrand Reinhold, 1989), 1392. See also Mitchell B. Boxer, Leslie C. Grammer, and Nicholas

Orfan, "Gutta-Percha Allergy in a Health Care Worker with Latex Allergy," *Journal of Allergy and Clinical Immunology* 93 (1994): 943–944.

25. For an early report on Galalith, see F. Schmitt, *Manuel du fabricant de boutons et peignes, articles en celluloid et en Galalithe* (Paris: J. Bailliére, 1923). Galalith listings on eBay are mostly for decorative pins (for example, "Gorgeous GALALITH FAUX CORAL BIRD PIN + PEARLS") and often hedge on the precise plastic composition among Bakelite, celluloid, and Galalith.

26. Primo Levi's writings relevant to Buna include *Survival in Auschwitz* (*If This Is a Man*) (New York: Collier Books, 1961) and *Periodic Table* (New York: Schocken Books, 1984), 211–233. Another literary source on Buna and neoprene can be found in the novel *The Weeping Wood,* by Vicki Baum, as quoted in Walter Gratzer, *The Longman Literary Companion to Science* (Harlow, U.K.: Longman, 1989), 400–402. As another contemporary example, see "Rubber: How Do We Stand?" the feature story for *Fortune* (June 1942), with cover illustration by Herbert Bayer based on the chemical structure of synthetic rubber.

27. Federal Security Agency, U.S. Public Health Service, *Clara Gives Benzol the Run Around,* Workers' Health Series no. 4 (Washington DC: U.S. Government Printing Office, 1941), unpaginated ten-page pamphlet. Other pamphlets in the series included *KO by CO Gas* and *Leonard's Appendix—and How It Burst.* The U.S. Public Health Service guidelines on distribution of these pamphlets ("Industrial Hygiene Education Materials," mimeographed sheets [Washington DC: U.S. Public Health Service, 1943]) state: "The pamphlets prepared by the Public Health Service deal with specific health problems of industrial workers. Distribute these at the close of meetings or in discussion groups. Place a few copies in the racks in the dispensary, union halls, recreation rooms, etc. Mail to the homes of workers so that the entire family may have the opportunity to read them."

28. For the initial synthesis of vinyl chloride ("ether hydrochlorique monochlorée"), see Henri Victor Regnault, *Annales de Chemie et Physique* 59 (1835): 358, as summarized in J. R. Parkington, *A History of Chemistry* (London: Macmillan & Co., 1964), vol. 4, 355. For Regnault's photographic contributions, see Laurie Virginia Dahlberg, *Victor Regnault and the Advance of Photography* (Princeton, NJ: Princeton University Press, 2005).

29. Morris G. Shepard, "Ostromislensky, Iwan Iwanowich," in *Dictionary of American Biography,* ed. Robert L. Schuyler and Edward T. James (New York: Charles Scribner's Sons, 1956), vol. 11, supplement 2, 505–506. See also I. I. Ostromuislenskii, "Synthesis of the Symmetrical Chloride and the Higher Chloride of Erythrene Caoutchouc: New Chlorides of Natural, Isoprene and Erythrene Caoutchoucs," *Journal of the Russian Physical Chemical Society* 48 (1916): 1132–1151.

30. The key Semon patent for B. F. Goodrich was U.S. Patent 1,929,453 (10 October 1933). See S. L. Brous and W. L. Semon, "Koroseal, a New Plastic," *Industrial and Engineering Chemistry* 27 (1935): 667–672. For biographical details on Semon, see Jon Marmor, "Waldo Semon—He Helped Save the World," *Columns: The University of Washington Alumni Magazine* (September 1999), www.washington.edu/alumni/columns/sept99/semon.html (15 May 2003). See also "Milestones," *Time*, vol. 153, 7 June 1999, 27.

31. Enrico C. Vigliani and Giulio Saita, "Benzene and Leukemia," *New England Journal of Medicine* 271 (1964): 872–876, quotation from 875. For biographical details on Vigliani, see the series of memorial comments that appeared as "La Scomparsa del Prof. Enrico Vigliani," *Medicina del Lavoro* 83 (1992): 4–17.

32. Ludwig Rehn, "Blasengeschwültse bei Fuchsin-Arbeitern," *Archiv für Klinische Chirurgie* 50 (1895): 588–600.

33. John L. Creech Jr., Maurice N. Johnson, Bradford Block, et al., "Angiosarcoma of Liver among Polyvinyl Chloride Workers—Kentucky," *Morbidity and Mortality Weekly Report (MMWR)*, original publication 9 February 1974; reprinted with additional editorial, *MMWR* 46 (7 February 1997): 97–101, quotation from 98. For Creech's earlier report on bone damage in vinyl chloride workers, see R. H. Wilson, W. E. McCormick, C. F. Tatum, and J. L. Creech, "Occupational Acroosteolysis: Report of 31 Cases," *JAMA* 201 (1967): 577–581.

34. John L. Creech and Maurice N. Johnson, "Angiosarcoma of the Liver in the Manufacture of Polyvinyl Chloride" (Special Communication), *Journal of Occupational Medicine* 16 (March 1974): 150–151, quotation from 150.

35. Ibid., "Special Communication: Editor's Note," 151. The details of Maltoni's laboratory research on vinyl chloride and the attempts of the Manufacturing Chemists' Association (MCA—the industry trade organization of petrochemical manufacturers) to contain information and minimize any regulatory response are provided in Gerald Markowitz and David Rosner, *Deceit and Denial: The Deadly Politics of Industrial Pollution* (Berkeley: University of California Press and the Milbank Memorial Fund Berkeley, 2002), 195–233. Markowitz and Rosner enriched their excellent analysis through access they gained to internal MCA documents. Nearly two years after the initial angiosarcoma outbreak, Joe Klein published a lengthy article on vinyl chloride ("The Plastic Coffin of Charlie Arthur," *Rolling Stone*, 15 January 1976, 43–47). Even at that time, Klein raised the issue of the American chemical companies' suppression of the Maltoni data, singling out B. F. Goodrich in particular. Goodrich vociferously objected, publishing its executive vice president's rebuttal to the Klein article, including a defense of the role of the Manufacturing Chemists' Association (Thomas B. Nantz, "PVC Controversy: The Company Line," *Rolling Stone*, 26 February 1976, 7–8). According to Klein, Goodrich was "so proud of their response that they've been circulating it to other chemical lobbyists on Capitol Hill" (letter from Joe Klein to me, 26 February 1976). The topic of data sup-

pression has been revisited in a more recent critique of the EPA's decision to discount any carcinogenic potential for vinyl chloride *other* than through angiosarcoma of the liver, despite evidence linking the chemical to cancer of other sites, especially the brain. Narrowing the parameters of its risk assessment could lead the EPA to lessen pollution controls on the carcinogen. See Jennifer Beth Sass, Barry Castleman, and David Wallinga, "Vinyl Chloride: A Case Study of Data Suppression and Misrepresentation," *Environmental Health Perspectives* 113 (2005): 809–812.

36. Henry Falk, John L. Creech Jr., Clark W. Heath Jr., Marice N. Johnson, and Marcus M. Key, "Hepatic Disease among Workers at a Vinyl Chloride Polymerization Plant," *JAMA* 230 (October 1974): 59–63, quotation from 59. As senior author, Dr. Key is listed last.

37. All *New York Times* articles on vinyl chloride in 1974. The articles appearing on 15 February, 13 March, and 1 June all carried the byline of Jane Brody. The coverage was capped in October 1974 in Alan Anderson Jr., "The Hidden Plague: Even the Families of Some Workers Are Endangered by Occupational Diseases," *New York Times Magazine,* 27 October 1974, 272–278. Additional articles related to vinyl chloride appeared in the *New York Times* during this period on 22 February, 28 February, 5 April, 16 April, 25 May, and 9 July. By the fall of 1974, public awareness of the vinyl chloride hazard had reached a point at which the Grateful Dead's Jerry Garcia was quoted as saying, "The making of records is an amazing bummer. It's a sweat-shop situation, one of the worst. . . . In a pressing plant there will be a dozen people in a poorly ventilated miserable place with hot vinyl fumes—the most monotonous, mindless kind of work and it's an awful situation in which to work. I really object to it. Vinyl chloride is poisonous, it's a carcinogen" (*Boston Phoenix [Boston after Dark],* 19 November 1974, section 2, 1).

38. International Agency for Research on Cancer (IARC), *IARC Monographs on the Evaluation of the Carcinogenic Risk of Chemicals to Man,* vol. 7 (Lyon, France: IARC, 1974).

39. *Industrial Union Department, AFL-CIO v. American Petroleum Institute et al.,* 448 U.S. 607, Supreme Court of the United States (1980), decided 2 July 1980.

40. International Agency for Research on Cancer, *IARC Monographs on the Evaluation of the Carcinogenic Risk of Chemicals to Man,* vol. 29 (Lyon, France: IARC, 1982); International Agency for Research on Cancer, *IARC Monographs on the Evaluation of the Carcinogenic Risk of Chemicals to Man: Overall Evaluations of Carcinogenicity: An Updating of IARC Monographs,* vols. 1–42, supplement 7 (Lyon, France: IARC, 1987), 127. See also Robert A. Rinsky, Alexander B. Smith, Richard Hornung, et al., "Benzene and Leukemia: An Epidemiologic Risk Assessment," *New England Journal of Medicine* 316 (1987): 1044–1050.

41. Yasuhiro Yamamura, "N-Hexane Polyneuropathy," *Folia Psychiatrica et Neurologica Japonica* 23 (1969): 45–57, quotation from 45.

42. Allan Herskowitz, Nobuyoshi Ishii, and Herbert Schaumburg, "N-Hexane Neuropathy: A Syndrome Occurring as a Result of Industrial Exposure," *New England Journal of Medicine* 285 (1971): 82–85.

43. Donald Katz, *Just Do It: The Nike Spirit in the Corporate World* (New York: Random House, 1994), 71. Bowerman's illness is misprinted in this source as a "narapathy."

44. Javad Towfighi et al., "Glue Sniffer's Neuropathy," *Neurology* 26 (1976): 238–243.

45. Shelby K. Kopp et al., "Asthma and Rhinitis Due to Ethylcyanoacrylate Instant Glue," *Annals of Internal Medicine* 102 (1985): 613–615. A remarkably similar case, also occurring in a model airplane hobbyist, was reported twenty years later, underscoring that these exposures continue to be a problem: Moan-Rita Yacoub, Catherine Lemiére, and Jean-Luc Malo, "Asthma Caused by Cyanoacrylate Used in a Leisure Activity," *Journal of Allergy and Clinical Immunology* 116 (2005): 462.

46. S. Lozewisc, A. G. Davison, A. Hopkirk, et al., "Occupational Asthma Due to Methyl Methacrylate and Cyanoacrylates," *Thorax* 40 (1985): 836–839. The initial health care worker case was reported in C. A. Pickering et al., "Occupational Asthma Due to Methyl Methacrylate in an Orthopaedic Theatre Sister," *British Medical Journal (Clinical Research Education)* 292 (1986): 1362–1363. A relatively new application of methacrylate, as a "glue" to re-expand collapsed vertebrae, has also been associated with asthma in medical personnel. See Brian S. Kirby, Azar Doyle, and Louis A. Gilula, "Acute Bronchospasm Due to Exposure to Polymethylmethacrylate Vapors during Percutaneous Vertebroplasty," *American Journal of Radiology* 180 (2003): 543–544.

47. R. Donelly, J. B. Buick, and J. Macmahon, "Occupational Asthma after Exposure to Plaster Casts Containing Methylene Diphenyl Diisocyanate," *Occupational Medicine* (London) 54 (2003): 432–434. I am indebted to Dr. Carrie Redlich of Yale University, a leading expert on isocyanate asthma, for calling to my attention the expanding end-market uses for these products.

48. For lung bleeding related to heating epoxies and other polymers, see Paul D. Blanc and Jeffrey A. Golden, "Unusual Occupational Disorders of the Lung: Case Reports and Literature Review," in *Unusual Occupational Diseases, Occupational Medicine State of the Art Reviews,* ed. Dennis J. Shusterman and Paul D. Blanc (Philadelphia: Hanley and Belfus, 1992), vol. 7, 403–422. For methacrylate fume in fax machine repair, see Lawrence W. Raymond, "Pulmonary Abnormalities and Serum Immunoglobulins in Facsimile Machine Repair Technicians Exposed to Butyl Methacrylate Fume," *Chest* 109 (1996): 1010–1018. For susceptors, see M. Sharman et al., "Detection of Residues of the Epoxy Adhesive Component Bisphenol A Diglycidyl Ether (BADGE) in Microwave Susceptors and Its Migration into Food," *Food Additives and Contaminants* 12 (1995): 779–787.

49. Scott P. Bruder and Alan B. Leahey, "Accidental Instillation of Cyano-acrylate Adhesive in the Eye," *Journal of the American Board of Family Practice* 8 (1995): 486–490, quotation from 488.

50. K. J. Blinder, W. Scott, and M. P. Lange, "Abuse of Cyanoacrylate in Child Abuse: Case Report," *Archives of Ophthalmology* 105 (1987): 1632–1633.

51. E. Martin Caravati and Toby L. Litovitz, "Pediatric Cyanide Intoxication and Death from an Acetonitrile-Containing Cosmetic," *JAMA* 260 (1988): 3470–3473.

52. For nitroethane causing methemoglobinemia, see Carl S. Hornfeldt and William H. Rabe III, "Nitroethane Poisoning from an Artificial Fingernail Remover," *Journal of Toxicology Clinical Toxicology* 32 (1994): 321–324; K. C. Osterhoudt et al., "Rebound Severe Methemoglobinemia from Ingestion of a Nitroethane Artificial-Fingernail Remover," *Journal of Pediatrics* 126 (1995): 819–821; and G. Shepherd, J. Grover, and W. Klein-Schwartz, "Prolonged Formation of Methemoglobin following Nitroethane Ingestion," *Journal of Toxicology Clinical Toxicology* 36 (1998): 613–616.

53. Artificial nail primers found to contain N,n-dimethyl-p-toluidine also cause methemoglobinemia. See Christopher H. Linden et al., "Corrosive Injury from Methacrylic Acid in Artificial Nail Primers: Another Hazard of Fingernail Products," *Pediatrics* 102 (1998): 979–984. This paper also contains an excellent discussion of the regulatory issues connected with the FDA and the Consumer Product Safety Commission in terms of these products.

54. U.S. Food and Drug Administration, Center for Food Safety and Applied Nutrition, Office of Cosmetics and Colors, "Update on Artificial Nail Removers," Fact Sheet, December 1999, revised 24 January 2003, and "Prohibited Ingredients and Related Safety Issues," Fact Sheet, 30 March 2000, revised May 2005, www.cfsan.fda.gov (9 October 2005).

55. Consumer Product Safety Commission, press releases: 73–014, "CPSC Bans Three Spray Adhesives—Asks Manufacturers of Others to Halt Production," 20 August 1973; 74–002, "CPSC Announces Intention to Lift Spray Adhesive Ban," 25 January 1974; 74–059, "CPSC Issues Ban on Vinyl Chloride in Aerosols," 16 August 1974; 77–121, "CPSC Bans Extremely Flammable Contact Adhesives," 9 December 1977; 78–002, "Paint Strippers to Display Sterner Warnings," 6 January 1978.

56. Consumer Product Safety Commission, press release 78–030, "CPSC Recommends Ban of Benzene in Consumer Products," 27 April 1978.

57. Consumer Product Safety Commission, press release 80–013, "CPSC Seeks Data on Levels of Benzene Found in Various Consumer Products," 16 April 1980.

58. Consumer Product Safety Commission, "Benzene-Containing Consumer Products; Proposed Withdrawal of Proposed Rule (16 CFR Part 1307),"

Federal Register 46 (13 January 1981): 3034–3036, quotation from 3035, and "Benzene-Containing Consumer Products; Withdrawal of Proposed Rule," 16 CFR parts 1145, 1307, 1500, and 1700, *Federal Register* 46 (22 May 1981): 27910–27911.

59. Consumer Product Safety Commission, "Benzene-Containing Consumer Products; Proposed Withdrawal of Proposed Rule," 3035.

60. Molly Sinclair, "Safety Watchdog Stays Rocky Course: Controversial CPSC Marks 10th Anniversary," *Washington Post,* 8 May 1983. By 1988, even George Will criticized the CPSC for its inaction. See George F. Will, "Lawn Darts and the Limits of Laissez Faire; They're Dangerous to Kids—So Do Something," *Washington Post,* 8 May 1988.

61. "Nominee to Head Safety Panel Withdraws," *New York Times,* 19 September 2001.

62. Don Colburn, "Art Supplies That Have Toxic Chemicals Must Carry Labels," *Washington Post,* 10 September 1991. See also "Arts and Crafts and Toxins," editorial, *Washington Post,* 28 September 1991.

63. Nail Systems International, D-Zolve, "Material Safety Data Sheet" (rev. 29 January 2001) and Web-based product information, www.nsinails.com (30 June 2003).

64. Elena H. Page et al., "Peripheral Neuropathy in Workers Exposed to Nitromethane," *American Journal of Industrial Medicine* 40 (2001): 107–113.

65. C. J. Booth et al., "Elevated Creatinine after Ingestion of Model Aviation Fuel: Interference with the Jaffe Reaction by Nitromethane," *Journal of Paediatrics and Child Health* 35 (1999): 503–504.

66. Jo E. Dyer and J. H. Reed, "Alkali Burns from Illicit Manufacture of GHB" (abstract), *Journal of Toxicology Clinical Toxicology* 35 (1997): 553.

67. Justin J. Brown and Charith S. Nanayakkara, "Acetone-Free Nail Polish Removers: Are They Safe?" *Clinical Toxicology* (Philadelphia) 43 (2005): 297–299.

68. Carlos Pastore et al., "Partial Conduction Blocks in N-Hexane Neuropathy," *Muscle Nerve* 26 (2002): 132–135.

69. "N-Hexane-Related Peripheral Neuropathy among Automotive Technicians—California, 1999–2000," *Morbidity and Mortality Weekly Report* 50 (2002): 1011–1013.

70. R. Lobo-Mendonça, "Tetrachloroethane—a Survey," *British Journal of Industrial Medicine* 20 (1963): 50–56.

71. James E. Norman Jr., C. Dennis Robinette, and Joseph F. Fraumeni, "The Mortality Experience of Army World War II Chemical Processing Companies," *Journal of Occupational Medicine* 23 (1981): 818–822. See also Howard A. Coyer, "Tetrachloroethane Poisoning," *Industrial Medicine* 13 (1944): 230–233.

72. Paul Garner, "Commentary: Industry Can Damage Your Health," *British Medical Journal* 314 (1 February 1997): 342.

73. William Belmont Parker, "Cooper, Peter," in *Dictionary of American Biography*, ed. Allen Johnson and Dumas Malone, vol. 2 (New York: Charles Scribner's Sons, 1958), 409–410.

74. For the *Seinfeld* episode in question, see Larry David, "The Invitations," originally broadcast 16 May 1996. In 1902, Thomas Oliver included among miscellaneous trade hazards "stamp-licker's tongue," describing it as "an infective process which generally yields to antiseptic treatment, such as weak carbolic acid, boric, or hyposulphite of soda mouth-wash." See Thomas Oliver, *Dangerous Trades* (London: John Murray, 1902), 803.

4. UNDER A GREEN SEA

1. Harris C. Faigel, "Mixtures of Household Cleaning Agents," *New England Journal of Medicine* 271 (1964): 618. The earliest medical report of a home bleach mixing misadventure appears to be a letter published in 1959: A. E. Bloomfield, "Domestic Chlorine Poisoning," *British Medical Journal* 2 (12 December 1959): 1332. Twenty years later, another letter to the same journal documented a case of deliberate exposure from repeated mixing with hypochlorite and intentional inhalation of the fumes. The patient would sometimes heat the mixture for a more potent effect and even spread the mixture on his skin. See P. Rafferty, "Voluntary Chlorine Inhalation: A New Form of Self-Abuse?" *British Medical Journal* 281 (1980): 1178–1179. For general information on the human toxicology of chlorine inhalation exposure, see Rupali Das and Paul D. Blanc, "Chlorine Gas Exposure and the Lung: A Review," *Toxicology and Industrial Health* 9 (1993): 439–455.

2. Frederick L. Jones, "Chlorine Poisoning from Mixing Household Cleaners," *JAMA* 222 (1972): 1312. Such cases continue to occur on a regular basis. See, for example: Rita Mrvos, Bonnie S. Dean, and Edward P. Krenzelok, "Home Exposures to Chlorine/Chloramine Gas: Review of 216 Cases," *Southern Medical Journal* 86 (1993): 654–657; and David A. Tanen, Kimberlie A. Graeme, and Robert Raschke, "Severe Lung Injury after Exposure to Chloramine Gas from Household Cleaners," *New England Journal of Medicine* 341 (1999): 848–849. Cases of bleach mishap numbering in the thousands are also tallied in annual published reports of the American Association of Poison Control Centers.

3. Suellen Hoy, *Chasing Dirt: The American Pursuit of Cleanliness* (New York: Oxford University Press, 1995), 100–110.

4. F. Racioppi, P. A. Daskaleros, N. Besbelli, et al., "Household Bleaches Based on Sodium Hypochlorite: Review of Acute Toxicology and Poison Control Center Experience," *Food and Chemical Toxicology* 32 (1994): 845–861. This publication is also the source for per capita household bleach consumption,

based on internal marketing reports from Procter and Gamble and from the Fédération internationale des associations de fabricants de produits d'entretien.

5. Masayasu Minami, Masao Katsumata, Kazumasa Miyake, et al., "Dangerous Mixture of Household Detergents in an Old-Style Toilet: A Case Report with Simulation Experiments of the Working Environment and Warning of Potential Hazard Relevant to the General Environment," *Human and Experimental Toxicology* 11 (1992): 27–34.

6. J. Naumovski et al., "Specter of Pulmonary Injuries after Inhalation of Irritative Fumes from Mixing Household Cleaners" (abstract), *American Journal of Respiratory and Critical Care Medicine* 159 (1999): A236. This experience was reported from the Clinic of Toxicology and Urgent Internal Medicine, Skopje, Macedonia.

7. An account of the historical background of chlorine bleaching is indebted to collaborative work with Dr. Kjell Torén, M.D., of the Department of Occupational and Environmental Medicine, Gothenburg University. See Kjell Torén and Paul D. Blanc, "The History of Pulp and Paper Bleaching: Respiratory-Health Effects," *Lancet* 349 (1997): 1316–1318.

8. Carl Scheele, "Om brunsten eller magnesia, och dess egenskaper," *Kongliga Svenska Vetenskaps Academiens Handlingar* 35 (1774): 89–116. Translated and extracted as "On Manganese and Its Properties," in Alembic Club Reprints no. 13, *The Early History of Chlorine* (Edinburgh: Alembic Club, 1905), 5–10, quotation from 5. The quotation in the original Swedish publication is, "Lik varm aqua regis," (94).

9. For Lavoisier's critique of Kirwin, see Richard Kirwin, *Essai sur le phlogistique: Avec notes de MM de Moreau, Lavoisier, de la Place, Monge, Berthollet & de Fourcroy* (Paris: Rue at Hotel Serpente, 1788). See also Henry Guerlac, "Lavoisier, Antoine-Laurent," in *Dictionary of Scientific Biography*, ed. Charles C. Gillispie, vol. 8 (New York: Charles Scribner's Sons, 1973), 66–91.

10. Humphry Davy, "The Bakerian Lecture: On Some of the Combinations of Oxymuriatic Gas and Oxygene and on the Chemical Relations of These Principles, to Inflammable Bodies"; and Humphry Davy, "On a Combination of Oxymuriatic Gas and Oxygene Gas," *Philosophical Transactions of the Royal Society of London* 101 (1811): 1–35 and 155–162, respectively. In the first article Davy details experiments on the properties of oxymuriatic gas, criticizing the logic of this nomenclature and suggesting the new term *chlorine*. The second paper describes additional related observations, including chlorine dioxide (not named as such) and its bleaching properties.

11. Claude-Louis Berthollet, "Memoir on Dephlogisticated Murine Acid, 1785," in Alembic Club Reprints no. 13, *The Early History of Chlorine*, 11–31.

12. Claude-Louis Berthollet, *Essay on the New Method of Bleaching: With an Account of the Nature, Preparation and Properties of Oxygenated Muriatic Acid, to which is Now Added, Observations and Experiments on the Art of Dying with Madder*, trans. with annotations from the French by R. Kerr, 2nd ed. (Edinburgh:

William Creech, 1791), 79. See also Satish C. Kapoor, "Berthollet, Claude Louis," in *Dictionary of Scientific Biography*, ed. Charles C. Gillispie, vol. 2 (New York: Charles Scribner's Sons, 1970), 73–82.

13. Interesting source material on bleaching before chlorine is provided in F. Home, *Experiments on Bleaching* (Edinburgh: Kincaid and Donaldson, 1756); and James Dunbar, *Smegmatologia, or the Art of Making Potashes and Soap and Bleaching Linen* (Edinburgh: printed for the author, 1736).

14. Jeremiah is quoted from the standard Hebrew text (English translation by Alexander Harkavy; New York: Hebrew Publishing Co., 1916). *Nitre* in this usage, for the Hebrew *neter* (נתר), refers to sodium carbonate, although *nitre* in other contexts can mean potassium nitrate (saltpeter) or, even more obscure, a sediment in refining maple syrup. The common translation *soap* is for the Hebrew *borit* (בורית). This refers to a substance made from the ashes of a wild shrub and used as a cleaning agent, that is, a form of potash.

15. The quotation attributed to Vespasian is based on Suetonius, *Lives of the Caesars*, trans. J. C. Rolfe, Loeb Classical Library (New York: Macmillan, 1914), 318–319 (book VIII, *Divus Vespianus*, chap. 23). For the proverbial "*non olet*," see "Money has no smell," in *The Concise Oxford Dictionary of Proverbs*, ed. J. A. Simpson (Oxford: Oxford University Press, 1982), 153. General information on the early history of bleaching, especially in the ancient world, is drawn from Franco Brunello, "Un po' di storia del candeggio," *Laniera* 76 (1963): 1423–1427; and Sidney Herbert Higgins, *A History of Bleaching* (London: Longmans, Green and Co., 1924). The annotated catalog of the Sidney Edelstein Collection is also a rich bibliographic resource on the subject: Moshe Ron, *Bibliotheca Tinctoria: Annotated Catalogue of the Sidney M. Edelstein Collection in the History of Bleaching, Dyeing, Finishing and Spot Removing* (Jerusalem: Jewish National and Hebrew Library, 1991). Additional details, including the citation for Pliny's *Natural History*, are drawn from Samuel Parkes, *Chemical Essays, Principally Relating to the Arts and Manufactures of the British Dominions*, 3rd ed. (London: Baldwin and Craddock, 1830), 387–420, "On Bleaching" (essay 12), quotation from 387.

16. Bernardino Ramazzini, *Diseases of Workers*, translation of the 1713 edition of *De Morbis Artificum* by Wilmer Cave Wright (Chicago: University of Chicago Press, 1940), 106–127, quotation from 111.

17. William Shakespeare, *The Winter's Tale*, IV, iii, 5–6: "The white sheet bleaching on the hedge, / With hey! the sweet birds, O how they sing!" *The Riverside Shakespeare* (Boston: Houghton Mifflin, 1974), 1586.

18. The bleaching fields of Haarlem were a recurring theme in Jacob von Ruisdael's paintings, from the 1640s through 1680s, ranging from small "cottage" operations to the industrial-scale bleaching grounds of Lucas de Clercq and "Del Mol," the massive operation owned by Michiel de Wael. The importance of the Haarlem fields is emphasized in Parkes, *Chemical Essays*, "On Bleaching" (essay 12).

19. The *"Golden Ass" of Apuleius*, trans. Robert Graves (New York: Pocket Books, 1952), 191–192.

20. Sulphur was also used as a fumigant. Godfrey Boyle, in commenting on the use of sulphur fumigation to eradicate bedbugs, noted in 1737, "This sulfur while burning will give a prodigiously strong funck and such as will kill all creatures in the universe." See Godfrey Boyle, *Miscellanea Vere Utilia or Miscellaneous Experiments and Observations on Various Subjects* (London: J. Robinson, 1737), 147. Sulphur fumigation continued to be used for certain bleaching applications (e.g., for wool and in bleaching straw used to make bonnets) well into the nineteenth century. See Charles Turner Thackrah, *The Effects of Arts, Trades, and Professions and of Civic States and Habits of Living on Health and Longevity: with Suggestions for the Removal of Many Agents which Produce Disease and Shorten the Duration of Life,* 2nd ed. (London: Longman, Rees, Orme, Brown, Green & Longman, 1832), 118–119.

21. Berthollet, "Memoir on Dephlogisticated Murine Acid, 1785." The information on the introduction of industrial bleaching in Great Britain is drawn from Parkes, "On Bleaching" (essay 12). Parkes was a contemporary acquaintance of many of the principal players involved. His essay on bleaching in the third edition was revised in light of criticism of his original essay on the subject, published in the first edition of 1815 and documented in a four-page response that he published in the following year. See Samuel Parkes, *Reply to Dr. Henry's Letter* (London: C. Baldwin, 1816).The true claim of priority in the introduction of chlorine bleaching has engendered historical debate ever since Parkes and Dr. Henry's public correspondence of the early nineteenth century. The most exhaustive examination of the question finds the weight of evidence in favor of Watts. See A. E. Munson and Eric Robinson, "The Introduction of Chlorine Bleaching," in *Science and Technology in the Industrial Revolution* (Manchester, U.K.: Manchester University Press, 1969), 252–337.

22. Robert Morris and James Kendryk, "Oxygenated Muriatic Acid," *The Edinburgh Medical and Physical Dictionary,* vol. 2 (Edinburgh: Bell and Bradfute, 1807), unpaginated.

23. Parkes, "On Bleaching," 398.

24. Walter Weldon, *On the Manufacture of Chlorine: A Lecture Delivered. . . . May 22nd 1874* (London: Thomas Scott, 1874). This thirty-six-page printed text of Weldon's lecture points out the drawbacks of early chlorine processes near the outset of his remarks, but devotes more of its attention to the virtues of chlorine. (See n. 34.) For additional background on the early bleach industry, see A. Clow and N. L. Clow, "The Chemical Industry: Interaction with the Industrial Revolution," in *A History of Technology,* vol. 4: *The Industrial Revolution,* ed. Charles Singer et al. (Oxford: Clarendon Press, 1958), 230–256.

25. Parkes, "On Bleaching," 400.

26. For Humphry's nomenclature for potassium and sodium, see Humphry Davy, "The Bakerian Lecture: On Some New Phenomena of Chemical Changes Produced by Electricity, Particularly the Decomposition of Fixed Alkalies," *Philosophical Transactions of the Royal Society of London* 98 (1808): 1–44, quotation from 32.

27. Clow and Clow, "The Chemical Industry." For additional details on Leblanc, see Robert Fox, "Leblanc, Nicolas," in *Dictionary of Scientific Biography*, ed. Charles Gillispie, vol. 8 (New York: Charles Scribner's Sons, 1973), 113–114.

28. A. P. Laurie, "The Chemical Trades," in *Dangerous Trades*, ed. Thomas Oliver (London: John Murray, 1902), 568–598, quotation from 571.

29. Weldon, *On the Manufacture of Chlorine*, comment near the outset of his lecture.

30. Great Britain, Noxious Vapours Commission, *Minutes of Evidence Taken Before the Royal Commission on Noxious Vapours; with an Appendix* (London: George Edward Eyre and William Spottiswood for Her Majesty's Stationery Office, 1878), 36. The commission took testimony from a wide range of witnesses, including laborers in the chemical industry.

31. Laurie, "The Chemical Trades," 571.

32. Arthur Vacher, "On the Origin of Disease: Occupation in Relation to Disease," in *Health Lectures Delivered in Manchester 1886–7*, 10th ser. (London: John Heyward, 1887), 23–24.

33. Laurie, "The Chemical Trades," 577.

34. Weldon, *On the Manufacture of Chlorine*, quotation from near the beginning of his lecture text.

35. For the life of Muspratt, see Philip Joseph Hartog, "Muspratt, James," in *Dictionary of National Biography*, ed. Leslie Stephen and Sidney Lee, vol. 13 (Oxford: Oxford University Press, 1959–60), 1330–1331.

36. See, for example, A. B., "Poisonous Inhalation of Chlorine," *Lancet* 39, no. 11 (27 April 1839): 194. This letter to the editor, dated 20 April 1839, is signed only as "A. B." In it, the author reports his accidental exposure as follows: "When preparing this gas for the purposes of experiment, the luting connecting the apparatus gave way, consequently a large quantity of chlorine escaped into the apartment." A. B. goes on to describe the severe cough and chest tightness that ensued.

37. Thackrah, *The Effects of Arts, Trades, and Professions*, 55–56.

38. For an analysis of Thomas Beddoes and the "pneumatic school," including their interest in the potential adverse effects of substances inhaled through occupational exposures, see Brian Dolan, "Conservative Politicians, Radical Philosophers and the Aerial Remedy for the Diseases of Civilization," *History of the Human Sciences* 15 (2002): 35–54.

39. Louis Bernard Guyton de Morveau, *Traité des moyens de désinfecter l'air, de prévenir la contagion, et d'en arrêter les progres*, 3rd ed. (Paris: Chez Bernard, 1805).

40. Jean-Nicolas Gannal, *Two Memoirs Read Before L'Academie Royale des Sciences, at Paris, on the Successful Inhalation of Dilute Chlorine, in the Early Stages of Pulmonary Consumption, as a Remedy Capable of Prolonging Life; . . . from the French of M. Gannal,* trans. William Horatio Potter (London: Callow and Wilson, 1830), 17.

41. Thackrah, *The Effects of Arts, Trades, and Professions,* 227. Thackrah's description of his use of chlorine inhalation occurs in the very last pages of the body of the text. His interest in gas inhalation preceded his focus on occupational disease. For example, in lectures given in 1823, he discussed "respiration of various gases; their effects on the animal economy." See Charles Turner Thackrah, *Outlines of a Course of Lectures on Physiology to be Delivered at the Philosophical Hall* (Leeds: Philosophical and Literary Society, Edward Baines, 1823), unpaginated.

42. William Wallace, *Researches Respecting the Medical Powers of Chlorine Gas Particularly in Diseases of the Liver,* 2nd ed. (London: Longman, Hurst, Rees, Orme, and Brown, 1824), 132–133. The frontispiece of Wallace's book illustrates a person in an exposure apparatus with his head out of the box.

43. Gannal, *Two Memoirs Read Before L'Academie Royale des Sciences at Paris,* 15.

44. Ibid. The (unpaginated) copy of the book that I examined included an inserted notice about obtaining a suitable apparatus from Perrins, Lea & Perrins in Worcester. Lea and Perrins Worcestershire sauce was first formulated in 1835. See R. W. Apple Jr., "Toque and Dagger: The Sauce Secrets of Worcester," *New York Times,* 21 June 2000.

45. James Hyatt, *The Elements of Chemistry* (New York: Clark, Austin & Smith, 1855). This 1855 text not only describes the procedure for inhaling chlorine but also provides an engraved "how to" illustration. It does also warn that overinhalation of the gas can be fatal. The engraving was based on a daguerreotype by Peter Welling of James Hyatt performing a chlorine inhalation maneuver. The daguerreotype image is currently in the Gillman Collection, Metropolitan Museum of Art, New York (see illustration credits). As late as the first decades of the twentieth century, the purported therapeutic benefits of chlorine gas inhalation were still being touted. A 1926 report on chronic lung disease in a paper mill worker exposed to bleach powder begins, "The recent advocacy of chlorine in the treatment of respiratory infections has tended to create the belief that industrial poisoning from low concentrations of this gas is improbable" (Carey P. McCord, "Industrial Poisoning from Low Concentrations of Chlorine Gas," *JAMA* 86 [1926]: 1687–1688).

46. The biographical details on Thackrah are drawn from Andrew Meiklejohn, *The Life, Work and Times of Charles Turner Thackrah* (Edinburgh: E. & S. Livingston, 1957). This publication also includes a facsimile of the second edition of Thackrah's *The Effects of Arts, Trades and Professions.*

47. Torén and Blanc, "The History of Pulp and Paper Bleaching."

48. For the early Chinese history of papermaking, see Ch'iao-Píng L., *The Chemical Arts of Old China* (Easton, PA: Journal of Chemical Education, 1948).

49. The German-based technical innovation of the Kraft process spread worldwide, but in the later part of the nineteenth century health concerns related to industrial bleach exposure were limited almost exclusively to the German medical literature. See, for example, Ludwig Hirt, *Die Gasinhalations-Krankheiten und die von ihnen besonders heimgesuchten Gewerbe- und Fabrikbetriebe* (Breslau and Leipzig: Hirt und Sohn, 1873), 95–100. By the twentieth century, the German toxicological literature was the most explicit in recognizing that "chronic chlorine poisoning" was associated with bronchitis among paper factory bleachers and others industrially exposed. See Ferdinand Flury and Franz Zernik, *Schädliche Gase: Dämpfe, Nebel, Rauch- und Staubarten* (Berlin: Julius Springer, 1931), 119–120. The American scientific literature, although muted, was not completely silent on the subject. In 1936, an anonymous physician from Wisconsin sent a query to *JAMA* requesting "any available data that you may have on the effect of so-called bleach gas, which is produced in the process of manufacture and bleaching paper." The correspondent was informed that this gas was likely to be chlorine. The response also noted, "The occurence of injurious effects from exposure to chlorine in a paper mill is well within the realm of possibility" (anonymous, "Injurious Effect of Chlorine in Paper Mill," *JAMA* 106 [1936]: 2024). See also McCord, "Industrial Poisoning from Low Concentrations of Chlorine Gas," in n. 45, above.

50. For early German industrial hygiene and experimental exposures to chlorine, see Karl B. Lehmann, "Experimentelle Studien über den Einflusz technisch und hygienisch wichtiger Gase und Dämpfe auf dem Organismus Theil III und IV: Chlor und Brom," *Archiv für Hygiene* 17 (1887): 231–285.

51. For much of the background on Haber I have largely relied on Hanspeter Witschi, "The Story of the Man Who Gave Us 'Haber's Law,' " *Inhalational Toxicology* 9 (1997): 201–209; and Hanspeter Witschi, "Fritz Haber: December 9, 1868—January 29, 1934," in "Fritz Haber and His Legacy to the Science of Toxicology," ed. H. P. Witschi, *Toxicology* 149 (2000): 3–15. A recent biography provides additional details of Haber's career: Daniel Charles, *Master Mind: The Rise and Fall of Fritz Haber, the Nobel Laureate Who Launched the Age of Chemical Warfare* (New York: HarperCollins, 2005). In the fall of 2005, an off-Broadway play about Haber opened. See Ken Gordon, "From a Scientist's Life, Art's Cautionary Tales," *New York Times,* 12 October 2005.

52. The Lewis Freeman quotation, based on material that originally appeared in the *Cornhill Magazine,* is cited from Arthur Hurst, "Gas Poisoning," in *Medical Diseases of the War,* 2nd ed. (London: Edward Arnold, 1918), 308–316, quotation from 311–312.

53. Wilfred Owen's "Dulce et Decorem Est" is frequently anthologized but perhaps not as carefully read as it might be in its specifics. See, for example, *The 100 Best Poems of All Time,* ed. Leslie Pockell (New York: Warner Books, 2001), 142–153.

54. Charles Lyell and Michael Faraday, *Report . . . on the Subject of the Explosion at the Haswell Collieries* (London: W. Clowes and Sons, 1844). For examples of early British writing on poisonous gases, see *Gentleman's Magazine and Historical Chronicle* 20 (1750): 225, 255, 312, 356–357, 454–456. "Sylvanus Urban" raises the original question regarding "poisons that can kill from a distance" in relation to recent deaths at Old Bailey and the history of the "Black Assize" (235), followed by various readers' responses (Edward Steele, 255; Paul Gemeage, 312; and John Hall, 356–357, 454–456).

55. For J. S. Haldane's work in the mines, including the anecdote on his son's recitation of Shakespeare, I have drawn on J. B. S. Haldane, "Some Adventures of a Physiologist," handwritten manuscript, 1945. This is an eleven-page manuscript for a radio broadcast memorializing his father on his death (author's collection). In an earlier radio broadcast on the dangers of warming air raid shelters with combustion sources (September 1940), J. B. S. Haldane also refers to his father's work in the mines, attributing to him the introduction of small birds to coal mines as an early warning system (which might also be used in shelters): "My father found that in air containing dangerous quantities of carbon monoxide birds fell off their perches long before he felt anything, though he was affected in the long run. So he introduced the use of birds as indicators for carbon monoxide after colliery explosions." See J. B. S. Haldane, *A Banned Broadcast and Other Essays* (London: Chatto and Windus, 1946), 160.

56. A. T. Sloggett, *Memorandum on Gas Poisoning in Warfare,* pamphlet, 32 pp., dated "1/4/18," Thomas Renton Elliot Archives, The Wellcome Library for the History and Understanding of Medicine.

57. Anonymous, *Soldier's Gas Notes, No. 7, Training Battalion (Drivers) RASC C Company,* Thomas Renton Elliot Archives, The Wellcome Institute for the History of Medicine. This eight-page pamphlet is composed of twenty-two questions and answers; the sixth item as quoted appears on its initial pages.

58. Haber's oversight of the deployment of war gas is fictionalized in André Malraux's *The Walnut Trees of Altenburg.* See Malraux's novel as excerpted in *The Longman Literary Companion to Science,* ed. Walter Gratzer (Harlow, U.K.: Longman, 1989), 395–397.

59. Witschi, "The Story of the Man Who Gave Us 'Haber's Law,'" quoted Haber text as reported and translated by Witschi, 203.

60. Witschi, "Fritz Haber: December 9, 1868–January 29, 1934," quoted Haber text as reported and translated by Witschi, 12.

61. For Haber and Weizmann, see Chaim Weizmann, *Trial and Error* (New York: Harper and Brothers, 1949), 353–354.

62. Davy, "On a Combination of Oxymuriatic Acid and Oxygene Gas," 155–162. Davy notes the bleaching power of what came to be known later as chlorine dioxide: "The compound destroys dry vegetable colors, but first gives them a tint of red" (161).

63. Nonetheless, there was relatively little published data on human exposures to chlorine dioxide, underscored by a 1954 publication reporting a single case of respiratory disease in a fifty-three-year-old industrial chemist ("Dr. Sch.") exposed in the production of the gas. See Heinz Petry, "Chlordioxyd— ein gefährliches Reizgas," *Archiv für Gewerbepathologie und Gewerbehygiene* 13 (1954): 363–369.

64. The report of the Brooklyn release was published three years after the actual event. See Herbert Chasis, John A. Zapp, James H. Bannon, et al., "Chlorine Accident in Brooklyn," *Occupational Medicine* 4 (1947), 152–176.

65. The release in La Barre was first described in Roy E. Joyner and Eugene G. Durel, "Accidental Liquid Chlorine Spill in a Rural Community," *Journal of Occupational Medicine* 4 (1962): 152–154. Joyner, then plant medical director for Union Carbide at Texas City, Texas, attempted to shift the blame for the eleven-month-old's death onto his family, noting that even though the infant's home was overcome with fumes from the nearby tank car, "most of this exposure occurred inside the home, but some (and possibly the critical portion) occurred when the father became frantic over the infant's choking and gasping and carried him outside into the even thicker cloud of gas" (153). The description is eerily reminiscent of World War I gas-attack narratives. Later follow-up of twelve cases from La Barre was reported in Hans Weill et al., "Late Evaluation of Pulmonary Function after Acute Exposure to Chlorine Gas," *American Review of Respiratory Disease* 99 (1969): 374–379. Just less than two months after the January 1961 derailment, on 28 March a second major chlorine transportation mishap occurred while a freighter unloaded gas tanks in Baltimore. Exposure sufficient to require treatment affected 156 longshoremen, at least 37 of whom were admitted to a hospital. Long-term follow-up of that cohort demonstrated a loss in lung function. See Theodore A. Kowitz et al., "Effects of Chlorine Gas upon Respiratory Function," *Archives of Environmental Health* 14 (1967): 545–558.

66. The release in Youngstown, Florida, was documented in later medical follow-up of the survivors, reported in Robert N. Jones et al., "Lung Function after Acute Chlorine Exposure," *American Review of Respiratory Disease* 134 (1986): 1190–1195.

67. J. Fleta, C. Calvo, J. Zuniga, et al., "Intoxication of 76 Children by Chlorine Gas," *Human Toxicology* 5 (1986): 99–100.

68. Yongyudh Ploysongsang, Billie C. Beach, and Ralph E. DiLisio, "Pulmonary Function Changes after Acute Inhalation of Chlorine Gas," *Southern Medical Journal* 75 (1982): 23–36.

69. Faysal M. Hasan, Adel Gehshan, and Farid J. D. Fuleihan, "Resolution of Pulmonary Dysfunction following Acute Chlorine Exposure," *Archives of Environmental Health* 38 (1983): 76–80.

70. The original modern description of reactive airways dysfunction syndrome following irritant exposure was by Brooks and coworkers. See Stephen M. Brooks, W. A. Weiss, and I. L. Bernstein, "Reactive Airways Dysfunction Syndrome (RADS): Persistent Asthma Syndrome after High Level Irritant Exposures," *Chest* 88 (1985): 376–384.

71. Brad B. Moore and Michael Sherman, "Chronic Reactive Airway Disease following Acute Chlorine Gas Exposure in an Asymptomatic Atopic Patient," *Chest* 100 (1991): 855–856.

72. Repeated "gassings" in the pulp paper industry leading to asthma and other adverse respiratory effects have been reported in British Columbia by Susan M. Kennedy et al., "Lung Health Consequences of Reported Accidental Chlorine Gas Exposures among Pulp Mill Workers," *American Review of Respiratory Diseases* 143 (1991): 74–79; in Quebec by Jean-Pierre Courteau, Robert Cushman, Françoise Bouchard, et al., "Survey of Construction Workers Repeatedly Exposed to Chlorine over a Three to Six Month Period in a Pulp Mill: I. Exposure and Symptomatology," *Occupational and Environmental Medicine* 151 (1994): 219–224; and in New Hampshire by Paul K. Henneberger, Michael B. Lax, and Benjamin G. Ferris, "Decrements in Spirometry Values Associated with Chlorine Gassing Events and Pulp Mill Work," *American Journal of Respiratory and Critical Care Medicine* 153 (1996): 225–231. An earlier study relevant to this subject was carried out among workers in an Alabama chlorine gas production facility: Edward H. Chester, David G. Gillespie, and Franklin D. Krause, "The Prevalence of Chronic Obstructive Pulmonary Disease in Chlorine Gas Workers," *American Review of Respiratory Disease* 99 (1969): 365–373. The study's conclusions were equivocal insofar as lung function is concerned, but the researchers documented that, of 139 workers in the plant, 55 (4 out of 10) had experienced one or more gassings intense enough to require oxygen therapy. The authors spent three days at the facility carrying out lung function testing; during that brief time alone, two workers were gassed, giving the researchers the opportunity to study chlorine's immediate effects.

73. Metin Gorguner et al., "Reactive Airways Dysfunction Syndrome in Housewives Due to a Bleach–Hydrochloric Acid Mixture," *Inhalation Toxicology* 16 (2004): 87–91.

74. J. Elliot Black, Elliot T. Glenny, and J. W. McNee, "Observations on 685 Cases of Poisoning by Noxious Gases Used by the Enemy," *British Medical Journal* (15 July 1915): 165–167.

75. Walter Broadbent, "Some Results of German Gas Poisoning," *British Medical Journal* (14 August 1915): 247–248, quoted passage from 247.

76. For the initial post–World War I U.S. follow-up at Camp Grant, see Robert S. Berghoff, "The More Common Gases: Their Effect on the Respiratory Tract; Observations on Two Thousand Cases," *Archives of Internal Medicine* 24 (1919): 678–684; "And in the face of these apparently normal findings" (683); "There is no apparent reason" (680). Even before the U.S. entry into the war, certain Americans were interested in the effects of chlorine gassing. See D. E. J. [Dennis E. Jackson], "The Pharmacological Action of Chlorine Gas," *Journal of Laboratory and Clinical Medicine* 1 (1916): 447–453. This lengthy editorial, in the journal's inaugural volume, reviews the animal toxicological data of Lehmann and others and the initial reports from the war, acknowledging the possibility of "permanent disability even if there is recovery from the immediate effects of the gas" (453).

77. M. C. Winternitz, *Collected Studies on the Pathology of War Gas Poisoning* (New Haven, CT: Yale University Press, 1920). A related volume of research was authored as Frank P. Underhill, *The Lethal War Gases: Physiology and Experimental Treatment* (New Haven, CT: Yale University Press, 1920).

78. Harry L. Gilchrist, "Residual Effects of Warfare Gases: The Use of Chlorine Gas, with Report of Cases," *Medical Bulletin of the Veterans' Administration* 9 (1933): 229–270; and Harry L. Gilchrist and P. H. Matz, *The Residual Effects of Warfare Gases, 1. Chlorine, 2. Mustard* (Washington DC: War Department, U.S. Government Printing Office, 1933).

79. For published medical analyses of Iranian survivors of mustard gas, see Ali Emad and Gholam Reza Rezaian, "The Diversity of the Effects of Sulfur Mustard Gas Inhalation on Respiratory System 10 Years after a Single, Heavy Exposure: Analysis of 197 Cases," *Chest* 112 (1997): 734–738; and Ali Emad and Gholam Reza Rezaian, "Characterization of Bronchoalveolar Lavage Fluid in Patients with Sulfur Mustard Gas–Induced Asthma or Chronic Bronchitis," *American Journal of Medicine* 106 (1999): 625–628. See also Paul D. Blanc, "The Legacy of War Gas," *American Journal of Medicine* 106 (1999): 689–690; and United Nations Security Council, *Report of the Mission Dispatched by the Secretary-General to Investigate Allegations of the Use of Chemical Weapons in the Conflict between the Islamic Republic of Iran and Iraq*, S/20060 (New York: United Nations, July 1988). Prior to its reemergence in the Middle East, the threat of mustard gas had receded to become little more than a metaphor. This status is underscored by Allen Ginsberg's lyric in *Howl and Other Poems* (San Francisco: City Lights Books, 1956), 14, "who were burned alive in their innocent flannel suits on Madison Avenue amid blasts of leaden verse. . . . & the mustard gas of sinister intelligent editors."

80. Alfred Gilman and Frederick S. Philips, "The Biological Actions and Therapeutic Applications of the B-Chloroethyl Amines and Sulfides," *Science* 103 (1946): 409–415, 436. When this article appeared on 5 April 1946, just before the first anniversary of VE Day, the authors were writing under the aegis of the

Edgewood Arsenal. A footer on the title page of the article notes that the paper has the approval of the following agencies: "Medical Division, Chemical Warfare Service, United States Army; Division 9, NDRC, and Division 5, Committee on Medical Research, OSRD; Committee on Treatment of Gas Casualties, Division of Medical Sciences, NRC; and the Chemical Warfare representative, British Commonwealth Scientific Office." The early history of this work is also recounted in Alfred Gilman, "The Initial Clinical Trial of Nitrogen Mustard," *American Journal of Surgery* 105 (1963): 574–578.

81. The ongoing concern over the chemical warfare agents is reflected in the continued appearance of high-profile medical reviews on this subject, such as Stefanos N. Kales and David C. Christiani, "Acute Chemical Emergencies," *New England Journal of Medicine* 350 (2004): 880–888.

82. Jonathan Borak and Werner F. Diller, "Phosgene Exposure: Mechanisms of Injury and Treatment Strategies," *Journal of Occupational and Environmental Medicine* 43 (2000): 110–119.

83. "Illness Associated with Drift of Chloropicrin Soil Fumigant into a Residential Area—Kern County, California, 2003," *MMWR* 53 (2004): 740–742.

84. Michael J. Burns and Christopher H. Linden, "Another Hot Tub Hazard: Toxicity Secondary to Bromine and Hydrobromic Acid Exposure," *Chest* 111 (1997): 816–819. "Hot tub lung," as opposed to bromine irritant injury, is an illness linked to microbial overgrowth in hot tubs. See Viktor Hanak et al., "Hot Tub Lung: Presenting Features and Clinical Course of 21 Patients," *Respiratory Medicine* 100 (2006): 610–615.

85. Anna-Carin Olin et al., "Prevalence of Asthma and Exhaled Nitric Oxide Are Increased in Bleachery Workers Exposed to Ozone," *European Respiratory Journal* 23 (2004): 87–92.

86. Ariel Hart and Matthew L. Wald, "Cloud of 'Green Stuff' Rising from Train Wreck, Then Death and a Ghost Town," *New York Times*, 8 January 2005.

87. "Public Health Consequences from Substances Released during Rail Transit—South Carolina, 2005; Selected States, 1999–2004," *MMWR* 54 (2005): 64–67.

88. A. Bernard et al., "Lung Hyperpermeability and Asthma Prevalence in School Children: Unexpected Associations with the Attendance at Indoor Chlorinated Swimming Pools," *Occupational Environmental Medicine* 60 (2003): 385–394.

89. "Homemade Chemical Bomb Events and Resulting Injuries—Selected States, January 1996–March 2003," *MMWR* 52 (2003): 662–664.

90. Christina Ng, Elise Stone, and Paul D. Blanc, "Prevention of Household Chemical Product Overexposure: Field Testing of an Educational Brochure," *Health Values* 18 (1994): 24–31.

91. James J. Jordan Jr., the advertising man who created the jingle "Ring around the collar" for Wisk detergent, was responsible for a number of well-

known slogans, including "Us Tareyton smokers would rather fight than switch." He died in 2004. See Stuart Elliott, "James J. Jordan Jr., Advertising Sloganeer, Is Dead at 73," *New York Times,* 6 February 2004.

5. GOING CRAZY AT WORK

1. Frederick Peterson, "Three Cases of Acute Mania from Inhaling Carbon Bisulphide," *Boston Medical and Surgical Journal* 128 (1892): 325–326, quotation from 325.

2. Some of the work presented in this chapter was presented at the 2nd International Conference on the History of Occupational Prevention, Norrköping, Sweden, September 2001, as Paul D. Blanc, "From Balloons to Artificial Silk: The History of Carbon Disulfide Toxicity."

3. Peterson, "Three Cases of Acute Mania from Inhaling Carbon Bisulphide," 326.

4. W. A. Lampadius, "Etwas über flüssigen Schwefel, und Schwefel-Leberluft," *Chemische Annalen* (Lorenz von Crell) 2 (1796): 136–137.

5. R. Chenevix, "On the Action of Platina and Mercury upon Each Other," *Philosophical Transactions of the Royal Society of London* 95 (1805): 104–130.

6. Humphry Davy, "New Analytical Researches on the Nature of Certain Bodies, Being an Appendix to the Bakerian Lecture for 1808," *Philosophical Transactions of the Royal Society London* 99 (1808): 450–470.

7. Henry M. Leicester, "Berzelius," in *Dictionary of Scientific Biography,* ed. Charles C. Gillispie, vol. 2 (New York: Charles Scribner's Sons, 1970), 90–97.

8. Jons Jacob Berzelius and Alexander Marcet, "Experiments on the Alcohol of Sulfur, or Sulphuret of Carbon," *Philosophical Transactions of the Royal Society London* 103 (1813): 171–199; Alexander Marcet, "Experiments on the Production of Cold by the Evaporation of Sulphuret of Carbon," *Philosophical Transactions of the Royal Society London* 103 (1813): 252–255.

9. Berzelius and Marcet, "Experiments on the Alcohol of Sulfur, or Sulphuret of Carbon," quoted footnote from 175.

10. Anselme Payen, *Précis de chimie industrielle á l'usage des écoles préparatoires aux professions industrielles et de fabricants* (Paris: Librarie de L. Hachette, 1849), 74. This, the first edition, relegates carbon disulfide to a single footnote.

11. Elizabeth Gaskell, *Cranford* (New York: Harper & Brothers, Publishers, 1853), 83 (in chapter 5, "Old Letters").

12. The Macintosh view of history is most clearly articulated by Thomas Hancock in his industrial memoir. See Thomas Hancock, *Personal Narrative of the Origin and Progress of the Caoutchouc or India-Rubber Manufacture in England* (London: Longman, Brown, Green, Longman & Roberts, 1857). A more neutral history is summarized in S. S. Pickles, "Production and Utilization of

Rubber," in *History of Technology*, vol. 5: *Late Nineteenth Century, c. 1850 to 1900*, ed. C. Singer et al. (Oxford: Clarendon Press, 1958), 752–775.

13. The biographic details on Parkes are drawn from R. B. Prosser, "Parkes, Alexander (1813–1890)," in *Dictionary of National Biography*, ed. Leslie Stephen and S. Lee, vol. 15 (London: Oxford University Press, 1959–60), 292–293.

14. Anselme Payen, *Précis de chimie industrielle á l'usage des écoles préparatoires aux professions industrielles et de fabricants et des agriculteurs*, 2nd ed. (Paris: Librarie de L. Hechette et cie, 1851), 675–689. This, the second edition of Payen's text, includes in its subtitle the words *"augm. de chapitres sur le sulfure de carbone."* In a new section on rubber, Payen discusses carbon disulfide vulcanization at length. He alludes to the danger of using carbon disulfide in enclosed spaces as a result of its vapors but does not specifically mention the toxic effects that may occur in these circumstances.

15. Guillaume-Benjamin Duchenne de Boulogne, "Étude comparée des lésions anatomiques dans l'atrophie musculaire progressive et dans la paralysie générale," *L'Union Médicale* 7, no. 51 (30 April 1853): 202–203 (203 misnumbered '303'). This report summarizes a paper Duchenne presented on 11 March and 8 April 1853. In calling attention to the similarity of carbon disulfide's symptoms with those of general paresis of the insane, Duchenne noted in particular a case he had observed on the service of Dr. (Gabriel) Andral at the Charité Hospital. He deferred detailing the case further, in the expectation that Andral would soon publish its details. Andral (1797–1876) was a leading clinician of the time and published widely on a number of subjects (he was the first to detail the hematological effects of lead poisoning in his "Essai d'hématologie patholo-gique," 1843), yet he does not appear to have independently published on carbon disulfide toxicity. Although he lived until 1876, he withdrew from active practice in 1866. See "Andral's Death" (obituary notice), *Boston Medical and Surgical Journal* 94 (1876): 313–314.

16. Credit for sounding the alarm on carbon disulfide clearly belongs to Auguste L. Dominique Delpech. Delpech's work on carbon disulfide first appeared in a medical publication in 1856. See "IV. Sociétés savantes . . . Académie de médecine," *Gazette Hebdomadaire de Médecine et de Chirurgie* 3 (18 January 1856): 40–41. This was a notice detailing a meeting of the Académie de médecine on 15 January 1856. Delpech's presentation was summarized in a single column length on page 41 and was noted as communicated by Michel Lévy, Grisolle, and Bouchardat. The last, Apollinaire Bouchardat, appears to have discussed the effects of carbon disulfide in his teaching as early as 1852 (which would have been one year before Duchenne's first report), but this was documented only years later. See Apollinaire Bouchardat, *Traité d'hygiéne publique et privée basée sur l'etiologie*, 2nd ed. (Paris: Balliére, 1883), 775. Bouchardat writes, "don mon course de 1852, j'ai exposé, d'aprés ce que j'ai observé dans la fabrique de Gavriel, les effets sur les ouvriers de inhalations contines du sulfure de carbone."

17. Auguste L. Delpech, "Accidens [*sic*] que développe chez les ouvriers en caoutchouc: L'inhalation du sulfure de carbone en vapeur," *L'Union Médicale* 10, no. 60 (31 May 1856): 265–267, quotation from 265: "Les désires vénériens et la érections étaient abolis."

18. See Delpech's 1846 University of Paris doctoral thesis: Auguste L. Delpech, "Des spasmes musculaires idiopathiques et de las paralysie nerveuse essentielle," Rignoux, Impremeur de la Faculté de Médecine, Paris, 1846. Although not directly related to chemical toxins, this documents Delpech's early interest in occupational etiology (on pp. 94–96, it contains a discussion of work-related palsies and cites Ramazzini).

19. A brief report of animal experiments that Delpech had performed with carbon disulfide, "detached" from his original 15 January Académie presentation, was also published as Auguste L. Delpech, "Accidents produits par l'inhalation du sulfure de carbone en vapeur: Expériences sur les animaux," *Gazette Hebdomadaire de Médecine et de Chirurgie* 3 (30 May 1856): 384–385. For Claude Bernard, see *Leçons sur les effets des substances toxiques et médicamenteuses* (Lessons on the effects of toxic substances) (Paris: J.-B. Balliére et Fils, 1857).

20. Auguste L. Delpech, *Mémoire sur les accidents que développe chez les ouvriers en caoutchouc; l'inhalation du sulfure de carbone en vapeur* (Paris: Labe, Libraire de la faculté de médecine, 1856). In this seventy-nine-page monograph (with a title similar to his *L'Union Médicale* article), Delpech explicitly acknowledges that Professor Bouchardat, in his lectures on hygiene at the Faculté, first called his attention to the illness among rubber workers (see n. 16 above).

21. The same year as Delpech's report, Professor E. Beaugrand published his own brief report. See E. Beaugrand, "Action du sulfure de carbone," *Gazette de Hôpitaux Civils et Militaires* 3 (1856): 331–332. He presents an analysis of the symptom complex of carbon disulfide poisoning organized in light of Delpech's findings.

22. Delpech's "magnum opus" on carbon disulfide toxicity was not published until 1863. See Auguste L. Delpech, "Industrie du caoutchouc soufflé: Recherches sur l'intoxication spécial que détermine le sulfure de carbone," *Annales d'Hygiéne Publique et de Médecine Légale* 19, ser. 2 (1863): 65–183.

23. Ibid., 68: "indique suffisamment l'usage, et qui est plus spécialement destiné á l'exportation."

24. Galignani (first name not stated), "Unhealthy Trades," *London Times,* 26 September 1863, 12.

25. Great Britain, Commissioners Appointed to Inquire into the Employment of Children and Yong Persons in Trades and Manufactures Not Already Regulated by Law, *First–Sixth Report of the Commissioners* (London: Her Majesty's Printing Office, 1863–67). The Fourth Report (1865) briefly addresses the conditions in the India rubber industry (pages 103–108), summarizing find-

ings from visits to five factories in 1863–64 that employed approximately thirteen hundred persons. H. W. Lord reports, "The children and young persons employed at Mssrs Macintosh & Co. seemed generally healthy and happy."

26. Ibid.; Herbert Birley's letter to the commissioners, dated 29 September 1863, is published on page 106 of the Fourth Report.

27. For details of the specific cases, see Delpech, *Annales d'Hygiéne Publique et de Médecine Légale.* Page 82 notes "excitation aphrodisiaque." Case XIX is also discussed on pages 81, 87, and 91; Case X, on pages 147–148.

28. On lead poisoning and mill-reeck, see J. E. D. Esquirol, *Mental Maladies: A Treatise on Insanity* (1845; reprint, New York: Hafner Publishing, 1965), 41.

29. An excellent analysis of the role of carbon disulfide in early French psychiatric thought is presented in R. R. O'Flynn and H. A. Waldron, "Delpech and the Origins of Occupational Psychiatry," *British Journal of Industrial Medicine* 47 (1990): 189–198.

30. Jean-Martin Charcot, *Leçons du mardi a la Salpêtriére: Policlinique 1888–1889, notes de cours de MM. Blin, Charcot, Henri Colin* (Paris: Progres Médical, 1889), 43–53, quotation from 43. The case of carbon disulfide intoxication was presented as the first of two cases of the third lesson of the series, Tuesday, 6 November 1888. Charcot acknowledges that Pierre Marie was the source of the clinical case.

31. An image of the photograph of Charcot inscribed to Sigmund Freud can be accessed on www.megapsy.com/Museum/pages/page101.htm (31 March 2006). The original is in the photography collection, Freud Museum, London (1N399). For the role of photography in this period, see Georges Didi-Huberman, *Invention of Hysteria: Charcot and the Photographic Iconography of the Salpêtriére,* trans. Alisa Hartz (Cambridge, MA: MIT Press, 2003).

32. The term *Charcot's carbon disulfide–hysteria* appears as late as 1943. See Karl B. Lehmann and Ferdinand Flury, *Toxicology and Hygiene of Industrial Solvents,* trans. Eleanor King and Henry F. Smyth Jr. (Baltimore: Williams & Wilkins, 1943), 303. (This edition was translated from the German text of 1938.)

33. By 1891, Georges Gilles de la Tourette published the definitive text on the subject of hysteria, with a brief preface by Professor Charcot. See Georges Gilles de la Tourette, *Traité clinique et thérapeutique de l'hystérie d'après l'enseignement de la Salpêtriére* (Paris: E. Plon, Nourrit et Cie, 1891), 101–109. In a section on "the role of intoxications as agent provocateurs of hysteria," Gilles de la Tourette devotes nine pages to the role of toxins in triggering the syndrome, including lead, alcohol, mercury, tobacco, and carbon disulfide. Gilles de la Tourette did have some independent interest in carbon disulfide, having earlier reported on the work of an Italian who investigated its toxicity. See G. Gilles de la Tourette, "De l'intoxication saraiguë par le sulfure de carbone: Researches expérimentales, par le Dr. Arrigo Tomassia, professeur de médecine legale á l'Université de Pavie," *Annales d'Hygiéne Publique et de Médecine Légale* 7, ser. 3 (1882):

292–297. Georges Guillain's work on carbon disulfide came somewhat later. See G. Guillain and V. Courtellemont, "Polynéurite sulfo-carbonée," *Revue Neurologique* 12 (1904): 120–123.

34. Marie's detailed report was published three days after the "lesson." See Pierre Marie, "Hysterie dans l'intoxication par le sulfure de carbone," *Bulletins et Mémoires de la Société Médicale des Hôpitaux de Paris* (9 November 1888): 1479–1480.

35. British medical writers had a particular interest in the adverse effects of carbon disulfide on the nerves of vision. This was first documented in a brief 1884 report: [Ophthalmological Society], "Reports of Societies: Ophthalmological Society of the United Kingdom. Nettleship. Amblyopia and Nervous Depression from Vapour of Bisulphide of Carbon and Chloride of Sulfur," *British Medical Journal* (18 October 1884): 760. In response to this presentation, the Ophthalmological Society appointed a committee (consisting of Drs. Nettleship, Adams, Frost, and Gunn) to investigate this problem further. A year later, that committee summarized findings from thirty-three cases of carbon disulfide poisoning, of which twenty-four involved the optic nerve. See "Ophthalmological Society," *Lancet* (17 January 1885). The next year, Hadden presented his work: W. B. Hadden, "A Case of Chronic Poisoning by Bisulphide of Carbon," *Proceedings of the Medical Society of London* 9 (1886): 115–117. Hadden's case had also developed ocular symptoms and was referred to Nettleship. This case report includes commentary by Benjamin Ward Richardson on the anesthetic properties of carbon disulfide and its use for the euthanasia of dogs (see below). Hadden's paper and Richardson's commentary were also summarized in *Lancet* (2 January 1886), 18. In 1889, a case manifest predominantly with peripheral nervous system damage was documented: A. M. Edge, "Peripheral Neuritis, Caused by the Inhalation of Bisulphide of Carbon," *Lancet* (7 December 1889): 1167–1168. This report referred to other British cases published in 1884 and 1887.

36. On the balloon makers, see Benjamin Ward Richardson, *On Health and Occupation* (London: Society for Promoting Christian Knowledge, 1879), 51.

37. Richardson provided details of this work on euthanasia of pets in B. W. Richardson, "Euthanasia for the Lower Creation—an Original Research and Practical Result," *Asclepiad* 1(1884): 260–275.

38. R. Eglesfeld Griffith, *A Universal Formulary* (Philadelphia: Blanchard and Lea, 1859), 451. This is also the source for the carbon disulfide–containing remedies that follow.

39. *Oxford English Dictionary,* 2nd ed., s.v. "gassed," citing the *Liverpool Daily Post* for the earliest printed appearance of this usage.

40. Thomas Oliver, "Indiarubber: Dangers Incidental to the Use of Bisulphide of Carbon and Naphtha," in *Dangerous Trades,* ed. Thomas Oliver (London: John Murray, 1902), 470–474, quotation from 472–473. Of note, early in his career Oliver had studied with Charcot.

41. For a comparison between the French and British approaches in the later part of the nineteenth century, see Edward Smith, *Handbook for Inspectors of Nuisances* (London: Knight and Co., 1873).

42. The Whitelegge rules are detailed in Oliver, ed., *Dangerous Trades,* "Appendix: Special Rules," 855–856.

43. The likelihood of ramie fiber use in Egypt is discounted in Alfred Lucas, *Ancient Egyptian Materials and Industries,* rev. J. E. Harris, 4th ed. (London: Histories and Mysteries of Man, Ltd., 1989), 149–150.

44. For the dating of cotton substitutes, I have relied on the relevant entries in the *Oxford English Dictionary,* 2nd ed.

45. For the flannelette citation and the dangers of children's sleepwear, see Thomas Oliver, *Diseases of Occupation from the Legislative, Social, and Medical Points of View* (London: Methuen and Co., 1908), 126. Unlike Oliver's 1902 text, which was an edited volume with chapters by various authors, Oliver's later book, which appeared in 1908, was written entirely by him. It was not until the 1960s that the public health implications of inflammable sleepwear were raised. Dr. George Crikelair, a plastic surgeon at Columbia University in New York, became a leader in this effort after caring for two children with clothing-related burns. See George F. Crikelair, "Flame Retardant Clothing," *Journal of Trauma* 6 (1966): 422–427; and his obituary notice: Jeremy Pearce, "Dr. G. F. Crikelair, 84; Set Fabric Safety Rules," *New York Times,* 3 March 2005.

46. A useful early industrial history of rayon can be found in W. D. Darby, *Rayon and Other Synthetic Fibers* (New York: Dry Goods Economists, 1929).

47. *Oxford English Dictionary,* 2nd ed., s.v. "glos," "rayon."

48. H. D. Jump and J. M. Cruice, "Chronic Poisoning from Bisulphide of Carbon," *University of Pennsylvania Medical Bulletin* 17 (1904–5): 193–196, quotation from 193.

49. A. P. Francine, "Acute Carbon Disulphide Poisoning," *American Medicine* 9 (1905): 871.

50. Anonymous, "Parliamentary Intelligence: Health Conditions in Artificial Silk Factories," *Lancet* (24 March 1928): 631.

51. Thomas M. Legge, *Industrial Maladies* (London: Humphrey Milford Oxford Press, Oxford Medical Publications, 1934), 120–122.

52. For an early muckraking of the international rayon cartel, see Grace Hutchins, *Labor and Silk* (New York: International Publishers, 1929).

53. *United States v. Du Pont,* 351 U.S. 377 (1956).

54. Alice Hamilton alluded to ongoing carbon disulfide exposure in the American artificial silk industry as early as 1925, discussing cases that were presented to her in 1923 by Dr. Richard Cameron in Buffalo, New York: Alice Hamilton, *Industrial Poisons in the United States* (New York: Macmillan, 1925), 368–369. She later discusses the issue at length in her autobiography, in which she also recounts her experiences presenting F. H. Lewy's work in Germany at

the International Congress on Occupational Health in 1938: Alice Hamilton, *Exploring the Dangerous Trades* (Boston: Little, Brown, 1943), 387–394. Hamilton uses the spelling "Lewey."

55. The major scientific paper arising from the investigation was F. H. Lewey *[sic]*, "Neurological, Medical and Biochemical Signs and Symptoms Indicating Chronic Industrial Carbon Disulphide Absorption," *Annals of Internal Medicine* 15 (1941): 869–883. The complete sixty-nine-page report of the investigation was published as Department of Labor and Industry, Commonwealth of Pennsylvania, *Survey of Carbon Disulphide and Hydrogen Sulphide Hazards in the Viscose Rayon Industry,* Occupational Disease Prevention Division Bulletin no. 46 (Harrisburg, PA: Commonwealth of Pennsylvania, August 1938). For additional biographical information on Lewy, see B. Holdorff, "Friedrich Heinrich Lewy (1885–1950) and His Work," *Journal of the History of the Neurosciences* 11 (2002): 19–28.

56. The information about the Belgian train cars used to segregate women carbon disulfide workers who were presumably lascivious was provided to me through personal communication with Dr. Eduard Kusters (University of Brussels) and Professor Michel Vanhoome (University of Ghent), Belgium (e-mail from Eduard Kusters, dated 8 January 2002).

57. The details of the Italian Fascist period draw heavily upon the work of Franco Carnevale and Alberto Baldesseroni, "La lotta di Mussolini contro le malattie professionali (1922–1943): I lavoratori e il primato Italiano nella produzione di seta artificiale," *Epidemiologia e Prevenzione* 27 (2003): 114–120. This work was presented in an earlier form as "The Italian Fascist Fight on Occupational Diseases" at the international conference "Occupational Health–Public Health: Lessons from the Past—Challenges for the Future," in Norrköping, Sweden, 6–9 September 2001.

58. Fedele Negro, "Les syndromes Parkinsoniens par intoxication sulfocarbonée," *Revue Neurologique* 2 (1930): 518–522.

59. Carnevale and Baldesseroni, "La lotta di Mussolini contro le malattie professionali."

60. Exposure data were published retrospectively after World War II in Enrico Vigliani, "Carbon Disulphide Poisoning in Viscose Rayon Factories," *British Journal of Industrial Medicine* 11 (1954): 235–241. Vigliani went on to become a leading investigator of benzene's link to leukemia (see chapter 3, n. 31).

61. The industrial base of Premnitz, Germany, was originally founded on munitions manufacturing. After that plant was taken apart in accordance with provisions of the 1918 Treaty of Versailles, the rayon staple industry was established in 1920 under the trade name Vistra. Rayon textile fiber (trade name Travis) came into production in 1928. See the Web site of the "Premnitz Industrial Park": www.premnitz.de (21 November 2004).

62. Hans Reiter, "Arbeitshygiene und Vierjahresplan" (Industrial hygiene and the four-year plan), in *Das Reichsgesundheitsamt 1933–1939: Sechs Jahre na-*

tionalsozialistische Führung (Berlin: Julius Springer, 1939), 243–252. Reiter notes, "In the newly established rayon staple *(Zellwollfrabriken)* we already were aware from various factories, especially from earlier experience in the precipitation baths, of the damage caused by hydrogen sulfide *(Schwefelwasserstoff)*, thus prevention by suction mechanisms has avoided the problem." Reiter's speech is cited in Robert N. Proctor, *The Nazi War against Cancer* (Princeton, NJ: Princeton University Press, 1999), 118, 313–314 (footnote). Proctor correctly translates *Schwefelwasserstoff* as "hydrogen sulfide." Although this substance can also be a hazard in this industry, it is more likely that a speechwriter, without specific technical expertise, used this word instead of *Schwefelkohlenstoff* (carbon disulfide), the more relevant toxin in this context. For the translation of the expanded text, I received the assistance of Dr. Martin Wangh.

63. Hans Schramm, "Chronische Schwefelkohlenstoff Vergiftungen in der Kunstseide- und Zellwollindustrie," *Deutsche Medizinische Wochenscrift* 66 (1940): 180–182. The title of this article makes the distinction between routine art silk *(Kunstseide)* and *Zellwolle* (rayon staple). Another, somewhat earlier German-language paper is also relevant to carbon disulfide and industrial health during the Fascist period: Juan Dantín-Gallego, "Erfahrungen über Schwefelkohlenstoffschädigungen bei der Olivenölbereitung in Andalusien, mit einigen diesbezüglichen Tierexperimenten," *Archiv für Gerbepathologie und Gewerbhygiene* 8 (1937): 124–138. This paper highlights an exposure source for carbon disulfide unrelated to rayon production—namely, the extraction of fats and oils, a longstanding, albeit minor, industrial application of carbon disulfide. Dantín-Gallego's report includes this statement: "I ask you to take into account that my work was written during the Spanish Civil War and therefore I had very limited scientific aids or literature at my disposal." Dantín-Gallego went on to become a leading figure in occupational medicine in Spain during the Franco years, beginning with a professorship in 1939; he died at the age of ninety in 1997. See Angel y Cols Bartolome Pineda, *Historia de la medicina del trabajo en España (1800–2000)* (Murcia, Spain: Diego Marin, 2004).

64. International Labour Office, *Occupation and Health: Encyclopaedia of Hygiene, Pathology and Social Welfare, Studied from the Point of View of Labour, Industry and Trades,* special supplement: *Industrial Health in Wartime* (Montreal: International Labour Office, 1944), 19–21.

65. Emil A. Paluch, "Two Outbreaks of Carbon Disulfide Poisoning in Rayon Staple Fiber Plants in Poland," *Journal of Industrial Hygiene and Toxicology* 30 (1948): 37–42. At least one other rayon staple plant (located in Wittenberg, Germany) was run with slave labor, in this instance from the Neuengamme concentration camp. See www.holocaust-education.de (21 November 2004).

66. Salient points of the Korean episode are documented in S. K. Cho et al., "Long-Term Neuropsychological Effects and MRI Findings in Patients with CS_2 Poisoning," *Acta Neurologica Scandinavica* 106 (2002): 269–275. Taiwan ap-

pears to have had a similar problem with exposures in the 150–300 part per million range. See C. C. Chu et al., "Polyneuropathy Induced by Carbon Disulphide in Viscose Rayon Workers," *Occupational and Environmental Medicine* 52 (1995): 404–407.

67. Recent data from the People's Republic of China through collaborative study with Belgian investigators are presented in Xiaodong Tan et al., "The Cross-Sectional Study of the Health Effects of Occupational Exposure to Carbon Disulfide in a Chinese Viscose Plant," *Environmental Toxicology* 16 (2001): 377–382.

68. For an example of other neurological damage from carbon disulfide, see Howard Frumkin, "Multiple System Atrophy following Chronic Carbon Disulfide Exposure," *Environmental Health Perspectives* 106 (1998): 611–613. The case report and literature review invoked a strongly critical letter to the editor and the author's counterreply: D. G. Graham, "Carbon Disulfide," *Environmental Health Perspectives* 108 (2000): A110–112. This exchange underscores the frequently contentious nature of such industrial injury cases.

69. The scientific literature pertaining to cardiovascular disease is reviewed in Agency for Toxic Substances Disease Registry, *Toxicological Profile for Carbon Disulfide* (Update) (1996–739–32) (Atlanta, GA: U.S. Department of Health and Human Services [ATSDR], 1996).

70. *United States v. Du Pont,* 351 U.S. 377 (1956), opinion by Justice Reed.

71. "Arnold N. Nawrocki, Cheese Innovator, 78," obituary, *New York Times,* 12 July 2002.

72. Anne T. Fidler and Michael S. Crandall, *HETA Report no. HETA-85–098-L1959, Teepak, Inc., Danville, Illinois* (Cincinnati: National Institute for Occupational Safety and Health, April 1989).

73. Ibid., 5.

74. R. M. Swift, "Drug Therapy for Alcohol Dependence," *New England Journal of Medicine* 340 (1999): 1482–1490.

75. M. J. Ellenhorn et al., *Ellenhorn's Medical Toxicology: Diagnosis and Treatment of Human Poisoning,* 2nd ed. (Baltimore: Williams & Wilkins, 1997), 1356–1362.

76. Carbon disulfide use in fumigation commonly occurred in combination with the liver toxin carbon tetrachloride as a so-called 80/20 fumigant. A NIOSH investigation before the ban found high peak levels of both toxins (carbon disulfide was at 327 parts per million) and concluded that "there is a serious potential health hazard due to high fumigant concentrations in treated grain in incoming rail cars." See S. H. Ahrenholz, *HETA Report no. HETA-83–375–1521, Federal Grain Service, USDA, Portland, Oregon* (Cincinnati: NIOSH [1973]). Health effects in exposed grain workers were indeed documented before the ban. See H. A. Peters, "Synergistic Neurotoxicity of Carbon Tetrachloride/Carbon Disulfide (80/20 Fumigants) and Other Pesticides in Grain Storage Workers," *Acta Pharmacologica Toxicol* (Copenhagen) 7 (1986): 535–546.

77. The metam sodium spill is thoroughly documented in James E. Cone et al., "Persistent Respiratory Health Effects after a Metam Sodium Pesticide Spill," *Chest* 106 (1994): 500–508. See also S. B. Pruett, L. P. Myers, and D. E. Keil, "Toxicology of Metam Sodium," *Journal of Toxicology and Environmental Health B Criteria Reviews* 4 (2001): 207–222.

78. U.S. Environmental Protection Agency, *2002 Toxics Release Inventory* (www.epa.gov/tri) (21 November 2004); and *1993 Toxics Release Inventory Public Data Release* (Washington DC: U.S. EPA, Office of Pollution Prevention and Toxics, 1995).

79. Philip J. Klemmer and Alexis A. Harris, "Carbon Disulfide Nephropathy," *American Journal of Kidney Diseases* 36 (2000): 626–629. See also the accompanying editorial: Richard P. Wedeen, "Occupational Renal Diseases," *American Journal of Kidney Diseases* 36 (2000): 644–645.

80. A three-page description of the Courtaulds rayon staple facility prior to initiation of NIOSH's initial study is contained in James H. Jones and Sherry G. Selevan, *Walk-Through Survey Report no. 75–16* (Cincinnati, OH: Industry-Wide Studies, NIOSH, 1975). A more complete descriptive report on the staple facility studied by NIOSH (not specifically identified but appearing to be the same Courtaulds plant), accompanied by industrial sampling data, was published as John Fajen, Bruce Albright, and Sanford S. Leffingwell, "A Cross-Sectional Medical and Industrial Hygiene Survey of Workers Exposed to Carbon Disulfide," *Scandinavian Journal of Work Environment and Health* 7, supplement 4 (1981): 20–27. Quoted statement on the need for further study is from this publication, 26.

81. The later data analysis was published as G. M. Egeland et al., "Effects of Exposure to Carbon Disulphide on Low Density Lipoprotein Cholesterol Concentration and Diastolic Blood Pressure," *British Journal of Industrial Medicine* 49 (1992): 287–293.

82. The aborted NIOSH Health Hazard Evaluation of the Courtaulds facility in the late 1990s was named "A Cross-Sectional Investigation of Health Effects in Carbon Disulfide Exposed and Non-Exposed Workers at a Viscose Rayon Factory" and was assigned the official NIOSH report number HETA 96–0114.

83. The data reanalysis sponsored by the carbon disulfide industry was published as Bertram Price et al., "A Benchmark Concentration for Carbon Disulfide: Analysis of the NIOSH Carbon Disulfide Exposure Database," *Regulatory Toxicology and Pharmacology* 24 (1996): 171–176.

84. One such Internet-marketed source, at least as late as 2006, was Make it Yours; see www.millenniumgeneralstore.com/classdemos/pg1.html (31 March 2006).

85. For a more complete *General Hospital* plot synopsis, see www.abc.go .com/daytime/generalhospital/episodes/19912.html (29 July 2005).

6. JOB FEVER

1. The welding exposure experiments are summarized in Paul D. Blanc et al., "Cytokines in Metal Fume Fever," *American Review of Respiratory Diseases* 147 (1993): 134–138.

2. Additional general background on metal fume fever is provided in Paul Blanc and Homer A. Boushey, "The Lung in Metal Fume Fever," *Seminars in Respiratory Medicine* 14 (1993): 212–225.

3. For zinc as a cold remedy, see "Zinc for the Common Cold," *Medical Letter on Drugs and Therapeutics* 39 (31 January 1997): 9–10; and R. B. Turner and W. E. Cetnarowski, "Effect of Treatment with Zinc Gluconate or Zinc Acetate on Experimental and Natural Colds," *Clinical Infectious Disease* 31 (2000): 1202–1208. The *Medical Letter on Drugs and Therapeutics* review is equivocal; the latter paper shows no zinc-related benefit.

4. For further information on endotoxin, see Cecile S. Rose and Paul D. Blanc, "Inhalation Fever," in *Environmental and Occupational Medicine,* ed. William N. Rom, 3rd ed. (Boston: Little, Brown, 1998), 467–480.

5. Andrew Meiklejohn, "Outbreak of Fever in Cotton Mills at Radcliffe, 1784," *British Journal of Industrial Medicine* 16 (1959): 68–69. This article includes the text of the original report by Thomas Percival, John Cowling, Alexander Eason, and Edward Chorley. See also Charles Webster, "Two-Hundredth Anniversary of the 1784 Report on Fever at Radcliffe Mill," *Society for the Social History of Medicine Bulletin* 36 (1985): 65–67.

6. For a contemporaneous history of the technology of the flying shuttle, spinning jenny, and water frame spinner, see Edward Baines, *History of the Cotton Manufacture in Great Britain* (London: H. Fisher, R. Fisher, and P. Jackson, 1835).

7. For an early general review summarizing the British view of byssinosis, see C. I. C. Gill, "Byssinosis in the Cotton Trade," *British Journal of Industrial Medicine* 4 (1947): 48–55; and, more recently, R. McL. Niven and C. A. Pickering, "Byssinosis: A Review," *Thorax* 51 (1996): 632–637.

8. Philibert Patissier, *Traité des maladies des artisans* (Paris: J.-B. Bailliére, 1822), 245. "Ces ouvriers inspirent continuellement un air chargé de débris cotonneux tréstenus qui excitent les bronches, provoquent la toux, et entretiennent dans les poumons une irritation perpétuelle. Ils sont souvent obligés de changer de profession pour prévenir la phthisie."

9. William Rathbone Greg, *An Enquiry into the State of the Manufacturing Population and the Causes and Cures of the Evils Therein Existing* (London: James Ridgeway, 1831), 15. The Greg family operation, the Quarry Bank Mill, was still operating outside Manchester well into the twentieth century. It was given to the British National Trust in 1939 and is now an industrial museum and favored picnic spot. See www.quarrybankmill.org.uk (11 March 2006).

10. James Phillips Kay, "Observations and Experiments Concerning Molecular Irritation of the Lungs as One Source of Tubercular Consumption; and on Spinners' Phthisis," *North of England Medical and Surgical Journal* I (February, 1831): 348–363, quotation from 359.

11. Charles Turner Thackrah, *The Effects of the Principal Arts, Trades, and Professions, and of the Civic States and Habits of Living on Health and Longevity: with a Particular Reference to the Trades and Manufactures of Leeds: and Suggestions for the Removal of Many of the Agents, which Produce Disease, and Shorten the Duration of Life* (London: Longman, Rees, Orme, Brown, and Green, 1831); Charles Turner Thackrah, *The Effects of Arts, Trades, and Professions, and of Civic States and Habits of Living on Health and Longevity, with Suggestions for the Removal of Many of the Agents which Promote Disease and Shorten the Duration of Life*, 2nd ed. (London: Longman, Rees, Orme, Brown, Green, and Longman, 1832), 68 (here and subsequently, the quotations are from the 2nd edition). As noted previously, a rich biographical note by Andrew Meiklejohn introduces a facsimile reprint of the 1832 text (Edinburgh: E. & S. Livingston, 1957).

12. Michael Sadler, "Speech in the House of Commons on the Second Reading of the Factories Regulation Bill (13 March 1832)" (excerpt), in *English Historical Documents 1833–1874*, ed. G. M. Young and W. D. Handcock (London: Eyre and Spottiswoode, 1956), 933–934. This brief excerpt does not give justice to Sadler's full speech, nor does it document his invocation of Thackrah. See Charles Wing, *Evils of the Factory System Demonstrated by the Parliamentary Evidence* (London: Sanders and Otky, 1837), 256–285. Wing dates the speech 16 March 1832.

13. *British Labourer's Protector, and Factory Child's Friend*, ed. George Stringer Bull and Charles Walker, issues 1–31, 21 September 1832–19 April 1833 (Leeds: R. Inchbold, printer). The parliamentary testimony related to the Ten Hour Bill is also at the core of Wing, *Evils of the Factory System Demonstrated by the Parliamentary Evidence*. Published after passage of the watered-down Factories Regulation Act in 1833, Wing's 498-page compendium argued for further legislation, ultimately realized in 1847.

14. Charles Turner Thackrah, "The Factory System (Opinion of Mr. Thackrah, Surgeon, Given at the Leeds Meeting)" [1832?], Goldsmiths'-Kress Library of Economic Literature no. 27554, University of London (one-page broadside from the Oastler collection of ephemera).

15. William Albert Samuel Hewins, "Oastler, Richard," and Michael Ernest Sadler, "Sadler, Michael Thomas," in *Dictionary of National Biography*, ed. Leslie Stephen and Sidney Lee, vol. 14, 738–740 (Oastler); vol. 17, 594–598 (Sadler).

16. *North of England Medical and Surgical Journal* (London: Whittaker, Treacher, and Arnot). The entire run was four issues, August 1830–May 1831. The first issue published the introductory essay cited (quotation from p. v). In addition to publishing Kay's article, during its short run the journal also published

Arnold Knight: "On the Grinders' Asthma," in two parts (issue 1, August, 85–91, and issue 2, November, 167–179). This was one of the first detailed reports of lung disease among Sheffield grinders. A highly positive review of Thackrah that appeared stated, "The subject is one of such great importance that we commend it to the attention of the profession" (issue 3, February 1831, 394–395).

17. James Phillips Kay, *The Moral and Physical Condition of the Working Classes Employed in the Cotton Manufacture in Manchester,* 2nd ed. enlarged (London: James Ridway, 1832), 90–92, quotation from 92.

18. Until recently the location of Thackrah's grave was unknown. See Graham Hardy, "Thackrah's Grave," *Occupational Medicine* 53 (2003): 505–506. This also provides a brief biographical synopsis of Thackrah largely informed by Meiklejohn's work (see n. 11 above).

19. Daniel Noble, *Facts and Observations Relative to the Influence of Manufactures Upon Health and Life* (London: John Churchill, 1843).

20. Edwin Chadwick, *Report to Her Majesty's Principal Secretary of State for the Home Department, from the Poor Law Commissioners on an Inquiry into the Sanitary Condition of the Labouring Population of Great Britain* (London: W. Clowes, 1842), "Instance of a superior moral and sanitary condition enjoyed by workers in a cotton factory," 236–238, quotation from 237. The only section specific to workplace exposures, "Employers' Influence on the Health of Workpeople by the Ventilation of Places of Work, and the Prevention of Noxious Fumes, Dust, &c.," spans only six pages (256–261) and largely blames workers' poor habits for overexposure. See chapter 7 text regarding Kyanization of wood and its related n. 31.

21. For relevant excerpts from Chadwick's report that helped to kill the Ten Hour Bill (coauthored by Thomas Tooke and Thomas Southwood Smith), see *English Historical Documents 1833–1874,* ed. G. M. Young and W. D. Handcock (London: Eyre and Spottiswoode, 1956), 941–949.

22. Elizabeth Gaskell, *North and South* (1854; London: Penguin Books, 1970), 146–147.

23. Louis-René Villermé, *Rapport à l'Académie des sciences morales et politiques sur l'état physique et morale des ouvriers employés dans les fabriques de soie, de coton, et de laine* (Paris: Académie des sciences morales et politiques, 1839), 148. "La toux est le premier symptôme d'une maladie lente et formidable de poitrine."

24. Daniel Joseph Mareska and Julian Heyman, *Enquête sur le travail et la condition physique et morale des ouvriers employés dans les manufactures de coton, a Gand* (Ghent, Belgium: F. et E. Gyselynck, 1845). This was published separately as an extract from the *Annales de la Société de Médecine de Gand,* vol. 16. To further underscore the acceptance in the French-language scientific literature that cotton dust caused lung disease, also see Jules Godfrain, "Quelques notes sur l'hygiéne des ouvriers des manufactures," M.D. thesis, Rignoux, Imprimeur de la Faculté de Médecine, Paris, 5 August 1852.

25. John Simon, *Public Health Reports,* ed. Edward Seaton, vol. 2 (London: Offices of the Sanitary Institute, 1887), 35–36. The quoted passage is from the *Fourth Report to the Privy Council, 1861,* and is based on Greenhow's field studies. Greenhow had also contributed to John Simon, *Third Report of the Medical Officer of the Privy Council, 1860* ([London]: Ordered, by the House of Commons, to be printed, 15 April 1861), appendix 6: "Dr. Greenhow's Report on Districts with Excessive Mortality from Lung-Diseases," 102–194.

26. Marx, *Das Kapital,* vol. 1, part 3, chap. 10, "The Production of Absolute Surplus-Value," sec. 3, "Branches of the English Industry without Legal Limits to Exploitation." Citing Greenhow's Privy Council report regarding the pottery trades, Marx concluded that they are so injurious as to be "a branch of industry by the side of which cotton-spinning appears an agreeable and healthful occupation" www.marxists.org/archive/marx/works/1867-cl/ch10 (16 March 2003).

27. Adrien Proust, *Traité d'hygiéne publique et privée* (Paris: G. Masson, 1877), 171.

28. Thomas Harris, "A Contribution to the Pathological Anatomy of Pneumokoniosis (Chalicosis Pulmonum)," *Journal of Anatomy and Physiology* 15 (1880–81): 395–404.

29. John T. Arlidge, *The Hygiene, Diseases, and Mortality of Occupations* (London: Percival and Company, 1892), 361.

30. Ibid., 407.

31. Ibid. In describing flock fever, Arlidge acknowledges his source as the work of "Dr. Parsons." This is Henry Franklin Parsons, who was a local medical officer active in the 1880s. In 1885 he reported on fever in the flock industry. See H. Franklin Parsons, "On the Manufacture of Rag Flock in Reference to the Possible Dissemination of Infectious Disease by this and Other Products of Woolen Rags," in *The 15th Annual Report of the Medical Officer of the Local Government Board for 1885[–1886]* (London: Her Majesty's Stationery Office [printed by Eyre & Spottiswoode], 1886), appendix A, no. 7, 61–72. Arlidge was quoting Parsons's text as it appears on 69.

32. Arlidge, *The Hygiene, Diseases, and Mortality of Occupations,* 375–376. For mill fever in linen making, see also John T. Arlidge, "On Occupations in their Relations to Health and Life (An Address Delivered at the Opening of the Section of Public Medicine, at the Annual Meeting of the British Medical Association, in Bath, August 1878)," *British Medical Journal* 2 (17 August 1878): 239–244. For information on the linen industry, Arlidge relied heavily on his colleague and fellow certifying medical officer Charles Nicholas Delacherois Purdon of Belfast. Arlidge was founding president of the Association of Certifying Medical Officers of Great Britain and Ireland; Purdon was one of its two vice-presidents. At the 1873 meeting of the association, Purdon presented the paper "The Mortality of Flax Mill & Factory Workers: As Compared with

Other Classes of the Community, the Diseases They Labour Under, and the Causes that Render the Death-Rate from Phthisis, &c. So High."

33. Edgar L. Collis, "The Occurrence of an Unusual Cough among Weavers of Cotton Cloth," *Proceedings of the Royal Society of Medicine* 8, part 2 (23 April 1915): 108–112, quotation from 112. In the same year, in his Milroy Lecture on the subject, Collis was unequivocal in linking dust from cotton stripping to "true asthma" and to mill fever. "Exposure to this dust has unpleasant effects for a chance visitor, who, not infrequently, suffers within twelve hours from an attack of mill fever, with sharp but transient febrile symptoms, but operatives soon become inured to such attacks." See Edgar L. Collis, "Industrial Pneumoconioses with Special Reference to Dust-Phthisis," *Public Health* 28 (1915): 260.

34. For these British governmental reports, see Austin Bradford Hill, *Artificial Humidification in the Cotton Weaving Industry: Its Effects upon Sickness Rate of Weaving Operatives* (London: Industrial Fatigue Research Board [Report 48], 1927); and C. Prausnitz, *Investigations on Respiratory Dust Disease in Operatives in the Cotton Industry*, Medical Research Council Special Report no. 212 (London: His Majesty's Stationery Office, 1936).

35. E. G. Davis, "Influence of Occupation on Health," *Boston Medical and Surgical Journal* 7 (1832–33): 251–253, 270–272, 288–289, 303–306, 315–316, 333–336, 366–368; 8 (1833): 13–14, 46–49, 155–159, 171–175, 189–193. Although appearing in sequentially numbered parts through XIII, the part beginning in volume 7 is numbered "IX," seemingly without a number VIII having appeared (thus twelve parts in total). The quoted passage on cotton mill work is discussed in part 10 of the series, 8 (1833): 47.

36. Benjamin W. McCready, "On the Influence of Trades, Professions and Occupations in the United States in the Production of Disease—Being the Prize Dissertation for 1837," *Transactions of the Medical Society of the State of New York* 3 (1836–37): 91–150, quotation from 109. A similar view from the same period holding that American mills were relatively disease-free is put forward by Charles A. Lee, "On the Effects of Arts, Trades, and Professions, as well as Habits of Living, on Health and Longevity," *Family Magazine* 8 (1840): 175–177, 212–215, 270–272, 302–305. The cotton industry is discussed on 304–305.

37. M. F. Trice, "Card-Room Fever: Strict Control of Dust Will Eliminate Health Hazard from Low-Grade Cotton," *Textile World* 60 (March 1940): 68.

38. Paul A. Neal, Roy Schneiter, and Barbara H. Caminita, "Report on Acute Illness among Rural Mattress Makers Using Low Grade, Stained Cotton," *JAMA* 119 (1942): 1074–1082. Another outbreak of mill fever in this period occurred when Danish cotton mills reopened in 1945, the labor force being exposed again after a long wartime hiatus (personal communication from Torben Sigsgaard, email dated 23 June 2006).

39. For additional background on the history of brass making and the emergence of metal fume fever, see Paul D. Blanc, "Metal Fume Fever from a His-

torical Perspective," in *Contributions to the History of Occupational and Environmental Prevention: 1st International Conference on the History of Occupational Prevention, Rome, Italy, 4–6 October 1998*, ed. A. Grieco, S. Iavicoli, and G. Berlinguer (Amsterdam: Elsevier, 1999), 211–221.

40. For Thackrah on the brass ague among the brass melters of Birmingham, see Thackrah, *The Effects of Arts, Trades, and Professions*, 2nd ed. Quotation from 101; brass button makers are discussed on 110.

41. Thackrah, *The Effects of the Principal Arts, Trades, and Professions, and of Civic States and Habits of Living*, 1st ed., 54.

42. *Pliny's Natural History*, trans. H. Rackam, Loeb Classical Library (Cambridge, MA: Harvard University Press, 1952). Quotation on cinnabar is from book 33, chap. 40, beginning line 123; cadmia is discussed in book 34.

43. The material on brass and related alloys in antiquity is drawn in part from Edward J. Cocks and B. Walters, *A History of the Zinc Smelting Industry in Britain* (London: George G. Harrap, 1968), 2–20; Leslie Aitchison, *A History of Metals*, vol. 2 (New York: Interscience Publishers, 1960), 322–327, 468–469; and F. W. Gibbs, "Extraction and Production of Metals: Non-ferrous Metals," in *A History of Technology: The Industrial Revolution*, vol. 4, ed. Charles Singer et al. (London: Oxford University Press, 1958), 118–147. See also David A. Scott, *Metallography and Microstructure of Ancient and Historic Metals* ([Marina del Rey, CA]: Getty Conservation Institute, 1991), 145; and John W. Humphrey, John P. Oleson, and Andres N. Sherwood, *Greek and Roman Technology: A Sourcebook* (London: Routledge, 1998), 223–224.

44. Ulrich Ellenbog, "On the Poisonous Evil Vapours," *Lancet* 1 (1932): 270–271. This translation is attributed to Cyril Barnard. In addition to this translated text, a facsimile of the German original was published in 1927 with an introduction by Friederich Zoepfl and Franz Koelsch: Ullrich Ellenbog, *Von den gifftigen besen Tempffen und Reuchen: Eine gewerbe-hygienische Schrift des XV Jahrhunderts* (Munich: Verlag der Münchner Drucke, 1927). The only extant copy of the 1524 original is preserved in the collection of the University of Texas, Galveston.

45. *Georgius Agricola De Re Metallica*, trans. Herbert Clark Hoover and Lou Henry Hoover (New York: Dover Publications, 1950), 112–113, 214–218, 354, 408–410, quotation from 214. See also Bern Dibner, *Agricola on Metals* (Norwalk, CT: Burndy Library, 1958). For another early description of zinc smelting, see Anneliese Grünhaldt Sisco and Cyril Stanely Smith, *Lazarus Ercker's Treatise on Ores and Assaying Translated from the German Edition of 1580* (Chicago: University of Chicago Press, 1951), nn. 271–272.

46. Alfred Boni, *Tutenag and Paktong: With Notes on Other Alloys in Domestic Use during the Eighteenth Century* (Oxford: Oxford University Press, 1924). Additional background on paktong can be found in David Kuhner, *The Bibliotheca Herbert Clark Hoover Collection of Metallica, Mining and Metallurgy*

(Claremont, CA: Libraries of the Claremont Colleges, 1980), xi (Cyril Stanley Smith), 139. Catalog item 583 is an anonymous journal of over seven hundred experiments carried out during 1700–1774 in an attempt to duplicate the composition of the Chinese alloy.

47. C. G. Ekeberg, "Underrattelse om tutanego," *Kongliga Svenska Vetenskaps Academiens Handlingar* 17 (1756): 316–317; translation as provided in Boni, *Tutenag and Paktong*, 10–11.

48. Song, Yingxing, *T'ien-kung K'ai-wu: Chinese Technology in the Seventeenth Century*, trans. E-tu Zen Sun and Shiou-chuan Sun (University Park and London: Pennsylvania State University Press, 1966), 242–247, quotation from 247. The Chinese title is rendered as "The Creations of Nature and Man" by the translators (preface, p. vii). In this translation, the author's name was transliterated as Ying-Hsing Sung.

49. W. Richardson, *Chemical Principles of the Metallic Arts, with an Account of the Principal Diseases Incident to Different Artificers, the Means of Prevention and Cure and a Concise Introduction to the Study of Chemistry* (Birmingham: Thomas Pearson, 1790), 169–170.

50. E. A. Blandet, "Colique de cuivre" and "Effets des vapeurs du zinc sur l'économie animale," *Annales d'Hygiéne Publique et Médecine Legale* 33 (1845): 461–462, 462–463 (two separate reports published sequentially).

51. Blandet followed up "Colique de cuivre" and "Effets des vapeurs du zinc sur l'économie animale" with the report "Du délire produit par l'inspiration des vapeurs d'oxyde de zinc," which was then followed by Guérard's refutation of a direct zinc effect in his "Sur les effets des vapeurs de zinc, opposés a ceux des boissons aqueuses, prises avec excés." See *Annales d'Hygiéne Publique Médecine Légale* 34 (1845): 222–223 (Blandet) and 224–226 (Guérard).

52. Augustus Kingsley Gardner, "An Account of a Disease Peculiar to Workmen in Brasscock Foundries," *New York Journal of Medicine* 10 (1848): 210–213.

53. Edward Headlam Greenhow, "On Brass-Founders' Ague," *Medical-Chirurgical Transactions* 54 (1862): 177–187, quotation from 177.

54. Lawrence Wright, *Warm and Snug: The History of the Bed* (London: Routledge & Kegan Paul, 1962).

55. Jeremy Brecher, Jerry Lombardi, and Jan Stackhouse, *Brass Valley: The Story of Working People's Lives and Struggles in an American Industrial Region* (Philadelphia: Temple University Press, 1982), 74–76.

56. For brass human exposure studies outside the United States, see Karl B. Lehmann, "Studien über technisch und hygienisch wichtige Gase und Dämpfe. 14. Das Giess- oder Zinkfieber," *Archiv für Hygiene* 72 (1910): 358–381. The experimental exposures Lehmann documents were carried out in 1906 but not published until 1910. See also Alfred Arnstein, "Beitrag zur Kenntnis des Giessfiebers," *Wiener Arbeiten aus dem Gebiete der Sozialen Medizin* 1 (1910): 49–58; E. Rost, "Zur Kenntnis des Giessfiebers, mit besonderer Berücksichtigung der Ausscheidungs-

verhältnisse der aufgenommenen Metalle Zink und Kupfer," *Arbeiten aus dem Reichsgesundheitsamte* 52 (1920): 1–40 (the exposures documented took place in 1911, although they were not published until 1920); and A. I. Burstein, "Lychoradka medno-lyteyeshkov" (Brass-founders' ague), *Gigiena Truda* 7 (1925): 17–41.

57. Drinker's initial exposure experiments were reported in Cyrus C. Sturgis, Philip Drinker, and Robert M. Thomson, "Metal Fume Fever. 1. Clinical Observations on the Effect of the Experimental Inhalation of Zinc Oxide by Two Apparently Normal Persons," *Journal of Industrial Hygiene* 9 (1927): 88–97, quotation from 88–89. Related publications include Philip Drinker, "Certain Aspects of the Problem of Zinc Toxicity," *Journal of Industrial Hygiene* 4 (1922): 177–197; and Philip Drinker, Robert M. Thomson, and Jane L. Flynn, "Metal Fume Fever: 4. Threshold Doses of Zinc Oxide, Preventive Measures, and the Chronic Effects of Repeated Exposures," *Journal of Industrial Hygiene* 9 (1927): 331–345.

58. Elsie de Wolfe, *The House in Good Taste* (New York: Century Company, 1913), 215–216.

59. Charles A. Pfender, "Brazier's Disease, Brass-Founder's Ague, or Acute Brass-Poisoning," *JAMA* 62 (1914): 296–297, quotation from 297.

60. A. C. Titus, Henry Warren, and Philip Drinker, "Electric Welding. 1. The Respiratory Hazard," *Journal of Industrial Hygiene* 17 (1935): 121–128, quotation from 121.

61. Philip Drinker, Henry Warren, and Richard Page, "Electric Welding. 3. Prevention of the Respiratory Hazard," *Journal of Industrial Hygiene* 17 (1935): 133–137, quotation from 135.

62. Joseph R. Kuh, Morris F. Cullen, and Clifford Kuh, "Metal Fume Fever," *Permanente Foundation Medical Bulletin* 4 (1946): 145–151.

63. Stephen F. Wintermeyer et al., "Pulmonary Responses after Wood Chip Mulch Exposure," *Journal of Occupational and Environmental Medicine* 39 (1997): 308–314.

64. William T. Brinton, Earl E. Vastbinder, John W. Greene, et al., "An Outbreak of Organic Dust Toxic Syndrome in a College Fraternity," *JAMA* 258 (1987): 1210–1212.

65. The term *inhalation fever* was first used in an unsigned *Lancet* editorial in 1978 ("Inhalation Fevers," *Lancet* 1, no. 8058 [4 February 1978]: 249–250); it was first proposed as a general term in Anna Rask-Anderson and David S. Pratt, "Inhalation Fever: A Proposed Unifying Term for Febrile Reactions to Inhalation of Noxious Substances," *British Journal of Industrial Medicine* 49 (1992): 40; with further follow-up as David S. Pratt and Anna Rask-Anderson, "Inhalation Fever: A Proposed Unifying Term for Febrile Reactions to Inhalation of Noxious Substances," *British Journal of Industrial Medicine* 50 (1993): 287–288.

66. Dennis J. Shusterman, "Polymer Fume Fever and Other Fluorocarbon Pyrolysis-Related Syndromes," *Occupational Medicine* 8 (1993): 519–531.

67. Thomas H. Glick et al., "Pontiac Fever: An Epidemic of Unknown Etiology in a Health Department. 1. Clinical and Epidemiologic Aspects," *American Journal of Epidemiology* 107 (1978): 149–160. The outbreak occurred in the office building of the Oakland County, Michigan, Department of Health, which may have facilitated the investigation.

68. "Respiratory Illness in Workers Exposed to Metalworking Fluid Contaminated with Nontuberculous Mycobacteria—Ohio, 2001," *MMWR* 51 (2002): 349–352.

69. Guo-chang Xing, "Some Opinions on Byssinosis in China," *American Journal of Industrial Medicine* 12 (1987): 737–742.

70. The "modern era" of byssinosis research in the United States began in the late 1960s with the work of Arend Bouhuys of Yale University. The first textile factory that he was able to gain access to study from the "inside" was a cotton mill run by the U.S. penitentiary at Atlanta, Georgia, where 25 percent of the prisoner labor force was symptomatic. See Arend Bouhuys, "Byssinosis in Textile Workers," in *Pneumoconiosis. Proceedings of the International Conference Johannesburg 1969*, ed. H. A. Shapiro (Capetown, South Africa: Oxford University Press, 1970), 412–416. For an example of the ongoing epidemiological literature delineating the nuances of byssinosis, see David C. Christiani, Xiao-Rong Wang, Lei-Da Pan, et al., "Longitudinal Changes in Pulmonary Function and Respiratory Symptoms in Cotton Textile Workers: A 15-Yr. Follow-Up Study," *American Journal of Respiratory and Critical Care Medicine* 163 (2001): 847–853. In 1987, a special issue of the *American Journal of Industrial Medicine* printed the proceedings of an international workshop, "Byssinosis in the Far East," underscoring the international importance of this problem (*American Journal of Industrial Medicine* 12, no. 6); this conference is the source of n. 69, above.

71. Gaskell, *North and South*, 147.

72. *American Textile Mfrs. Inst. v. Donovan*, 452 U.S. 490 (1981). Opinion by Justice Brennan; joined by White, Marshall, Blackmun, and Stevens. Justices Rehnquist, Burger, and Stewart dissented; Justice Powell did not take part. Robert H. Bork argued for the textile manufacturers. For worker testimony, see fn. 9. See also William J. Curran and Leslie I. Boden, "Occupational Health Values in the Supreme Court: Cost-Benefit Analysis," *American Journal of Public Health* 71 (1981): 1264–1265.

73. Juliana Hatfield, "Metal Fume Fever," © 2000 Juliana Hatfield Music (BMI). All rights for the world on behalf of Juliana Hatfield Music (BMI) administered by Zomba Songs, Inc. (BMI). Used by permission.

7. EMERGING TOXINS

1. For the early history of anthrax-caused wool-sorters' disease, see T. Carter, "The Dissemination of Anthrax from Imported Wool: Kidderminster 1900–

1914," *Occupational and Environmental Medicine* 61 (2004): 103–107; and N. Metcalfe, "The History of Woolsorters' Disease: A Yorkshire Beginning with an International Future?" *Occupational Medicine* (London) 54 (2004): 489–493. The first "naturally occurring" case in the United States in thirty years occurred in 2006. See Sewell Chan, "New York City Man Has Inhalation Anthrax, Officials Say," *New York Times,* 23 February 2006 and "Inhalation Anthrax Associated with Dried Animal Hides—Pennsylvania and New York City, 2006," *MMWR* 55 (2006): 280–282.

2. Amanda Hesser, "An Old-Fashioned, Versatile Treat," *New York Times,* 3 October 2001.

3. Jonathan Eig, "Butter Flavoring May Pose a Risk to Food Workers," *Wall Street Journal,* 3 October 2001. See also "Claims Are Settled in Suit Involving Popcorn Plant," *Wall Street Journal,* 6 October 2005. The case involved fifteen injured workers.

4. "Fixed Obstructive Lung Disease in Workers at a Microwave Popcorn Factory—Missouri, 2000–2002," *MMWR* 51 (2002): 345–347; and Kathleen Kreiss et al., "Clinical Bronchiolitis Obliterans in Workers at a Microwave-Popcorn Plant," *New England Journal of Medicine* 347 (2002): 330–338. Cases of lung disease related to butter flavoring continue to be reported, leading to criticism of government oversight and of the industry trade group involved, the Flavor and Extract Manufacturing Association, a group also known by the same initials as the federal agency FEMA. See Andrew Schneider, "Disease Is Swift, Response Is Slow. Government Lets Flavoring Industry Police Itself despite Damage to Workers' Lungs," *Baltimore Sun,* 23 April 2006.

5. In 1956, three major journals published, nearly simultaneously, a series of cases of silo-filler's disease. See Leo T. Delaney Jr., Herbert W. Schmidt, and Charles F. Stroebel, "Silo-Filler's Disease," *Proceedings of the Staff Meetings of the Mayo Clinic* 31 (4 April 1956): 189–198; R. R. Grayson, "Silage Gas Poisoning: Nitrogen Dioxide Pneumonia, a New Disease in Agricultural Workers," *Annals of Internal Medicine* 45 (September 1956): 393–408; and Thomas Lowry and Leonard M. Schuman, "'Silo-Filler's Disease'—a Syndrome Caused by Nitrogen Dioxide," *JAMA* 163 (15 September 1956): 153–160. The last article was preceded in date by a brief editorial by Lowry: Thomas Lowry, "'Silo-Filler's Disease': A Newly Recognized Syndrome," *Bulletin of the University of Minnesota Hospitals and Minnesota Medical Foundation* 27 (1 April 1956): 203. This editorial marks the first appearance (three days earlier than Delaney's 4 April article) of the term *silo-filler's disease.* Although all three investigations pinpointed nitrogen oxide as the culprit in acute lung injury, only Lowry and Schuman clearly described an indolent course consistent with progressive bronchiolitis. Given that metal silos were introduced in U.S. agriculture in the later part of the nineteenth century, it is curious that nitrogen dioxide emerged as a toxin so much

later if enclosed metal silos alone are the driving risk factor for exposure. Sporadic silo-filling deaths indeed were documented prior to the 1950s, for example in a 1914 report of four "trustees" overcome on the hospital farm of the Athens Ohio State Hospital. See E. R. Hayhurst and Ernest Scott, "Four Cases of Sudden Death in a Silo," *JAMA* 58 (1914): 1570–1572. These four deaths were ascribed to carbon dioxide fermentation with fairly convincing laboratory data in support of this view, although nitrogen dioxide was possibly also present. Lowry and Schuman noted a likely explanation for the sudden recognition of a "new" syndrome emerging in the 1950s: "A trend in modern farming methods toward increasing use of organic nitrates in fertilizing mixtures and also other commercial chemical compounds containing nitrogen appears to favor increasingly high nitrate concentrations in crops generally" (158). Silo-filler's disease remains an ongoing risk from corn silage. See James F. Leavey et al., "Silo-Filler's Disease, the Acute Respiratory Distress Syndrome, and Oxides of Nitrogen," *Annals of Internal Medicine* 141 (2004): 410–411.

6. David G. Kern et al., "Flock Worker's Lung: Chronic Interstitial Lung Disease in the Nylon Flocking Industry," *Annals of Internal Medicine* 129 (1998): 261–272.

7. William L. Eschenbacher et al., "Nylon Flock–Associated Interstitial Lung Disease," *American Journal of Respiratory and Critical Care Medicine* 159 (1999): 2003–2008.

8. Sibel Atis et al., "The Respiratory Effects of Occupational Polypropylene Flock Exposure," *European Respiratory Journal* 25 (2005): 110–117.

9. For the earlier U.S. outbreaks, see "Severe Respiratory Illness Linked to Use of Shoe Sprays—Colorado, November 1993," *MMWR* 42 (1993): 885–887; and Michael F. Caron and C. Michael White, "Pneumonitis following Inhalation of a Commercially Available Water Repellent," *Journal of Toxicology Clinical Toxicology* 39 (2001): 179–180. For the outbreaks in Europe, see R. Heinzer et al., "Recurrence of Acute Respiratory Failure following Use of Waterproofing Sprays," *Thorax* 59 (2004): 541–542; and R. de Groot, I. de Vries, and J. I. Meulenbelt, "Sudden Increase of Acute Respiratory Illness after Using a Spray Product to Waterproof Clothing and Shoes" (abstract), *Journal of Toxicology Clinical Toxicology* 42 (2004): 443. For the 2005–2006 U.S. outbreak, see "Respiratory Illness Associated with Boot Sealant Products—Five States, 2005–2006," *MMWR* 55 (2006): 488–490.

10. Yih-Leong Chang et al., "Segmental Necrosis of Small Bronchi after Prolonged Intakes of Sauropus Androgynus in Taiwan," *American Journal of Respiratory and Critical Care Medicine* 157 (1998): 594–598.

11. Joëlle L. Nortier et al., "Urothelial Carcinoma Associated with the Use of a Chinese Herb (Aristolochia Fangchi)," *New England Journal of Medicine* 342 (2000): 1686–1692. See also California Department of Health Services, 17 No-

vember 2004, "State Public Health Officer Warns Consumers about Herbal Products," press release www.applications.dhs.ca.gov/pressreleases/store/Press Releases/04–73.html.

12. T. L. Kurt et al., "Dinitrophenol in Weight Loss: The Poison Center and Public Health Safety," *Veterinary and Human Toxicology* 28 (1986): 574–575.

13. "The Anabolic Steroid Guide, Profile: DNP (Dinitrophenol)," www .fitness-x.co.uk (10 October 2005). This site suggests contacting www .elitefitness.com. In 2002, George Spellwin, the research director of Elite Fitness, published on the Internet an open letter to *Business Week* in anticipation of a negative profile concerning the death of one its discussion forum members, Eric Perin, a.k.a. YoungNHugeGuns. The FDA was reportedly investigating the death in relation to DNP use. www.elitefitness.com/articledata/efn/072202b .html (10 October 2005). For a medical report of DNP poisoning in a body-builder who obtained the substance on the Internet, see H. Mustonen, R. Kuosa, and K. Hoppu, "Severe Poisoning by a Fat-Burning Dietary Substance" (abstract), *Journal of Toxicology Clinical Toxicology* 42 (2004): 546–547. A case of a fatal DNP overdose in a seventeen-year-old is presented in Allen L. Hsiao et al., "Pediatric Fatality following Ingestion of Dinitrophenol: Postmortem Identification of a 'Dietary Supplement,'" *Clinical Toxicology* 43 (2005): 281–285.

14. Robert Sullivan, "Home Remedy Dept.: A Case of the Blues," *New Yorker*, 11 November 2002, 70–71.

15. K. Hori et al., "Believe It or Not: Silver Still Poisons" (abstract), *Journal of Toxicology Clinical Toxicology* 40 (2002): 394–395.

16. John Butter, *Remarks on the Irritative Fever Commonly Called the Plymouth Dock-Yard Disease; with Mr. Dryden's Detailed Account of the Fatal Cases, including That of the Lamented Surgeon, Dr. Bell* (Devonport: Congdon and Heale, 1825), 134–136; quoted excerpts are from a continuous section of the text.

17. For examples of early sources on the uses of pine products, see Pierre Belon, *De Arboribus Coniferis* (Paris: Apud Preuost, 1553), 16; and A. J. Axt, *Tactatus de Arboribus Coniferis et Pice Conficienda* (Jena: Johannis Bielkii, 1679). Although mineral pitch (bitumen)—as opposed to pine pitch—has been employed since antiquity in sealing watercraft (e.g., the "pitch" of Noah's ark), this use was restricted to the Near East, where natural sources of this commodity can be found.

18. Samuel Pepys, in his navy memoranda of the seventeenth century, already commented on the advantages of oak and its shortages: "Memorandum. That both Captain Priestman and his lieutenant, Fairborn, by their letters, the former the 17th of May and the latter the 28th of December 1685, enclosing a sample, do observe that the upper part of the Bonadventure's plank under water, being oak, is not touched at all with the worm, while the lower next to the keel, being of beech, is very dangerously eaten, this sample being taken from the 3rd stake next the keel." Elsewhere in his notes, Pepys mentions of his acquaintance and fellow diarist that "Mr. Evelyn in discourse tells me that want of

timber has always been complained of in England." See *Publications of the Naval Records Society,* vol. 60: *Samuel Pepys's Naval Minutes,* ed. J. R. Tanner (London: Naval Records Society, 1926), 234, 249.

19. The Royal Society for the Encouragement of Arts, Manufactures and Commerce (The Royal Society of Arts), *Abstract of the Premiums Offered by the Society* (London: John Nichols, 1784).

20. Anonymous, *Some Observations on that Distemper in Timber Called the Dry Rot* (London: J. Johnson, 1795). This pamphlet is cited as the first appearance of "dry rot" in print (*Oxford English Dictionary,* 2nd ed., s.v. "dry-rot"), although the use of the term in the 1784 Royal Society for the Encouragement of Arts, Manufactures and Commerce premium list (n. 19, above) appears to have precedence.

21. Ambrose Bowden, *A Treatise on Dry Rot; in which are Described the Nature and Causes of that Disease in Ships, Houses, Mills, Ec. Ec. with the Methods of Prevention and Cure . . .* (London: Burton and Briggs, 1815).

22. Robert Finlayson, *An Essay Addressed to Captains of the Royal Navy, and those of the Merchant's Service; on the Means of Preserving the Health of their Crews: with Directions for the Preservation of Dry Rot in Ships* (London: Thomas and George Underwood, 1824), 53. A publication of the same page length appeared one year earlier as Robert Finlayson, *An Essay on the Baneful Influence of so Frequently Washing Decks in His Majesty's Ships on the Health of British Seamen, with Observations on the Prevention of Dry Rot in the Royal Navy* (London: Egerton, 1823).

23. Michael Faraday, *On the Practical Prevention of Dry Rot in Timber; Being the Substance of a Lecture Delivered by Professor Faraday at the Royal Institution, February 22, 1833* (London: J. and C. Allard, 1834).

24. The toxicity of corrosive sublimate was well recognized long before its introduction as a wood preservative. See, for example, W. Broomfield, *An Account of the English Nightshades and their Effects (Also Practical Observations on the Use of Corrosive Sublimate)* (London: R. Baldwin, 1757); and Pierre Toussaint Navier, *Contre-poisons de l'arsenic, du sublimé corrosif, du verd-de-gris et du plomb* (Paris: n.p., 1777). The earliest clinical case report of the oral use of charcoal as a poison treatment was for inadvertent ingestion of corrosive sublimate. See William P. Hort, "Case of Poisoning with Corrosive Sublimate, in which the Administration of Charcoal Afforded Great Relief," *American Journal of Medical Sciences* 6 (1830): 540–541. A contemporaneous report notes that the poison corrosive sublimate was present in the house of another victim for the purpose of destroying maggots in sheep. See Archibald Blacklock, "Case of Poisoning with Corrosive Sublimate," *Edinburgh Medical and Surgical Journal* 36 (1831): 92–94.

25. Michael Faraday, "On Dry Rot," manuscript notes dated 22 February 1833, Collection of the Royal Institution of Great Britain, London, RI MS F4 D, pp. A13–14, quotation from A14.

26. Faraday, *On the Practical Prevention of Dry Rot in Timber,* quotation from his introductory remarks.

27. George Birkbeck, *A Lecture on the Preservation of Timber by Kyan's Patent for the Prevention of Dry Rot* (London: John Weale, 1835), 27–28.

28. Kyan's patent 3764 (of 31 March 1832) was "for a new mode of preserving certain vegetable substances from decay." A subsequent patent, 4508 (of 11 February 1836), served "to extend only to His Majesty's colonies and plantations abroad." See Andrew Pritchard, *A List for all the Patents and Inventions in the Arts and Manufactures* (London: Whittaker and Co., 1841). United States Senate bill 125, introduced 26 January 1835, authorized letters of patent to be issued to Kyan, waving a requirement that otherwise was in place for two years' residence in the United States by an alien seeking a U.S. patent. See S 125, 23rd Cong., 2nd sess.

29. Richard Bissell Prosser, "Kyan, John Howard," in *National Dictionary of Biography,* ed. Leslie Stephen and Sidney Lee, vol. 31, 347–348. This is also the source for the laudatory song about Kyan.

30. Cram's 1838 adverse experience with Kyanizing was first reported only in 1885. See Octave Chanute, "The Preservation of Timber: Report of the Committee on the Preservation of Timber, Presented and Accepted at the Annual Convention, June 25th, 1885," *Transactions of the American Society of Civil Engineers* 14 (1885): 254.

31. Edwin Chadwick, *Report to Her Majesty's Principal Secretary of State for the Home Department, from the Poor Law Commissioners on an Inquiry into the Sanitary Condition of the Labouring Population of Great Britain* (London: W. Clowes, 1842), 258–259.

32. Sir William Burnett's patent, 5249 (26 July 1838), was "for improvements in preserving wood, and other vegetable matters, from decay." See Pritchard, *A List for all the Patents for Inventions in the Arts and Manufactures.* See also William Burnett, *Reports on the Solution of Chloride of Zinc* (London: William Clowes, 1848); and anonymous, *Sir W. Burnett's Patent Process for the Preservation of Timber, Canvas, Cordage, Cotton, Woolen &c. from Dry Rot, Mildew, and C.* (London: Prepared by the Manufactory of the patentees [circa 1850]).

33. Anonymous, *Burnettizing or the Process for Preventing the Rapid Decay of Timber* (Cambridge, MA: Allen and Farnham, 1856).

34. See the following twelve-page promotional brochure: Charles Payne, *Memoir Descriptive of Payne's Patent Process for the Preservation and Improvement of Wood & Other Vegetable Substances from Wet and Dry Rot, Fire, the Ravages of Worms, &c. and also the Means of the Patent Creosoting Process, as the Processes are Employed by the Timber Preserving Companies of London and New York* (Melbourne, Australia: Lucas Brothers, 1858).

35. Jeffrey Oaks, *Date Nails and Railroad Tie Preservation,* University of Indianapolis Archeology and Forensics Laboratory Special Report no. 3, Vol. 1 (Indianapolis, IN: University of Indianapolis, 2002). Kyanization did continue to

have certain uses well into the twentieth century. Its principal modern promoter (for example, in treating telephone poles) was a German engineer, Friedrich Moll. See Kurt Mauel, "Moll, Friedrich Rudolf Heinrich Carl," in *Dictionary of Scientific Biography*, ed. Charles C. Gillispie, vol. 9 (New York: Charles Scribner's Sons, 1974), 458–459.

36. Sir John Barrow, *The Life of George Lord Anson, Admiral of the Fleet; Vice-Admiral of Great Britain; and First Lord Commissioner of the Admiralty, Previous to, and During, the Seven-Years' War* (London: John Murray, 1839), 448–451, quotation from 450. Barrow appends to his biography of Lord Anson a supplementary chapter, beginning on page 421 (dated 1 December 1838), concerning the state of the contemporary British navy, including the physical condition of its ships. This supplement contains, inter alia, his comments on dry rot and wood preservatives. Barrow's criticism of the mercuric chloride process motivated Kyan to write his only published writing on his invention, a fourteen-page polemic (with a supplemental testimonial): John Howard Kyan, *An Answer to the Supplemental Chapter in Lord Anson's Life (by Sir John Barrow, Bart.) in Reference to the Preservation of Timber for the Navy* (London: printed for the author by W. H. Cox, 1839). Kyan's only other published work of note was a book on optics and light: John Howard Kyan, *On the Elements of Light* (London: Longman, Orme, Brown, Green & Longman, 1838). In its introduction, in which he lauds Faraday, he acknowledges that he is known only for "the preservation of timber from Dry Rot."

37. John Elliston, *On the Medicinal Properties of Creosote* (London: G. Woodfall, 1835), offprint of *Medico-Chirurgical Transactions* 19, n.s. (1835). Elliston was the first to report on creosote in English.

38. John Rose Cormack, *A Treatise on the Chemical, Medicinal, and Physiological Properties of Creosote Illustrated by Experiments on the Lower Animals* (Edinburgh: J. Carfrae & Son, 1836). Cormack's 154-page work includes a summary of the original synthesis of creosote by the German scientist Karl Ludwig von Resichenbach in 1830.

39. Payne, *Memoir Descriptive of Payne's Patent Process*, 5.

40. Percivall Pott's original report of scrotal cancer appeared as a short (five-page) chapter in a larger work. See Percivall Pott, *The Chirurgical Works of Percivall Pott*, (London: Hawes Clark and Collins, 1775), vol. 5, 50–54. Near the beginning of his brief essay Pott notes, "Every body is acquainted with the disorders to which painters, plumbers, glaziers, and the workers in white lead, are liable: but there is a disease as peculiar to a certain set of people, which has not, at least to my knowledge, been publicly noticed; I mean the chimney-sweepers' cancer" (50). In 1808, James Earle published a revised edition of the *Chirurgical Works* (Pott had been his father-in-law and colleague), expanded with his own observations. The chapter on cancer of the scrotum is rich in annotations, which include a report of cancer of the facial skin of a chimney sweep

(Pott had limited his comments to the scrotum and testis) and a lengthy description of a case of cancer of the hand in a gardener who had been contaminated by repeatedly strewing soot from a bucket in order to kill slugs. See James Earle, *The Chirurgical Works of Percivall Pott, F.R.S. Surgeon to St. Bartholomew's Hospital* (London: J. Johnson, 1808), vol. 3, 177–183.

41. Henry T. Butlin, *On Cancer of the Scrotum in Chimney-sweeps and Others: Three Lectures Delivered at the Royal College of Surgeons of England* (London: British Medical Association, 1892).

42. Stephen Mackenzie, "A Case of Tar Eruption," *British Journal of Dermatology* 10 (1898): 417. This was one of two cases Mackenzie "exhibited" to fellow dermatologists and was reported in the "Society Intelligence" column, a regular feature of the journal.

43. Thomas Oliver, *Diseases of Occupation from the Legislative, Social, and Medical Points of View* (London: Methuen and Co., 1908), 383–385.

44. Hugh Campbell Ross, John Westray Cropper, and H. Bayon, *The Problem of the Gasworks Pitch Industries and Cancer*, The John Howard McFadden Researches (London: John Murray, 1912). This monograph subsumes two papers: H. C. Ross, J. W. Cropper, and W. J. Atkinson Butterfield, "The Problem of the Gasworks Pitch Industries and Cancer"; and H. Bayon, "Epithelial Cell-Proliferation Induced by the Injection of Gasworks Tar."

45. Thomas M. Legge, *Industrial Maladies*, Oxford Medical Publications (London: Oxford University Press, Humphrey Milford, 1934), 15, table 6. Legge documents that skin cancer related to coal tar was not added to the list of notifiable occupational diseases in Britain until 1920; through 1931, 693 skin cancer cases related to pitch and tar (including patent fuel production) were documented, including 94 fatalities.

46. W. J. O'Donovan, "Epitheliomatous Ulceration among Tar Workers" (in two parts), *British Journal of Dermatology and Syphilis* 32 (July 1920): 215–228; 32 (August–September 1920): 245–252. Quotation is from 216; the J. R. case is described on 223.

47. H. A. Cookson, "Epithelioma of the Skin after Prolonged Exposure to Creosote," *British Medical Journal* (1 March 1924): 368 and plate.

48. The information on the chronology of the use of creosote in the railroads is derived largely from Oaks, *Date Nails and Railroad Tie Preservation*.

49. Norman Lenson, "Multiple Cutaneous Carcinoma after Creosote Exposure," *New England Journal of Medicine* 254 (1956): 520–522. This marks the first U.S. recognition of cancer risk specific to creosote. Although skin cancer from many other coal tar derivatives had already become better appreciated by the 1930s (as already stated, the United Kingdom listed coal tar skin cancer as an official occupational disease in 1920), industrial exposures to coal tars as a class were not well controlled in this period in the United States. In 1940, the executive director of the Steel Workers Organizing Committee in Birmingham, Al-

abama, wrote to Florence Perkins (then secretary of labor), "Recently I have run across a condition wherein the victims are not so numerous, nevertheless it is causing serious suffering to workers, namely, cancer, due to spraying casters, structural steel and pipes with coal tar. During the past few months there have been called to my attention four different cases of men having skin cancer, allegedly due to this work in the Central Foundry Company in Bessemer, Alabama. I believe that a study should be made of this condition since, perhaps, it is prevailing in other plants and that something should be done to force employers to furnish proper clothing and equipment to prevent this chemical continually coming in contact with the flesh of men." Letter published in Gerald Markowitz and David Rosner, *"Slaves of the Depression": Workers' Letters about Life on the Job* (Ithaca, NY: Cornell University Press, 1987), 148–149.

50. Peyton Rous, "Influence of Hereditary Malformations on Carcinogenesis in 'Crew' Mice and Deer Mice of Hairless Strains" (abstract), *Proceedings of the American Association for Cancer Research* 2 (April 1956): 143. As a parenthetical aside, Rous notes, "(Mr. Wentworth Cumming of Carworth Farms generously provided the tumor mice and those for breeding also. Use of the wood preservative was discontinued at the Farms.)"

51. Philip J. Landrigan [and Mauro A. Tumolo], "Health Risks of Creosotes" (Questions and Answers), *JAMA* 269 (1993): 1309.

52. Anonymous, "Eruptions in Lumber Workers" (Queries and Minor Notes), *JAMA* 106 (1936): 2092.

53. Allen D. Lazenby, "Pentachlorphenol" (Queries and Minor Notes), *JAMA* 110 (1938): 229. The initial term *pentachlorphenol* was later replaced by *pentachlorophenol*.

54. Karl Herxheimer, "Ueber Chlorakne," *Münchener Medicinische Wochenschrift* 46, no. 9 (28 February 1899): 278. A brief biographic note on Herxheimer, after whom a well-known immune reaction is named, can be found in B. G. Firkin and J. A. Whitworth, *Dictionary of Medical Eponyms,* 2nd ed. (New York: Parthenon Publishing Group, 1996).

55. Ludwig Teleky, "Die Pernakrankheit (Chloracne)," *Klinische Wochenschrift* 6 (1927): 845–848, 897–901. For a biography of Teleky, see Andreas Wulf, *Der Sozialmediziner Ludwig Teleky (1872–1957) und die Entwicklung der Gewerbehygiene zur Arbeitsmedizin* (Frankfurt am Main: Mabuse-Verlag, 2001). On Teleky's immigration to the United States, he was professionally assisted by the anthropologist Franz Boas through the Emergency Committee in Aid of Displaced Foreign Medical Scientists. Related correspondence is preserved in the Boas Archives, American Philosophical Society, Philadelphia.

56. For early U.S. reports on chloracne from chlorinated insulation materials, see W. B. Fulton and J. L. Matthews, *A Preliminary Report of the Dermatological and Systemic Effects of Exposure to Hexachloro-naphthalene and Chlorodiphenyl,* Special Bulletin no. 43 (Harrisburg, PA: Pennsylvania Department of

Labor, Bureau of Industrial Standards, 1936); and Cecil K. Drinker, Madeleine Field Warren, and Granville A. Bennett, "The Problem of Possible Systemic Effects from Certain Chlorinated Hydrocarbons," *Journal of Industrial Hygiene and Toxicology* 19 (1937): 263–299.

57. Karl O. Stingily, "A New Industrial Chemical Dermatitis," *Southern Medical Journal* 33 (1940): 1268–1272, quotation from 1269.

58. William M. Gafafer, *Manual of Industrial Hygiene and Medical Service in War Industries* (Philadelphia: W. B. Saunders Company, 1943), 176–177.

59. Louis Schwartz, "Dermatitis from Creosote-Treated Wooden Floors," *Industrial Medicine* 11 (1942): 387.

60. Ernst W. Baader and H. J. Bauer, "Industrial Intoxication Due to Pentachlorophenol," *Industrial Medicine and Surgery* 20 (1951): 286–290. This was Baader's first non-German-language publication after World War II. Baader was an important figure in German occupational medicine during the 1933–45 period and after. Robert Proctor documents that Baader joined the Nazi Party on 1 May 1933 and was active in the Nazi apparatus. See Robert Proctor, *The Nazi War on Cancer* (Princeton, NJ: Princeton University Press, 1999), 302, fn. 24. Baader also authored a textbook on occupational medicine, the first edition of which appeared in 1931, with second and third editions appearing during the war years, and new editions continuing to be published after World War II. In addition, Baader served as a coauthor for *Die körperliche Erziehung zum Soldaten: Handbuch für die körperliche Erziehung der Jugend als Vorbereitung für den Dienst in der Wermacht* (Physical education for the soldier: Manual for the physical education of youth as preparation for the Wermacht) (Berlin: W. Limpert-Verlag, 1936). An obituary notice for Baader, by Franz Koelsch (another occupational medicine figure of the period), jumps directly from 1933 to the postwar period; see F. Koelsch, "Prof. Dr. med. Dr. Dr. h.c. Ernst Baader geb. 14.5.1892—gest. 1.11.1962" (Prof. Ernst Baader, M.D., Dr. h.c., born 14 May 1892—died 1 November 1962), *Münchener Medizinische Wochenschrift* 104 (1962): 2521–2522. By 1954, Baader was sufficiently rehabilitated to join the exiled Ludwig Teleky (see n. 55 above) and Heinrich Zangger (a Swiss scientist and close friend of Einstein's) on the masthead of the reestablished journal *Archiv für Gewerbepathologie und Gewerbehygiene,* whose publication had been suspended since 1945. A biannual E. W. Baader Prize of five thousand euros, endowed by the Baader family, is now awarded by the German Society for Industrial Medicine to a young and promising practitioner of occupational medicine from Germany or "a German-language foreign country."

61. Anonymous, "Occupational Acne" (Questions and Answers), *JAMA* 188 (20 April 1964): 336.

62. Jacob Bleiberg and Roger H. Brodkin, "New Weed Killers Produce Chloracne" (letter), *JAMA* 189 (6 July 1964): 66–67.

63. In addition to the *JAMA* reference to self-administration of 2,4,5-T, I confirmed this directly with Dr. Key himself, the public health physician in-

volved (e-mail, 6 November 2004). Dr. Key went on to become the first director of NIOSH when that agency was founded in 1970. Key presented a related abstract on his work (then at the forerunner of NIOSH, the Division of Occupational Health, U.S. Public Health Service, Cincinnati) at the 15th International Congress of Occupational Health in Vienna, Austria. See Marcus M. Key, "Occupational Chloracne," in section AIII of *Occupational Diseases and Toxicology* (Abstract AIII-163), *15th International Congress of Occupational Health Abstract Book* (Vienna: Permanent Commission and International Association on Occupational Health, 1966), 301–302.

64. Extensive documentation of the history of Agent Orange, its application, and the toxicity of dioxin can be found in Committee to Review the Health Effects in Vietnam Veterans of Exposure to Herbicides, Institute of Medicine, *Veterans and Agent Orange* (Washington, DC: National Academy Press, 1994).

65. U.S. Congress, *Joint Resolution of Congress, H.J. Res. 1145,* 88th Cong., 2nd sess., 7 August 1964 (Gulf of Tonkin Resolution).

66. Jacob Bleiberg et al., "Industrially Acquired Porphyria," *Archives of Dermatology* 89 (1964): 793–797.

67. I gathered additional information from a telephone interview with Dr. Roger Brodkin (31 October 2004), who had been one of the principal treating dermatologists in the outbreak.

68. The cleanup of the former herbicide manufacturing plant has been one of the most expensive and controversial EPA efforts. See "Giant Harbor Project Collides with Dioxin-Laced Superfund Site in Newark Bay: Army Corps, Port Authority Ignore Warnings, Fail to Plan for Health and Environmental Danger," Natural Resources Defense Council, press release (4 January 2005).

69. Committee to Review the Health Effects in Vietnam Veterans of Exposure to Herbicides, Institute of Medicine, *Veterans and Agent Orange.*

70. Elizabeth Rosenthal, "Liberal Leader from Ukraine Was Poisoned," *New York Times,* 12 December 2004.

71. Alexandra Geusau et al., "Severe 2,3,7,8-Terachlorodibenzo-p-Dioxin (TCDD) Intoxication: Kinetics and Trial to Enhance Elimination in Two Patients," *Archives of Toxicology* 76 (2002): 316–325.

72. Bowden, *A Treatise on Dry Rot;* quoted passage from p. 164.

73. For railroad use of arsenic, see Oaks, *Date Nails and Railroad Tie Preservation.* For playground use, see Adam Liptak, "The Poison Is Arsenic, and the Suspect Wood," *New York Times,* 26 June 2002; John Leland, "Treated-Wood Precautions," *New York Times,* 4 July 2002; (Associated Press), "Agreement Reached on Use of a Pesticide," *New York Times,* 18 March 2003; and Elizabeth Olson, "Hidden Arsenic in Older Play Sets," *New York Times,* 25 November 2003.

74. The chronology of U.S. EPA action on wood preservatives is derived from Jay Feldman and Terry Shistar (National Coalition against the Misuse of

Pesticides), "Poison Poles—a Report about Their Toxic Trail and Safer Alternatives," www.beyondpesticides.org/wood/pubs/poisonpoles/ (31 March 2006).

75. Stephen Wood et al., "Pentachlorophenol Poisoning," *Journal of Occupational Medicine* 25 (1983): 527–530. The fatality due to jackhammering pentachlorophenol is also reported in Ronald E. Gray et al., "Pentachlorophenol Intoxication: Report of a Fatal Case, with Comments on the Clinical Course and Pathologic Anatomy," *Archives of Environmental Health* 40 (1985): 161–164. I gathered additional information in a brief telephone interview with Dr. Stephen Wood (19 August 2005).

76. Chris Carlsten, Stephen Carl Hunt, and Joel D. Kaufman, "Squamous Cell Carcinoma of the Skin and Coal Tar Creosote Exposure in a Railroad Worker," *Environmental Health Perspectives* 113 (2005): 96–97.

77. H. J. Roberts, "Aplastic Anemia Due to Pentachlorophenol," *New England Journal of Medicine* (letter), 305 (1981): 1650–1651; and H. J. Roberts, "Aplastic Anemia and Red Cell Aplasia Due to Pentachlorophenol," *Southern Medical Journal* 76 (1983): 45–48. Both of these reports include the case of a twenty-seven-year-old physician-in-training who, on weekends off from the hospital, had been building a log cabin. He brushed pentachlorophenol directly onto the logs as well as soaking the insulation between them. Seven months into the project, he developed aplastic anemia and died six months later. I became aware of this case only after a medical student whom I had supervised in clinical duties at my hospital shared the story with me. The victim, who had been his father, died shortly before he was born. His son, the current medical student, was unaware of the published case reports about his father.

78. Ryan Reed, "Trick or Treated? CCA Alternatives More Corrosive and Expensive," Buildernews online, www.buildernewsmag.com (July 2004). The herbicide market has been far from static as well. Even within the line of chlorinated phenoxyherbicides for which 2,4,5-T was the progenitor, the closely related toxin 2,4-D has been joined by MCPP (also known as mecoprop) and MCPA. Although not contaminated by dioxin, these herbicides carry their own toxicities. See Darren M. Roberts et al., "Intentional Self-Poisoning with the Chlorophenoxy Herbicide 4-chloro-2-methylphenoxyacetic Acid (MCPA)," *Annals of Emergency Medicine* 46 (2005): 275–284. Meanwhile, 2,4-D continues to be linked to workers' deaths through exposure to its manufacturing precursor, 2,4-dichlorophenol, an exceedingly potent toxin. See Morbidity and Mortality Weekly Report, "Occupational Fatalities Associated with 2,4-Chlorophenol (2,3-DCP) Exposure, 1980–1998," *MMWR* 49 (2000): 516–518.

79. Wolmanized Natural Select Treated Wood and Lumber, *Material Safety Data Sheet*, Brewer Lumber, Saint Clair, Minnesota (1 October 2003); Naturewood Amine Based Treated Wood, *Material Safety Data Sheet*, Osmose, Inc., Buffalo, New York (11 August 2003).

80. Fiberon Deck Board, *Material Safety Data Sheet*, Fiber Composites, LLC, New London, North Carolina (10 October 2001); TREX Wood-Polymer Lumber Products—Woodland Brown, *Material Safety Data Sheet*, Trex Company, LLC, Winchester, Virginia (27 January 2003).

81. "Deportee (Plane Wreck at Los Gatos)," words by Woody Guthrie, music by Martin Hoffman, TRO-© Copyright 1961 (Renewed), 1963 (Renewed), Ludlow Music, Inc., New York, NY. Used by permission. Elsewhere Guthrie described "the dumped oranges and peaches and grapes and cherries rotting and running down into little streams of creosote poisoned juices." See Woody Guthrie, *Pastures of Plenty: A Self-Portrait* (New York: Harper and Row, 1990), 7.

82. Anthony E. Lang and Andres M. Lozano, "Parkinson's Disease," *New England Journal of Medicine* 339 (1998): 1044–1053, 1130–1143.

83. *James Parkinson (1755–1824), A Bicentenary Volume of Papers Dealing with Parkinson's Disease, Incorporating the Original "Essay on the Shaking Palsy,"* ed. Macdonald Critchley (London: Macmillan, 1955), quotations regarding Case III from 163–164 (pp. 11–12 of original essay); Case I from 162 (p. 10 of original essay); Case II from 163 (p. 11 of original essay).

84. James Parkinson, *Revolutions without Bloodshed; or, Reformation Preferable to Revolt* (London: Eaton and Smith, 1794). See also James Parkinson, *The Villager's Friend and Physician*, 2nd ed. (London: C. Whittingham, 1804). In this book, aimed at self-help for the general public, Parkinson cites an aphorism that I have not been able to trace otherwise: "He gets little for his pains who sad disease by labour gains" (7). A brief overview and listing of Parkinson's radical writings can be found in Kenneth L. Tyler and H. Richard Tyler, "The Secret Life of James Parkinson (1755–1824): The Writings of Old Hubert," *Neurology* 36 (1986): 222–224.

85. James Parkinson, *Hints for the Improvement of Trusses Intended to Render Their Use Less Inconvenient, and to Prevent the Necessity of an Understrap. With the Description of a Truss of Easy Construction and Slight Expence for the Use of Labouring Poor* (London: C. Whittingham for H. D. Symonds, 1802).

86. Caroline M. Tanner, "Occupational and Environmental Causes of Parkinsonism," in *Unusual Occupational Diseases, Occupational Medicine State of the Art Reviews*, ed. Dennis J. Shusterman and Paul D. Blanc, (Philadelphia: Hanley and Belfus, 1992), vol. 7, 503–513.

87. For a case documenting dementia pugilistica, see (Robert E. Scully), "Case Records of the Massachusetts General Hospital Weekly Clinicopathological Exercises, Case 12–1999, a 67-Year-Old Man with Three Years of Dementia," *New England Journal of Medicine* 340 (1999): 1269–1277.

88. Peter S. Spencer et al., "Guam Amyotrophic Lateral Sclerosis-Parkinsonism-Dementia Linked to a Plant Excitant Neurotoxin," *Science* 237 (1987): 517–522, quotation from 518.

89. Richard Stone, "Guam: Deadly Disease Dying Out," *Science* 261 (1993): 424–426.

90. Susan J. Murch, Paul Alan Cox, and Sandra Anne Banack, "A Mechanism for Slow Release of Biomagnified Cyanobacterial Neurotoxins and Neurodegenerative Disease in Guam," *Proceedings of the National Academy of Sciences* 101 (2004): 12228–12231. See also Paul Alan Cox and Oliver W. Sacks, "Cycad Neurotoxins, Consumption of Flying Foxes, and ALS-PDC Disease in Guam," *Neurology* 58 (2002): 956–959.

91. R. Stanley Burns et al., "The Clinical Syndrome of Striatal Dopamine Deficiency: Parkinsonism Induced by 1-methyl-4-phenyl-1,2,3,6-tetrahydropyridine (MPTP)," *New England Journal of Medicine* 312 (1985): 1418–1421.

92. For background on copper and iron, see Matthew J. Ellenhorn et al., *Ellenhorn's Medical Toxicology: Diagnosis and Treatment of Human Poisoning*, 2nd ed. (Baltimore: Williams & Wilkins, 1997), 1554–1556, 1558–1562.

93. Lawrence C. Erway and Sidney E. Mitchell, "Prevention of Otolith Defect in Pastel Mink by Manganese Supplementation," *Journal of Heredity* 64 (1973): 111–119 (including figure; the journal's cover illustration for that issue was captioned " 'Screw Neck' Pastel Mink: An Otolith Defect").

94. John Couper, "On the Effects of Black Oxide of Manganese When Inhaled into the Lungs," *British Annals of Medicine, Pharmacy, Vital Statistics and General Science* 1 (1837): 41–42, quotations from 41. Couper's article appeared in a French translation the same year, although this version inexplicably deleted Couper's concluding paragraphs, in which he emphasizes early identification of cases and removal from further exposure and is unequivocal in finding that manganese is the cause of the injury. See John Couper, "Note sur les effets du peroxide de manganese," *Journal de Chemie Médicale, de Pharmacie, de Toxicologie, et Revue des Nouvelles Scientifiques Nationales et Étrangeres* 3, ser. 2 (1837): 233–235. The French translation has sometimes led to confusion about the location of this initial outbreak of manganese poisoning, in Great Britain or France. See, for example, Lloyd B. Tepper, "Hazards to Health: Manganese," *New England Journal of Medicine* 264 (1961): 347–348. Couper, who was a professor at the University of Glasgow, makes clear that the cases he described occurred among bleaching powder workers employed by Charles Tennant and Co., in Scotland.

95. George Eliot, *Quarry for Middlemarch*, ed. Anna Theresa Kitchel (Berkeley and Los Angeles: University of California Press, 1950), 35.

96. H. R. Shubert, "The Steel Industry," in *A History of Technology*, vol. 5: *The Late Nineteenth Century*, ed. Charles Singer et al. (New York and London: Oxford University Press, 1958), 53–71.

97. The key initial report is Heinrich Embden, "Zur Kenntniss der metallischen Nervengifte: Ueber die chronische Manganvergiftung der Braunsteinmüller," *Deutsche Medicinische Wochenschrift* 27 (14 November 1901): 795–796. Dr. Embden's report summarizes a clinical presentation made on 15

October 1901 in Hamburg and also discusses a simultaneous case report (9 October 1901) by Dr. Rudolf von Jaksch of Prague, which appeared in the *Wiener Klinischen Rundschau*. Embden correctly attributed his cases to manganese, but von Jaksch, apparently unaware of Couper's original work, at first suspected that heat exposure might explain the etiology of the neurological illness that he observed. For the German-language reports, I have drawn on the review and translation in David L. Edsall, F. P. Wilbur, and Cecil K. Drinker, "The Occurrence, Course and Prevention of Chronic Manganese Poisoning," *Journal of Industrial Hygiene* 1 (1919): 183–193. This is the source of the description of M. J., von Jaksch's initial case of 1901.

98. Louis Casamajor, "An Unusual Form of Mineral Poisoning Affecting the Nervous System: Manganese?" *JAMA* 60 (1913): 646–649, quotation from 646.

99. David L. Edsall, F. P. Wilbur, and Cecil K. Drinker, "The Occurrence, Course and Prevention of Chronic Manganese Poisoning," *Journal of Industrial Hygiene* 1 (1919): 183–193, quotations from 186, 190, and 189, in the order presented. This paper documents a further investigation of the same cohort reported by Casamajor in 1913, expanded with additional cases.

100. Ibid., quotation from 198.

101. For a Cuban manganese report, see Rafael Penalver, "Manganese Poisoning," *Industrial Medicine and Surgery* 24 (1955): 1–7. The mines of Chile were particularly known for causing manganese madness. See John Donaldson, "The Physiopathologic Significance of Manganese in Brain: Its Relation to Schizophrenia and Neurodegenerative Disorders," *NeuroToxicology* 8 (1987): 451–462. Japanese manganese mines near Kyoto, a key part of Japan's World War II steel industry, were dependent largely on a conscripted Korean labor force. See James Sterngold, "One Man's Struggle to Preserve a Bitter Memory," *New York Times,* 5 December 1989. For Taiwan, see Chin-Song Lu et al., "Levodopa Failure in Chronic Manganism," *Neurology* 44 (1994): 1600–1602.

102. Ahmed H. Sadek, Ronald Rausch, and Paul E. Schultz, "Parkinsonism Due to Manganism in a Welder," *International Journal of Toxicology* 22 (2003): 393–401.

103. Hugo Mella, "The Experimental Production of Basal Ganglion Symptomatology in Macacus Rhesus," *Archives of Neurology and Psychiatry* 11 (1924): 405–417.

104. H. B. Ferraz et al., "Chronic Exposure to the Fungicide Maneb May Produce Symptoms and Signs of CNS Manganese Intoxication," *Neurology* 38 (1988): 550–553.

105. Giuseppe Meco et al., "Parkinsonism after Chronic Exposure to the Fungicide Maneb (Manganese Ethylene-Bis-Dithiocarbamate)," *Scandinavian Journal of Work Environment and Health* 20 (1994): 301–305. For information on current usage of Maneb and Mancozeb and the evolving body of evidence relating to their toxicity, see Y. Zhou et al., "Proteasomal Inhibition Induced by

Manganese Ethylene *Bis*-Dithiocarbamate: Relevance to Parkinson's Disease," *Neuroscience* 128 (2004): 281–291. As a class, pesticides have been suspect as an environmental factor in Parkinsonism, although specific associations have been difficult to establish beyond Maneb and Mancozeb. Recently, however, a Parkinson's disease outbreak has been reported among Swedish mill workers who produced paper impregnated with a chemical antimildew agent called diphenyl. The diphenyl-treated paper, which was marketed to wrap oranges, was produced at the Swedish plant from 1954 through 1970. See Gunilla Wastensson et al., "Parkinson's Disease in Diphenyl-Exposed Workers—a Causal Association?" *Parkinsonism & Related Disorders* 12 (2006): 29–34.

106. For manganese absorption into the body via the nose, see Hans Tjalve and Jorgen Henrikson, "Uptake of Metals in the Brain via Olfactory Pathways," in "Manganese: Are There Effects from Long-Term, Low-Level Exposure?" ed. Joan Cranmer, Donna Mergler, and Mildred Williams-Johnson, *Neuro Toxicology* 20 (1999): 181–195. This 1999 special issue of the journal *Neuro Toxicology* was devoted entirely to manganese in follow-up to an international conference held in Little Rock, Arkansas (26–29 October 1997).

107. Robert A. Yokel and Janelle S. Crossgrove, *Manganese Toxicokinetics at the Blood-Brain Barrier*, Research Report, Health Effects Institute 119 (Boston: Health Effects Institute, 2004).

108. American Chemical Society, "'Green' Detergent Catalysts Herald Cleaner, Brighter 21st Century," in *What's Happening in Chemistry* (Washington DC: American Chemical Society, 1995), 39–40.

109. Ronald Hage et al., "Efficient Manganese Catalysts for Low-Temperature Bleaching," *Nature* (London) 369 (1994): 637–639. See also Vikki Chin Quee-Smith et al., "Synthesis, Structure, and Characterization of a Novel Manganese(IV) Monomer, [Mn^{IV}(Me$_3$TACN)(OMe)$_3$] (PF$_6$)(Me$_3$TACN = N,N'N'–Trimethyl-1,4,7-triazacyclononane), and Its Activity toward Olefin Oxidation with Hydrogen Pyroxide," *Inorganic Chemistry* 35 (1996): 6461–6465. Both publications stemmed from research at Unilever Laboratories.

110. Patricia Layman, "Unilever Rolls Out 'New Generation' Detergent," *Chemical and Engineering News,* 16 May 1994, 35; and Michael Freemantle, "Chemistry of Disputed Detergent Unveiled," *Chemical and Engineering News,* 27 June 1994, 5–6. See also Gavriella Stern, "Unilever, Responding to Critics, Alters Formula for Much Touted Detergent," *Wall Street Journal,* 7 June 1994. Manganese bleach has not been entirely abandoned. See Kevin F. Sibbons, Kirtida Shastri, and Michael Watkinson, "The Application of Manganese Complexes of Ligands Derived from 1,4,7-Triazacyclononane in Oxidative Catalysis," *Dalton Transactions* (7 February 2006): 645–661. Referring to manganese bleach, the authors note, "To date there has only been modest success in this regard, but . . . it is likely that there will be viable applications for these systems in the near future" (645).

111. Hamilton, *Exploring the Dangerous Trades,* 415–416.

112. For additional background on the introduction of tetraethyl lead, see Christopher C. Sellers, *Hazards of the Job* (Chapel Hill: University of North Carolina Press, 1970).

113. See, for example, "Blood Lead Levels—United States, 1999–2002," *MMWR* 54 (2005): 513–516. This report documents the dramatic 88 percent fall in the percentage of U.S. children with elevated blood lead values following the removal of lead from gasoline, combined with stricter controls on lead-based paint.

114. Ethyl Corporation, *Ethyl 1995 Annual Report* (Richmond, VA: Ethyl Corporation, 1995); Ethyl Corporation, *Ethyl Corporation 2001 Annual Report on Form 10-K* (Richmond, VA: Ethyl Corporation, 2001); Ethyl Corporation, "About Ethyl," www.ethyl.com (June 2000).

115. Joseph Zayed et al., "Occupational and Environmental Exposure of Garage Workers and Taxi Drivers to Airborne Manganese Arising from the Use of Methylcyclopentadienyl Manganese Tricarbonyl in Unleaded Gasoline," *American Industrial Hygiene Association Journal* 55 (1994): 53–58; and Joseph Zayed et al., "Airborne Manganese Particles and Methylcyclopentadienyl Manganese Tricarbonyl (MMT) at Selected Outdoor Sites in Montreal," *Neuro Toxicology* 20 (1999): 151–157.

116. U.S. Environmental Protection Agency, "Comments on the Gasoline Additive MMT (Methylcyclopentadienyl Manganese Tricarbonyl)," www.epa .gov (updated 28 June 2002).

117. For Ethyl-sponsored comment on monkeys, see D. R. Lyman et al., "Environmental Assessment of MMT Fuel Additive," *Science of the Total Environment* 93 (1990): 107–114, quotation from 108. For other Ethyl-sponsored publications, see G. L. Ter Haar et al., "Methylcyclopentadienyl Manganese Tricarbonyl as an Antiknock: Composition and Fate of Manganese Exhaust Products," *Journal of the Air Pollution Control Association* 24 (1975): 858–860; and W. Clark Cooper, "The Health Implications of Increased Manganese in the Environment Resulting from the Combustion of Fuel Additives: A Review of the Literature," *Journal of Toxicology and Environmental Health* 14 (1984): 23–26.

118. Ethyl Corporation, "Ethyl Corporation Wants to Remove Millions of Pounds of Smog-Related Pollutants per Year from the Environment," paid advertisement, *New York Times,* 7 March 1996.

119. John H. Cushman Jr., "E.P.A. Accuses a Company of Distortion," *New York Times,* 8 March 1996.

120. Ethyl Corporation, "MMT and Public Health: *Separating Fact from Fiction,*" briefing materials (14 May 1996), quotation from 21. This is a twenty-one-page unbound text.

121. See the following *Wall Street Journal* items: John Urquhart, "Ethyl Acts to Avert Losses If Canada Bans Fuel Additive," 11 September 1996; John

Urquhart, "Canada's House of Commons Is Expected to Vote Ban of Ethyl Fuel Additive," 28 October 1996; "Canadian House Votes Ban on Ethyl Corp. Additive," 3 December 1996; "Ban on Ethyl's Additive Voted by Canadian Senate," 10 April 1997; John Urquhart, "Canada Lifts Ban on Ethyl's Additive; U.S. Firm to Terminate Its Legal Fight," 21 July 1998.

122. Howard Frumkin and Gina Solomon, "Manganese in the U.S. Gasoline Supply," *American Journal of Industrial Medicine* 31 (1997): 107–115. See also James M. Lyznicki, Mitchell S. Karlan, and Mohamed Khaleem Khan, for the Council on Scientific Affairs, American Medical Association, "Manganese in Gasoline," *Journal of Occupational and Environmental Medicine* 41 (1999): 140–143.

123. "MTBE Waiver Benefits Texas Oil Refiners, Enviros Say," *Environmental News Service,* 22 October 2003. See also Carl Hulse, "Congressional Negotiators Are Nearing Agreement on Broad Energy Measure," *New York Times,* 25 July 2005.

124. U.S. Environmental Protection Agency, "Notification Letter to Donald R. Lynam, Vice President, Air Conservation, Ethyl Corporation Requiring Alternative Tier 2 Testing Requirements for the Fuel Additive MMT, from Margo T. Oge, Director, Office of Transportation and Air Quality," 11 May 2000, forty-four pages, including attachments.

125. For the Web sites described, see www.aftonchemical.com and www.newmarket.com (28 July 2005). Robert Burns's poem "Afton Water" was composed in 1791.

126. Following Ethyl's submission of data, the EPA's review will require at least a year, and if further long-term animal toxicology studies are needed (primate studies are likely in that event), these would require several more years, along with other "modeling" of manganese effects requiring possibly two to three additional years (personal communication, Joe Sopata, EPA chemist, e-mails, 28 July 2005 and 8 March 2006).

127. Herbert L. Needleman and Philip J. Landrigan, "Toxins at the Pump," *New York Times,* 13 March 1996. See also Philip J. Landrigan, "MMT, Déjà Vu and National Security" (editorial), *American Journal of Industrial Diseases* 39 (2001): 434–435.

CONCLUSION

1. Jennifer Lee, "White House Minimized the Risks of Mercury in Proposed Rules, Scientists Say," *New York Times,* 7 April 2004.

2. David Barstow, "A Trench Caves In; a Young Worker Is Dead. Is It a Crime? When Workers Die—First of Three Articles: The Plumber's Apprentice," *New York Times,* 21 December 2003. The courts have also played a role in downgrading health and safety violations. For example, in 2005 an administra-

tive law judge in Alabama reduced a fine charged to the Federal Mine Safety Administration for a 2001 accident killing thirteen people. The fine had cited improper roof supports and failure to prevent a buildup of explosive gases; the judge found that the violations were "minor" and reduced the fine from $435,000 to $3,000. See "National Briefing: Alabama: Fine Reduced in Fatal Mine Explosions," *New York Times*, 3 November 2005.

3. Chemical terrorism has also diverted resources from the Centers for Disease Control's National Center for Environmental Health. For example, in 2005 this particular CDC center published a twenty-five-page supplement to the *Morbidity and Mortality Weekly Report:* Martin G. Belson, Joshua G. Schier, and Manesh M. Patel, "Case Definitions for Chemical Poisoning," *MMWR Recommendations and Reports* 54 (14 January 2005): RR-1–24. It states, "The case definitions in this report should be used by clinicians and public health officials in two settings: 1) after a credible threat of a chemical release or 2) after a known chemical release. The list of chemicals that have potential for use as a terrorist weapon is extensive."

4. Tara Parker-Pope, "Score One for the Couch Potatoes: New Studies Link Bicycling to Impotence," *Wall Street Journal*, 15 October 2002.

5. Steven M. Schrader, Michael Breitenstein, and Brian Lowe, *Health Hazard Evaluation Report HETA 2000–0305–2848; City of Long Beach Police Department; Long Beach, California, May 2001* (Cincinnati, OH: NIOSH, 2002).

6. NIOSH, "Prolonged Riding Linked to Decrease in Erectile Measure in Bicycle Patrol Officers," *NIOSH Update*, 18 October 2002. Another example of NIOSH promoting findings that are unlikely to be alarming to the industrial sector can be found in NIOSH, "Medical Interns' Risk for Car Crashes Linked with Extended Shifts in NIOSH-Funded Study," *NIOSH Update*, 3 January 2005.

7. Leonard J. Goldwater, "From Hippocrates to Ramazzini: Early History of Industrial Medicine," *Annals of Medical History New Series* 8 (1936): 27–35.

8. "Brief Report: Lead Poisoning from Ingestion of a Toy Necklace—Oregon, 2003," *MMWR* 53 (18 July 2004): 509–511.

9. Stephen Lebaton, "150 Million Pieces of Toy Jewelry Are Cited for Lead Content in Largest Government Recall," *New York Times*, 8 July 2004.

10. U.S. Congress, Senate, Committee on Commerce, Science and Transportation, "Testimony of Ms. Nancy Nord," 190th Cong., 1st sess., 12 April 2005. See also John Files, "Senate Approves Consumer Nominee," *New York Times*, 30 April 2005.

11. See, for example, Susan Okie, "What Ails the FDA?" *New England Journal of Medicine* 352 (2005): 1063–1066.

12. Murray Chass, "Varied Factors Caused Pitcher's Death," *New York Times*, 19 February 2003; Robert Pear and Denise Grady, "Government Moves to Curtail the Use of Diet Supplement," *New York Times*, 1 March 2003; U.S. Depart-

ment of Health and Human Services, "FDA Announces Plans to Prohibit Sales of Dietary Supplements Containing Ephedra," press release, 30 September 2003.

13. Maria R. Lucarelli et al., "Toxicity of Food Drug and Cosmetic Blue No. 1 Dye in Critically Ill Patients," *Chest* 125 (2004): 793–795.

14. U.S. Food and Drug Administration, "FD&C Blue No. 1 (Blue 1) in Enteral Feeding Solutions," *Public Health Advisory* (29 September 2003).

15. For a series of letters on the subject of osteonecrosis of the jaw linked to bisphosphonates, along with the response from Novartis Pharmaceuticals, see (1) Brian G. M. Durie, Michael Katz, and John Cowley, (2) Sook-Bin Woo, Karen Hande, and Paul G. Richardson, (3) Marie Maerevoet, Charlotte Martin, and Lionel Duck, and (4) Peter Tarasoff and Yong-jiang Hei (response), in "Osteonecrosis of the Jaw and Bisphosphonates," *New England Journal of Medicine* 353 (7 July 2005): 99–102.

16. "Update: Hydrogen Cyanamide–Related Illness—Italy 2002–2004," *MMWR* 54 (29 April 2005): 405–408.

17. Multiple reports have documented a link between artificial nails and hospital-acquired infections. See, for example, A. Gupta et al., "Outbreak of Extended-Spectrum Beta-Lactamase-Producing Klebsiella Pneumoniae in a Neonatal Intensive Care Unit Linked to Artificial Nails," *Infection Control Hospital Epidemiology* 25 (2004): 210–215. In that study, babies were approximately eight times more likely to be infected if exposed to a health care worker with artificial nails.

18. The suspect chemical component of flame retardants is addressed in Thomas A. McDonald, "A Perspective on the Potential Health Risks of PBDEs," *Chemosphere* 46 (2002): 745–755.

19. Michael Eddleston and Michael R. Phillips, "Self-Poisoning with Pesticides," *British Medical Journal* 328 (2004): 42–44.

20. Stephen Frost, "A Sketch of China's Coal Industry," *CSR China Weekly* 1, week 8 (2005): 1–4. See also Erik Khoum, "Dangerous Coal Mines Take Human Toll in China," *New York Times*, 19 June 2000. The recent record in the United States has been poor in relative terms. See "Tolerating Death in the Mines" (editorial), *New York Times*, 5 February 2006. Also nearer to home than China, the Mexican coal mine disaster of 19 February 2006 underscores the persistent, international nature of this problem. See James C. McKinley Jr., "With 65 Still Entombed at Mexican Mine, Ache Deepens," *New York Times*, 3 March 2006.

21. Metin Akgun et al., "Silicosis Caused by Sandblasting of Jeans in Turkey: A Report of Two Concomitant Cases," *Journal of Occupational Health* 47 (2005): 346–349. See also Aygun Gur et al., "Silicosis Is in Denim Sandblasting Workers (Two Case Reports)" (abstract), *European Respiratory Journal* 26, supplement (2005): 147.

22. Hannah More, *Patient Joe or the Newcastle Collier* (Bath: S. Hazard, 1795), a one-page broadside (36.5 × 52.5 cm). More, although now obscure, was

a famous Christian do-gooder and promoter of the family values of her day. *Patient Joe* was published in the context of More's numerous Cheap Respiratory Tracts (for example, the 1798 pamphlet *The History of Mary Wood, the House-Maid; or The Danger of False Excuses*). Elizabeth Denlinger, in her catalog of the New York Public Library exhibition Before Victoria: Extraordinary Women of the British Romantic Era, juxtaposes More, as one extreme of the era, with her contemporary Mary Wollstonecraft, the early feminist and social progressive. Elizabeth Denlinger, *Before Victoria: Extraordinary Women of the British Romantic Era* (New York: New York Public Library/Columbia University Press, 2005).

23. Frost, "A Sketch of China's Coal Industry." Li Yang's 2003 film *Blind Shaft (Mang jing)* was banned in China for its harsh realism and inherent social critique. See also Manohla Dargis, review of *Blind Shaft, Los Angeles Times,* 19 March 2004.

24. L. J. Henderson and Elton Mayo, "Effects of the Social Environment," in *The Environment and Its Effect upon Man* (Boston: Harvard School of Public Health, 1937), 1–16, quotation from 7.

25. Matteo Giulio Bartoli, *Il Dalmatico: Resti di un'antica lingua romanza da Veglia a Ragusa e sua collocazione nella Romania Apennino-Balcanica* (Rome: Istituto della Enciclopedia Italiana, 2000), 11; (originally published in German under the title *Dal Dalmatische*) (Vienna: A. Hölder, 1906). See also Martin Maiden, "Into the Past: Morphological Change in the Dying Years of Dalmatian," *Diachronica* 21 (2004): 85–111.

26. *Samuel Wood Whose Arm with the Shoulder blade was torn off by a Mill y^e, 15th of Aug: 1737. He was brought to St. Thomas's Hospital ye next day where he was Cured by Mr. Ferne,* etching, plate mark 23.5 × 18.6 cm (London: published by Samuel Wood according to an act of Parliament, 1 November 1737), in the author's collection. The Wellcome Institute for Medical Research also possesses a print.

27. Ernst Pawel, *The Nightmare of Reason: A Life of Franz Kafka* (New York: Farrar Straus Giroux, 1984). For a time, Kafka also worked at his uncle's asbestos factory in Prague.

28. W. G. Sebald, *Austerlitz,* trans. Anthea Bell (New York: Modern Library, 2001), 13. In the novel's text, Austerlitz makes this comment in French: "Combien des ouvriers périrent, lors de la manufacture de tels miroirs, de maligne et funestes affectations á la suite de l'inhalation de vapeurs de mercure et de cyanide."

29. George Bernard Shaw, *Mrs. Warren's Profession: A Play in Four Acts* (London: Grant Richards, 1902), 193–194. Mrs. Warren speaks of her sister's death in act 2. The paralysis of the hands to which Shaw refers, also called wristdrop, was a common sign of advanced lead poisoning. Benjamin Franklin, in a 1786 letter, describes his own experiences as a young printer when coworkers suffered from the ill effects of lead with the loss of use of their hands, a condition that Franklin

refers to as "the dangles." See "Franklin on Bifocals and Lead Poisoning, 1785–1786," in *Classics in Medical Literature from the University of Pennsylvania, 1765–1965* (Philadelphia: Medical Affairs, 1965), 26–27.

30. William Dodd, "A Voice from the Factories," in *The Laboring Classes of England, Especially Those Engaged in Agriculture and Manufactures; in a Series of Letters. By an Englishman. Also, a Voice from the Factories, a Poem, in Serious Verse* (Boston: John Putnam, 1847), 155, from stanza 18. Dodd also authored *The Factory System Illustrated; In a Series of Letters to the Right Hon. Lord Ashley, M.P., Etc. Etc.* (London: John Murray, 1842).

31. Muriel Rukeyser, "Book of the Dead," in *U.S. 1* (New York: Covici Friede, 1938), 70–71.

INDEX

cadmia, 197–200
cadmium inhalation, 174
caisson disease, 118
California: benzene-related aplastic anemia in, 288n22; bicycle policemen in, 263; hexane neuropathy in, 98; metal fume fever in, 209–10; metam sodium in, 165–66, 170; MMT (gas additive) banned in, 259
Cameron, Richard, 312n54
Caminita, Barbara, 196
Canada: MMT (gas additive) in, 256, 258–59; RADS cases in, 124
cancer: asbestos exposure and, 16; of bladder, 70; calcium-lowering treatment drugs for, 265; chemotherapy for, 61–62, 127; coal tar linked to, 228–30, 331n40, 332n45, 332n49; from herbal diet aid, 218; radiation exposure linked to, 70–71; of scrotum, 228–29, 331n40; vinyl chloride linked to, 71–74, 290–91n35. *See also* leukemia; liver diseases; radiation exposure
canning factory: sealants in, 56–57, 288n22
carbon: manganese linked to, 252–53
carbon dioxide: as choke damp, 118
carbon disulfide: as air contaminant, 166–67; as Antabuse by-product, 165, 170, 265; cyclical use and concerns of, 134, 152, 167–71; diverse applications of, 134–35; as fumigant, 165, 315n76; history of, 135–37; in metam sodium, 165–66, 170; properties of, 135, 137–38; in vulcanization process, 138–40, 164–65; warnings about, 141, 149–50, 308n14
carbon disulfide poisoning: cases described, 132–34, 141–43, 144; from cellophane manufacturing, 157–58, 163–64; Charcot on, 146–48; dismissal of, 157; of grain workers, 315n76; hospitals for, 163; hysteria linked to, 144–49, 310n32; Parkinson's disease linked to, 160, 163, 244; in rayon manufacturing, 154–64, 313–14n62; treatment of, 156; unabated threat of, 167–71; vision effects of, 149, 311n35; warnings

about, 149–50; work speedup linked to, 160
carbon monoxide: as after damp, 118; warning systems for, 22, 302n55
carbon tetrachloride, 135, 315n76
cardiovascular disease: carbon disulfide exposure linked to, 164, 169–70
carpal tunnel syndrome: characteristics of, 17; current frequency of, 16; history of, 18–20; workers at risk for, 1, 16, 17, 20
Carson, Rachel, 8–9, 26, 273n6
casein, 64–65
Castleman, Barry, 277n34
CCA (chromated copper arsenate), 238–40, 260
CDC. *See* Centers for Disease Control (CDC)
Cellon, 59–60
cellophane manufacturing, 157–58, 163–64
Cellophane société anonyme, 157–58
cellulose: definition of, 49–50; in polymer sealants, 58–59. *See also* viscose method
cellulose acetate: development of, 58–60; new markets for, 62–63; recycling of, 89
cellulose wool manufacturing, 161–62
Centers for Disease Control (CDC): emerging pathogens research of, 215–16; on mildew preventive in latex paint, 272n2; NIOSH marginalized by, 263. *See also* Morbidity and Mortality Weekly Report (MMWR, CDC publication)
Chadwick, Edwin, 187–88, 224–25, 319n20
Chamber of Commerce, 20, 278n44
Chamorro people, 244
charcoal, 329n24
Charcot, Jean-Martin: on carbon disulfide case, 146–48; on hysteria, 145–46, 149, 310n32; image of, 148–49; students of, 148, 311n40
Charcot-Marie-Tooth disease, 146
Charles Macintosh and Company, 139, 140, 144, 307n12
cheese packaging, 164
Chekhov, Anton, 36

coal tar and coal gas manufacturing: by-products of, 53–55, 226–27; cancer linked to, 228–30, 331n40, 332n45, 332n49; ecological effect of, 286n9; in WWI era, 58

coatings: chloronaphthalene as, 232–33; DMF as, 87–88; heat and, 81; use of term, 46. *See also* insulation

collagen, 49, 50–51

College of Physicians (U.S.), 155–56

Collis, Edgar, 193, 321n33

Combustion Improver No. 2 (gas additive), 256

Commissioners Appointed to Inquire into the Employment of Children and Young Persons in Trades and Manufactures Not Already Regulated by Law, 144, 309n25

Commissioners for the Employment of Children, 282n10, 283n15

condom micromanufacturing, 143

Connecticut: brass making in, 206. *See also* Yale University

Consumer Product Safety Commission (CPSC): arsenic-treated wood and, 240; artificial nail products and, 85, 293n53; benzene investigation of, 85–86; inaction of, 86–87, 263–64, 294n60; interagency cooperation and, 90

consumption. *See* tuberculosis

contact cement, 86. *See also* rubber cement

Cooke, W. E., 275–76n27, 276n30

Cooper, Peter, 91

Copland (professor), 103

copper: biological function of, 246; in brass making, 197–200, 202, 203–5; in wood preservative, 225

copper azole (CA), 240

copper boron azole (CBA), 240

copper sulfate, 225

Cormack, John Rose, 227

corporate responsibility concept, 91

corrosive sublimate: alternatives to, 225–26; in Kyanization, 223–26; toxicity of, 329n24. *See also* mercuric chloride

cotton mills: belated U.S. recognition of diseases in, 193–96; cotton dust exposure standards and, 212–13; early conditions in, 180–82; lung diseases from working in, 178–81, 189–93, 211–12, 321n33; mechanized carding in, 177–78; prison-run, 325n70

cotton phthisis: use of term, 189

Council of the Royal Society (Britain), 10

Couper, John, 338n94

Courtauld, Samuel, 164

Courtaulds Fibers, Inc., 156, 164, 169, 170, 316n80

CPSC. *See* Consumer Product Safety Commission (CPSC)

Cram, Gen. T. J., 224

Creech, John L., Jr., 71–72

creosote: alternative to, 240; cancer linked to, 228–30, 331n40, 332n45, 332n49; continued use of, 230, 239; declining use of, 231; EPA proposals on, 238–39; irritant dermatitis linked to, 234; questions about, 230–37; as wood treatment, 226–27

Crikelair, George, 312n45

Cuba: manganese Parkinsonism in, 250

Cullen, Morris, 209–10

CVC Capital Partners, 170

cyanide poisoning: from acetonitrile, 83–84; dinitrophenol (DNP) compared with, 218; at film recovery plant, 40–42; literature about, 269. *See also* hydrogen cyanide gas; Zyklon

cyanoacrylate glues, 80, 88, 292n45

cycad (false sago palm), 244–45, 246

cytokines, 210

Dantín-Gallego, Juan, 314n63

Darwin, Erasmus, 111

data suppression, 290–91n35

Davis, E. G., 193–94, 321n35

Davy, Humphry: carbon disulfide studies of, 136; chlorine dioxide synthesized by, 98, 122, 303n62; on corrosive sublimate, 223; on oxymuriatic gas and oxygene, 296n10; on potash and soda ash, 106; safety lamp of, 98, 118

DDT, 8–9

DEA (Drug Enforcement Agency), 89

Death of a Salesman (Miller), 23

Degesch (Deutsche Gesellschaft für Schädlingsbekämpfung, German Society for Pest Control), 121
Delacroix, Victor, 142
Delay, Tom, 259
Delpech, Auguste L. Dominique: carbon disulfide studies of, 141–42, 143–45, 156, 308n16, 309nn19–20; Charcot on, 146; medical context of, 144–45; recommendations of, 150, 168
dementia pugilistica, 244
Democratic Party (U.S.), 258
Denlinger, Elizabeth, 344n22
Denmark: match industry in, 37; mill fever in, 321n38
De Re Metallica (Agricola), 199–200
diacetyl, 217
Diamond Match Company, 39
Diamond Shamrock facility, 236–37, 335n68
Dickens, Charles, 31–32
dietary supplements: deaths from, 328n13; disease outbreaks from, 217–18; manganese as, 245–47; zinc as, 174
dimethylformamide (DMF), 87–88
dinitrophenol (DNP), 218, 328n13
dioxin (TCDD), 236–40
diphenyl, 339n105
Direction for the Health of Magistrates and Studentes, A (Gratarolo), 24
Dire Straits (band), 1–2, 4
Disease of Workers (Ramazzini), 30, 31
diseases: naming of, 2, 18–19
disulfiram, 165, 170, 265
DNA, 127
Docker's Union, 229
docks, 219–20, 303n65
Dodd, William, 269–70
Donohue, Thomas, 278n44
dope (doping): use of term, 59–60
Dow Chemical Company, 71, 231, 235
Dowicide: use of term, 231
Dreiser, Theodore, 16
Drinker, Cecil, 333n56, 339n99
Drinker, Philip, 12, 207, 209
dry cleaning agents, 135

dry rot: texts on, 221–22, 238; use of term, 329n20. See also wood preservative treatments
Dry Rot (anon.), 221–22
Duchenne de Boulogne, Guillaume-Benjamin, 141, 308n15
DuPont company, 156, 158, 163, 164
dye making, synthetic: benzene in, 52–55, 286n11, 287n14; bladder cancer linked to, 70; manganese-based, 248
dyes, food, 265
D-Zolve Tip Blender, 88

Earle, James, 331n40
Earth Day, 7
East Jersey Match Company, 39
Eastman, George, 58–59
economics: of benzene production, 55, 60–61, 69; of cellophane manufacturing, 158; of chlorine bleach, 110–11; laissez faire approach to, 34–39, 40; of papermaking, 114; of pentachlorophenol, 235; of rayon manufacturing, 156; in regulation evasions, 31–32; regulations and solutions subsumed to, 34–39; of synthetic dyestuffs, 53–54, 57; of wood preservative treatments, 221, 224
EDF (Environmental Defense Fund), 257–58
Edinburgh Medical and Physical Dictionary, The, 103–4
Edward II, King of England, 14
Effects of Arts, Trades and Professions on Health and Longevity (Thackrah), 113, 182–84, 300n41
Egypt (ancient): creosote use in mummification in, 227; glue use in, 47; repetive strains in, 19; textile industry in, 153
Ehrlich, Anne, 273n4
Ehrlich, Paul, 273n4
eighteenth century: air pollution in, 14, 30; bleaching in, 101–2; brass founding in, 201–3; burnout in, 24–25; cancer in chimney sweeps, 228; carbon disulfide synthesis in, 135; chlorine use in,

fire hazards: carbon disulfide and, 141; in fighter aircraft, 59; of flannelette sleepwear, 154, 312n45; in sweatshop industries and low-wage workplaces, 42–44

Fisheries Preservation Association (Britain), 11

flame retardants: debates on, 265; iron sulfate, 225; sleepwear, 154, 312n45

flannel, 153–54, 312n45

flock fever, 192, 217, 320n31

Florida: chlorine gas spill in, 123

fluorine gas, 130

fluorocarbons, 210–11, 217

food: dyes for, 265; packaging of, 82, 164, 169, 170

formaldehyde, 64–65

Fortune magazine, 289n26

France: benzene-induced aplastic anemia and leukemia in, 61–62, 74–75, 286n11; carbon disulfide poisoning in, 135–36, 141–43, 146–49, 308nn14–16, 309n20; cellophane in, 157–58; chlorine and bleaching in, 104; chlorine fumigation in, 111; chlorine inhalation in, 112; cotton dust inhalation problems in, 180–81, 189; dye industry of, 57; eighteenth-century chemists of, 96–98; impressionism and pollution, 13; match industry in, 36, 38, 39; metal fume fever in, 204; public health text in, 190; rayon manufacturing in, 159; soda manufacturing in, 106; synthetic silk in, 154; vinyl chloride monomer developed in, 67–68; vulcanization in, 140–41; wood preservative in, 225; workplace hazard categories in, 151

Franklin, Benjamin, 345n29

Fred Fear Match Company, 39

Freedman, Rose, 285n25

Freeman, Lewis, 116–17

free markets. *See* economics

Freese, Barbara, 286n9

freon, 166, 210–11. *See also* fluorocarbons

Freud, Sigmund, 148

Friedrich Engels Chemical-Fiber Works, 162

fuller's trade, 99–101, 102

fume fever. *See* metal fume fever

Fumifugium (Evelyn), 14

fumigants: carbon disulfide as, 165, 315n76; chlorine as, 111; chloropicrin as, 128; corrosive sublimate as, 223, 329n24; cyanide as, 121; metam sodium as, 165–66, 170; sulfur as, 298n20

fungicides: manganese Parkinsonism linked to, 251–53, 339n105; in wood preservative treatments, 231–34. *See also* bacteria and fungi; pest control; pesticides and pesticide manufacturing

furniture making and repair: glues in, 47, 48; hexane in, 77; metal beds and, 205–6; methylene chloride in strippers for, 87. *See also* wood preservative treatments

Gabrilowich, Bessie (later, Cohen), 42–43

Gaines, M. Toulmin, 234

Galalith (plastic), 64–65, 289n25

Gall, Mary, 86–87

Gallimore, John, 108–9

galvanized steel: described, 173; fume fever from welding, 173–75, 208–10

gamma butyrolactone, 88–89

Gannal, J.-N. (author), 112

Garcia, Jerry, 291n37

Gardner, Augustus, 204

gas: use of term, 117–18

Gaskell, Elizabeth, 188–89, 212, 307n11

gasoline: cracking of, to yield benzene, 69; leaded, 254–57; reformulated, 259

gasoline additives: antiknock, 241; ethyl in, 254–57; MTBE as, 259–60; nitromethane in, 88; organic manganese in, 255–61; Parkinsonism linked to, 241–42

gassed: use of term, 150

gasworks pitch industry, 229–30

Gay-Lussac, Joseph-Louis, 96

Gazio, Antonio, 21–22

General Artificial Silk Works, 155–56

General Hospital (TV show), 170

Georgia: prison textile mill in, 325n70

German Democratic Republic (GDR): rayon manufacturing of, 162

Mariana Islands: Parkinsonism epidemic centered in, 244–45
Marie, Pierre, 146, 149, 310n30
Markowitz, Gerald, 290–91n35
Marshall, Thurgood, 75
Martineau, Harriet, 31–32
Marx, Karl, 30, 31, 190, 281n3, 320n26
Maryland: benzene poisoning cases in, 56–57; chlorine gas poisoning in, 303n65; Kyanized railroad ties in, 224–25
Massachusetts: Boston Poison Information Center in, 92–93
match industry, 35–39, 282n13
mattress making program, 195–96, 210
MCA (Manufacturing Chemists' Association), 273n6, 290–91n35
McCready, Benjamin W., 194
McGrigor, James, 103
MCPA, 336n78
MCPP (mecoprop), 336n78
Medical-Surgical Society of Paris, 141
medical treatments: anesthesia, 59, 137, 150; artificial nails and, 265, 344n17; carbon disulfide in, 150; chlorine in, 111–13, 300n45; creosote in, 227, 230; disease outbreaks from alternative, 217–18, 328n13; FD&C Blue no. 1 in, 265; glues in, 47, 80–81, 292n46; manganese in, 248; MDI-based casts in, 81; superglue emergencies and, 82–83; surveillance in, 216–17
medieval period: brass making in, 200; glues in, 47–48; Jewish liturgy on working dangers, 272n6; papermaking in, 113; resins used in, 52
Meikleham, Robert Stuart, 279n50
melancholy, 24–25
Memorandum on Gas Poisoning in Warfare (pamphlet), 119
mental hospitals: carbon disulfide cases in, 132–34
mental illness. *See* carbon disulfide poisoning; insanity
mercuric chloride, 223–26
mercury: biological effects of, 5–6, 245–46; cleanup of, 272n2; EPA standards on, 262; health dangers understood in, 197, 199; literature about, 269; medicinal uses of, 5–6, 272–73n3; in mildew preventive, 6–7; poisonous properties of, 329n24; use of in felt hat industry, 9. *See also* corrosive sublimate
mercury poisoning: of hat makers/milliners, 9; history of, 5–7; insanity due to, 145; from Kyanization, 224–25; palsy from, 243; Renaissance lawsuit concerning, 30
metal: bedsteads of, 205–6; galvanization of, 173–75, 208–10; manganese in processing, 249–50; silos of, 217, 326–27n5
metal fume fever: among brass workers, 196–97, 203–5, 206–8; cytokines in, 210; endotoxin and, 175; experimental approach to, 172–73; historical context of, 180; human experimental studies of, 172–73, 206–7, 210, 214; self-limiting nature of, 173–74, 175; song lyrics on, 213; from welding galvanized material, 173–75, 208–10
metallic zinc, 201, 202, 203–5
metalworking: health dangers understood in, 197–200; silica exposure in, 33–34, 281–82n8, 282n10, 318–19n16. *See also* brass and brass making; welding
metam sodium, 165–67, 170
methacrylic acid, 293n53
methane gas, 118, 135
methylcyclopentadienyl manganese tricarbonyl (MMT), 255–61
methylene chloride, 87
methylene diphenyl diisocyanate (MDI), 81
methyl ethyl ketone, 78
methyl isothiocyanate, 166
methyl methacrylates, 80–81, 84, 88, 292n46
methyl tertiary butyl ether (MTBE), 259–60
Mexico: coal mining deaths in, 344n20; folk treatments in, 5–6
Michigan: inhalation fever in, 211, 325n67; mercury exposure from paint in, 6

microwave cooking: packaging for, 82; popcorn, 217

Middle East: bitumen sources in 328n17, laundering processes in, 99; paper-making in, 113

Middlemarch (Eliot), 248

milk protein (casein), 64–65

mill fever: belated U.S. recognition of, 193–96; in Britain vs. U.S., 193–96; first documented, 183; history of, 180–82; occasional outbreaks of, 211–12; persistence of, 210–14; redis-covery of, 191–93; role of flax in, 192, 320–21n32; symptoms of, 176–77. *See also* byssinosis (brown lung); job fever; Monday morning fever; cotton mills

mineral tar, 220, 222

miners and mining: advice for, 32; birds as warning systems for, 302n55; Davy safety lamp for, 98, 118; diseases of, 117–19; downgrading of violations in, 342n2; explosions in, 118, 135, 266, 268, 342n2; occupational text on, 199–200; voices of, 267, 344n22

mink, screw-neck, 246–47

Mississippi: chloracne in, 233–34; wood preservatives in, 231

Missouri: chlorine gas spill in, 129; mi-crowave popcorn lung in, 216–17

Mitchell, S. Weir, 25–26

Miyake, Issey, 81

MMT (methylcyclopentadienyl manganese tricarbonyl), 255–61

model airplane building, 80, 88, 292n45

molecules, aromatic, 54

Moll, Friedrich, 330n35

Monday morning fever, 173, 175, 176, 177, 206, 210. *See also* metal fume fever; mill fever; zinc oxide inhalation

monkey pox, 215, 216

Monsanto company, 235

Moody, Gilbert, 60

Moral and Physical Condition of the Work-ing Classes, The (Kay), 186

Morbidity and Mortality Weekly Report (*MMWR*, CDC publication), 6, 72, 272n2, 290n33, 341n113, 343n3

More, Hannah, 267, 344n22

Morgagni, Giovanni (anatomist), 180

Morocco: manganese Parkinsonism in, 250

Moroni, Giovanni, 269

motion pictures. *See* film and cinema

MPTP (heroin substitute), 245, 246

Mosley, Stephen, 275n19

MTBE (methyl tertiary butyl ether), 259–60

mundic (arsenic), 238

munitions manufacturing, 58, 127

muriatic acid. *See* hydrochloric acid

Muspratt, James, 107, 108, 111

mustard gas weapons, 120–21, 126–27, 305n79

NAFTA (North American Free Trade Agreement), 259

nail polish removers, 83, 89. *See also* artifi-cial nails

naphtha odor, 144

National Academy of Sciences (Institute of Medicine), 20, 278n45, 335n64

National Association of Factory Occupiers (England), 31

National Cancer Institute (NCI), 89–90

National Institute for Occupational Safety and Health (NIOSH): angiosarcoma studies and, 73; on carbon disulfide, 164, 168–70, 315n76; cotton dust ex-posure standards of, 212–13; on cumu-lative trauma injuries, 20; on homi-cides and burnout, 279n53; inaction of, 262–63; on nitromethane expo-sure, 88; personnel of, 334n63; un-alarming reports of, 263, 343n6

National Institutes of Health (NIH), 195–96. *See also* National Cancer In-stitute

National Museum of American History, 44

National Retail Dry Goods Association of America, 155

Nature (journal), 253

Naturewood Amine Base Treated Wood, 240

Nawrocki, Arnold N., 164

Nazi Germany: Haber exiled from, 121–22; occupational medicine in, 159, 234, 312n54, 334n60; rayon manufacturing of, 160–62, 313n61, 313–14n62; slave labor used by, 66, 161–62, 289n26, 314n65

Neal, Paul, 196

Needleman, Herbert, 260

Neolithic period: repetitive strain injuries in, 19

neoprene, 65, 67, 289n26

Netherlands: deaths from mixing household cleaners in, 94; early bleaching in, 101, 297n18; manganese bleach catalyst in, 253

neurological diseases: fuel additives linked to, 241–42; hexane linked to, 76–77; nitromethane linked to, 88; tetraethyl lead linked to, 254–55. *See also* carbon disulfide poisoning; carpal tunnel syndrome; Parkinson's disease

neurotoxicology, 145

neurotransmitters, 243, 246, 251

Nevada: chloracne case in, 235

New England Journal of Medicine: on benzene and leukemia, 69–70; on carbon disulfide cases, 134; on creosote-related cancer, 230; on mixing household cleaners, 93; on osteonecrosis of the jaw, 344n15

New Hampshire: RADS cases in, 124

New Jersey: asbestos processing in, 16; chloracne and porphyria cases in, 235–37; Superfund site in, 335n68

NewMarket Corporation, 260

New York City: chlorine gas poisoning in, 122–23; Triangle Shirtwaist fire in, 42–44

New York State: airplane doping in, 287n19; carbon disulfide poisoning in, 321n54; Love Canal, 7, 273n7

New York Journal of Medicine, 283n14

New York Times: on angiosarcoma, 73–74, 291n37; ergonomics at, 40; on MMT (gas additive), 260; MMT (gas additive) ad in, 257–58; on popcorn, 216; on worker deaths, 263, 342n2

nickel, 202

Nightingale, Florence, 281n5

NIH (National Institutes of Health), 195–96

Nike Corp., 77

nineteenth-century period: air concerns in, 13–14, 22–23; asbestos in, 15; brass making in, 196–97, 204–6; burnout in, 25–26, 280n61; carbon disulfide cases in, 132–34, 135–37, 141–43, 146–48, 149–50, 308nn14–16; carpal tunnel syndrome in, 18–19, 277n37; chlorine dioxide synthesized in, 122, 303n62; chlorine gas discovered in, 98; chlorine's uses in, 103–5, 111–13; coal gas manufacturing in, 53; coal tar hazards in, 228–30; cotton mill work in, 180–82; dock-yard disease in, 219–20; glues in, 48; labor reform in, 184–87; manganese disease in, 247–48; mining studies in, 117–18; occupational health text in, 182–84, 187; papermaking in, 113–14, 301n49; Parkinsonism in, 242–43; public vs. occupational health in, 187–91; rubber in, 52; social Darwinism in, 35, 39–40; soda manufacturing in, 107–10; steel manufacturing in, 249; victim blaming in, 31–32; vulcanization in, 138–40; wood preservative treatments in, 222–26; workers subsumed to technology in, 32–34

NIOSH. *See* National Institute for Occupational Safety and Health (NIOSH)

nitric acid, 97

nitrocellulose, 58–59, 62

nitroethane, 84–85, 90

nitrogen, 118, 136

nitrogen dioxide, 217, 326–27n5

nitrogen mustards, 127

nitromethane, 88

Noble, Daniel, 187

Nord, Nancy, 264

North American Free Trade Agreement (NAFTA), 259

North and South (Gaskell), 188–89, 212

plastics industry; polyvinyl chloride (PVC)

polypropylene, 163

polyurethane, 81

polyvinyl chloride (PVC): in aerosol sprays, 73–74; as cancer-causing agent, 71–74, 290–91n35; CPSC's investigation of, 85; development of, 67–69

popcorn factory, 216–17

popholyx, 198

popular culture. *See* advertising; arts; film and cinema; literature; song lyrics; television

porphyria, 236–37

Portugal: bleach use in, 94

potash, 106

Pott, Percivall, 331n40

pottery industry, 320n26

PPG, 167

Proctor, Robert, 334n60

Proctor and Gamble, 253

professionals: burnout of, 23–25

Proust, Adrien, 190

public health: chemical risk assessment of, 121; emerging pathogens and, 215–16; emerging toxins ignored in, 216–19; flannelette sleepwear and, 154, 312n45; household chlorine use as threat to, 129–30; laissez faire economics and, 35–39; occupational health ignored in, 187–91, 194; reform movement for, 187–88; text on, 190. *See also* regulatory evasions

Public Interest Research Group, 87

public policy: historical patterns critical to making, 3, 4, 9–10, 57. *See also* regulations; *specific agencies*

pulmometer, 183, 212

Purdon, Charles Nicholas Delacherois, 320–21n32

PVC. *See* polyvinyl chloride (PVC)

Quarry Bank Mill (Manchester), 317n9

Quebec: RADS cases in, 124

quicksilver, 5–6. *See also* mercury

radiation exposure: benzene compared with, 57, 61–62, 287n13; cancer linked to, 70–71; protection against, 150; radium, 270

RADS. *See* reactive airway dysfunction syndrome (RADS)

railroad accidents: chlorine gas spills in, 123, 129; metam sodium spill in, 165–66, 170

railroads: chlorine gas transport via, 122; creosoted ties for, 227, 228–30, 336n76; date nails of, 226, 238; Kyanized ties for, 224–25

Ramazzini, Bernardino: on fuller's trade, 100–101; on lawsuit against manufacturer, 30; references to, 31, 180, 281n3

Rambousek, Joseph, 287n14

ramie fiber, 153, 312n43

rayon industry: carbon disulfide poisonings in, 158–62; carbon disulfide unabated in, 170–71; development of, 154–57; failed controls in, 168; post-WWII period in, 162–64; rayon staple production in, 160–62, 168, 313n61, 313–14n62, 316n80; slave labor used in, 161–62, 314n65

reactive airway dysfunction syndrome (RADS): described, 124, 304n72; hot tub disinfector's lung symptoms and, 128; Iranian victims of, 127; ozone gas and, 129; WWI victims of, 125–26

Reagan, Ronald, 43, 86

record industry, 291n37

Redlich, Carrie, 292n47

red phosphorous, 36–39

Regnault, Henri Victor, 67–68

regulations: attacks on, 8; on cumulative trauma injuries, 20, 278n44; deferred enforcement of, 42–44; denial, anger, bargaining, and acceptance pattern in, 29; failure to enforce, 168–69; inaction in, 87–89; on industrial chlorine uses, 129; jurisdictional squabbles and, 84–87; political struggles over, 262–70; recommendations on, 90–91; in rubber industry, 152; shutdown and murder prosecution for violating, 41–42, 43. *See also* workplace safety rules

SARS, 215, 216
Saussure (professor), 103
scabies treatment, 248
Scandinavian countries: papermaking in,
    114, 129; pine tar production in, 221
Scanlon, Terrence, 86
Scattergood, Thomas, 13
Scheele, Carl, 95–96, 98
Schneiter, Roy, 196
Schorr, A., 285n26
Schuman, Leonard M., 326–27n5
Science of the Total Environment, 257
Scotland: chlorine and bleaching in, 103,
    104–6, 338n94; lead-induced insanity
    in, 145; soda manufacturing in, 107–8
Scott, Ernest, 326–27n5
scrotal cancer, 228–29, 331n40
sculptured nails. *See* artificial nails
sealants: benzene in, 56–57; cellulose based,
    in WWI, 58–59; chemical solvents in,
    46–48, 52; polyurethane in, 81; use of
    term, 46
Sebald, W. G., 269, 345n28
Seinfeld (TV show), 91, 295n74
Semon, Waldo Lonsbury, 68, 79
sewage treatment plant, 124
sexual impotence or overexcitation: bicycle
    riding and, 263; from carbon disulfide
    exposure, 142, 143, 144–45, 149, 156
Shakespeare, William, 101, 118, 297n17
Shaw, George Bernard, 269, 345n29
Sherman Anti-Trust Act, 163
shipbuilding: early treatments in, 222; gal-
    vanized welding in, 209–10; gas tar
    and scrotal cancer in, 228–29; Ply-
    mouth dock-yard disease in, 219–20;
    water-repellant resins in, 220–21. *See
    also* wood preservative treatments
shoddy fever, 183, 191–92
shoemaker's polyneuropathy, 77, 89
shoe manufacturing: benzene exposure in,
    66–67, 69–70; as cottage industry,
    90–91; hexane exposure in, 77
Shul'tsev, G. P., 283n13
Shuttleworth, James Kay. *See* Kay, James
    Phillips
sick building syndrome, 21–23
Silent Spring (Carson), 8–9, 26, 273n6

silicosis: chlorine gas poisoning compared
    with, 125; etymology of term, 190;
    outbreaks of, 4, 266–67; silica expo-
    sure linked to, 33–34, 281–82n8,
    282n10, 318–19n16
silk, synthetic, 154–57
Silkwood, Karen, 273n7
silo-filler's disease, 217, 326–27n5
silver: silver nitrate in carbon disulfide, 139;
    toxic effects of, 218
Simon, John, 189–90, 283n15
skin diseases: chlorine-related, 232–35; coal
    tar–related, 228–30, 331n40, 332n45,
    332n49; herbicide-related, 235–37;
    irritant dermatitis, 234, 334n60;
    pentachlorophenol-related, 231–32,
    237, 239–40
Slaves of the Needle (Grindrod), 18
Sleeper (film), 8
sleepwear, 86
Smith, Adam, 35
Smith, R. Angus, 275n20
smithsonite, 198
smog and fog episodes, 11–13, 274n15
smokestack scrubbing devices, 107–8
soap making, 99, 297n14
social Darwinism, 35, 39–40
Society of American Wood Preservers, 238
soda ash manufacturing: papermaking and,
    114; pollution by, 107–9; process of,
    106–7; workers' exposure in, 108–11
sodium chloride (salt), 95–97, 106. *See also*
    soda ash manufacturing
sodium sulfate, 106–7
Soldier's Gas Notes (pamphlet), 119
solvents: aromatic molecules as, 54–55;
    characteristics of, 51; continued haz-
    ards of, 89–90; gamma butyrolactone
    as, 88–89; as glue catalysts, 79–80; in-
    dustrial demand for, 76; labeling of,
    86; nitromethane as, 88; in polymer-
    ization process, 69; in resin product,
    46–48; in rubber cement, 52–55; for
    superglue removal, 83–84; used in
    developing economies, 89, 90–91.
    See also benzene; carbon disulfide;
    hexane; methylethyl ketone; toluene;
    turpentine

song lyrics: cleanliness obsession reflected in, 131, 306n91; on creosote-poisoned fruit (Guthrie), 241, 337n81; on industrial disease (Knopfler, White), 1–2, 4; on Kyanization, 224; on metal fume fever (Hatfield), 213; on repetitive strain injuries, 277n37; on Triangle Shirtwaist fire (Schorr and Rumshinsky), 285n26

"Song of the Shirt," 18, 20

South Carolina: chlorine gas spill in, 129

Southern Medical Association, 233–34

Southern Medical Journal, 123

Southern Pacific Railroad, 230

Soviet Union (USSR): metal fume studies in, 207; Tajikistan weavers, 18, 277n37. *See also* Russia

Spain: bleach use in, 93–94; carbon disulfide use in, 314n63; chlorine gas poisoning in, 123

Spellwin, George, 328n13

spelter (metal), 201–2

spelter shakes, 206

spinner's phthisis, 181–82, 187

spirometer (earlier, pulmometer), 183, 212

spray painting, 81

spun acetate (acetate silk), 62–63, 288n23

Sri Lanka, pesticide regulation in, 266

stamp-licker's tongue, 91, 295n74

steam power, 33–34

steel manufacturing, 248–50. *See also* galvanized steel

Steorts, Nancy Harvey, 86, 264

"Steppe, The" (Chekhov), 36

stethoscope, 183

Stingily, Karl O., 233–34

Stratton, Hal, 264

styrene, 65

sublimate, 30

suicides, 143, 151, 266

sulfite process, 114

sulfur, 52, 136, 152, 298n20

sulfur dioxide, 13–14

sulfuric acid: in bleaching process, 101–2; in breaking down salt, 106–7; as runoff from soda manufacturing, 108

sulfur mustard weapons, 120–21, 126–27

Superfund sites, 335n68

superglues: asthma linked to, 80–82; development of, 78–80; emergency room visits linked to, 82–83; misuse of, 47; reactions to, 79–82, 292n45; recommendation on, 83, 90; removal agents for, 83–84

susceptors, 82

Sweden: benzene poisoning in, 56, 286n11; match industry in, 37, 38; paper industry of, 129; Parkinsonism and antimildew agent in, 339n105

swimming pools, 122, 123, 130

syphilis treatment, 232

tachyphylaxis, 175

Taiwan: herbal diet aid disease in, 217; rayon manufacturing in, 314–15n66

Tajikistan: tarsal tunnel syndrome in, 18, 277n37

tannery processes, 271n2

tarsal tunnel syndrome, 18, 277n37

technological changes: in brass making, 173–75, 203–5; by-products of, 55; carpal tunnel syndrome and, 18–19; in glue making, 78–82; modern match industry and, 35–39; in papermaking, 114; in rubber industry, 138–40; in textile and clothing industry, 152–54, 177–78, 182; in welding, 173–75, 208–10; workers' concerns subsumed to, 32–34. *See also* carbon disulfide poisoning

Teepak, Inc., 164, 169, 170

Teflon, 210–11, 214

Teleky, Ludwig, 233, 234, 284n17, 333n55

telephone/telegraph poles, 227, 330n35

television: on carbon disulfide, 170; commercial jingle on stains, 130–31; on glue toxicity, 91, 295n74

Tenant, James, 105–6

Ten Hour Bill (Britain), 184–87, 188

Tennant, Charles, 107, 338n94

terrorist attacks: fears of, 215–19; resources diverted to concerns about, 263, 343n3; Sarin used in, 127. *See also* chemical weapons

tetrachloroethane, 59, 89–90

workaholic: use of term, 25

workplace safety rules: on benzene surveillance, 66–67; decompression tables in, 118; failures of, 40–44; pamphlets on, 66–67, 69, 289n27; on phosphorous, 37; protective bars and, 31–32; state-by-state determination of, 159; for vulcanization, 151–52

World Health Organization, 121

World War I: benzene distribution interrupted by, 57–58; chlorine gas as weapon in, 115–19, 126; gases in, 126–28; manganese Parkinsonism in, 250; mustard gas as weapon in, 120–21; phosgene gas as weapon in, 120, 128; RADS cases from, 125–26

World War II: chemical weapon development in, 127; chloracne ignored in, 234; chlorine after, 122–23; food shortage in western Pacific in, 244–45; galvanized welding in, 209–10; German occupational medicine in, 159, 312n54, 333–34n60; radiation exposure studies after, 70–71; rayon manufacturing in, 158–62; slave labor used in, 161–62, 314n65; synthetic insulation for wiring in, 67; synthetic rubber development in, 65–66; tetrachloroethane exposure in, 89–90

Wright, Lawrence, 205–6

Wynter, Andrew, 282nn9,10

X-rays. *See* radiation exposure

xylene, 54

Yale University, 126, 292n47, 325n70

"Yellow Wallpaper, The" (Gilman), 26, 280n61

Ying-xing Song, 201

youth. *See* children and youth

Yperite (sulfur mustard), 120–21

Yugoslavia (former): bleach in, 94; industrial explosion in, 268

Yushchenko, Viktor, 237

Zangger, Heinrich, 333–34n60

zellwolle (German). *See* rayon industry, rayon staple in

zinc: in brass making, 197–208; as dietary supplement, 174; terms for, 201. *See also* metallic zinc; zinc oxide inhalation

zinc chloride: as wood preservative, 225, 226, 230

zinc oxide inhalation: early mention of, 201; endotoxin compared with, 175; human experimental studies of, 172–73, 206–7, 210, 214; from industrial distillation of zinc, 203–5; from welding galvanized material, 173–75, 208–10. *See also* metal fume fever

Zyklon, 121

Text:	11.25/13.5 Adobe Garamond
Display:	Garamond
Compositor:	Sheridan Books, Inc.
Indexer:	Margie Towery
Printer and binder:	Sheridan Books, Inc.